Lecture Notes of the Institute for Computer Sciences, Social Informatics and Telecommunications Engineering 150

More information about this series at http://www.springer.com/series/8197

Raffaele Giaffreda · Radu-Laurentiu Vieriu
Edna Pasher · Gabriel Bendersky
Antonio J. Jara · Joel J.P.C. Rodrigues
Eliezer Dekel · Benny Mandler (Eds.)

Internet of Things

User-Centric IoT

First International Summit, IoT360 2014
Rome, Italy, October 27–28, 2014
Revised Selected Papers, Part I

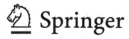 Springer

Editors

Raffaele Giaffreda
CREATE-NET
Trento
Italy

Radu-Laurentiu Vieriu
University of Trento
Trento
Italy

Edna Pasher
Management Consultant
Edna Pasher Ph.D & Associates
Tel Aviv
Israel

Gabriel Bendersky
Management Consultant
Edna Pasher Ph.D & Associates
Tel Aviv
Israel

Antonio J. Jara
University of Applied Sciences
Institute of Information Systems
Delémont
Switzerland

Joel J.P.C. Rodrigues
University of Beira Interior
Covilhã
Portugal

Eliezer Dekel
IBM Research Laboratory
Haifa
Israel

Benny Mandler
IBM Research
Haifa
Israel

ISSN 1867-8211   ISSN 1867-822X (electronic)
Lecture Notes of the Institute for Computer Sciences, Social Informatics
and Telecommunications Engineering
ISBN 978-3-319-19655-8   ISBN 978-3-319-19656-5 (eBook)
DOI 10.1007/978-3-319-19656-5

Library of Congress Control Number: 2015940419

Springer Cham Heidelberg New York Dordrecht London

Printed on acid-free paper

Springer International Publishing AG Switzerland is part of Springer Science+Business Media
(www.springer.com)

IOT360 2014 - User-Centric IoT

Preface

This volume includes the proceedings of four conferences dedicated to the role the Internet of Things (IoT) plays in user-centric technologies and applications in different domains. The 44 revised full papers in this volume were carefully reviewed and selected from a total of 67 submissions. The conferences also featured six special contributions from recognized experts in the field.

The first conference, COIOTE, focused mainly on artificial intelligence techniques for the ever-growing field of the IoT, a field expected to produce deep transformations on physical things as their virtual counterparts become more and more capable of autonomous behavior.

The second one, PERGAMES, focused on how to best leverage on IoT-gathered data in many application domains, leading to the design and deployment of pervasive games for various sectors, such as health and well-being, ambient-assisted living, smart cities/societies, education, cultural heritage, tourism and more.

The third conference, HealthyIoT, provided the health-related flavor of IoT, relating to the use of more widely available and adopted wearables.

The fourth conference focused mainly on the integration of smart objects and on the most advanced operational technology trend of cloud-based "Everything as a Service" where an appropriate cloud should support a high level of "as a service" paradigm. This deployment paradigm will enable the easy adoption of IoT-based services and applications by end users, while calling for smart object providers as well as platform middleware providers to architect their solutions accordingly.

April 2015   Raffaele Giaffreda

First International Conference on Cognitive Internet of Things Technologies – COIOTE 2014
Rome – October 27, 2014

Preface

The First Conference on Cognitive Internet of Things Technologies, COIOTE 2014, took place on October 27 at the NH Leonardo Da Vinci hotel in Rome, Italy. The main focus of the conference was on artificial intelligence techniques for the ever-growing field of the Internet of Things (IoT), a field expected to produce deep transformations on physical things by making them more intelligent. We are pleased to confirm that the whole experience including delegates from industry and academia was very fruitful, with many interesting new ideas and technical discussions.

Our Technical Program Committee, co-chaired by Professors Artur Arsénio and Erik Mannens, assembled an excellent technical program consisting of 11 papers in the main track, including several invited submissions from top researchers in the field. Additionally, four other papers were grouped into a Special Session entitled "Affordance in the Internet of Things (AIoT)".

Upon reviewing various successful stories of intelligent machines adding value and comfort to the human existence, Dr. Artur Arsénio highlighted in his keynote presentation the irrefutable benefits of bringing intelligence into objects, a topic that was highly appreciated among the attendees.

In the same agenda we included a COIOTE Panel session, organized by Dr. Franck Le Gall from Easy Global Market, on an interesting topic about the relations between IoT and the fields of cognitive sciences, nanotechnologies, and biotechnologies.

On behalf of the Organizing Committee of COIOTE 2014, we would like to thank all the authors who contributed their valuable work to the conference, and the TPC members and reviewers for maintaining the quality of the technical program. We would also like to thank our keynote speaker and panelists for contributing with their time, knowledge, and wisdom. We thank the organizers of the AIoT special session, Alice Ruggeri, Luigi Di Caro, and Alessio Antonini, for the added value to the conference. COIOTE 2014 would have not been possible without the dedicated work of all abovementioned individuals.

This event was part of the IoT360 summit, endorsed and organized by the European Alliance for Innovation (EAI) and technically sponsored by CREATE-NET. We are grateful to the EAI staff, particularly to Ms. Giorgia Nisi, who tirelessly looked after every detail in making this conference possible.

We hope that the papers included in these proceedings will serve as valuable reference for topics related to artificial intelligence in the context of the IoT.

Frederik Santens
Radu-Laurentiu Vieriu

International Conference on Pervasive Games PERGAMES 2014
Rome, Italy, 26 October 2014

Preface

PERGAMES 2014, the First International Conference on Pervasive Games, was held at LUISS Enlabs, Rome, on October 27, 2014, as a co-located event with the IoT360 Summit of EAI.

The conference focus was on understanding how to best design and deploy pervasive games for various sectors, such as health and well-being, ambient-assisted living, smart cities/societies, education, cultural heritage, tourism and more. It aimed at bringing together international researchers, IoT and game developers, as well as industry delegates to address issues and trends, research, and technological advances in the world of pervasive games for different application fields.

The conference was structured as a single-track, multi-session event. To encourage active participation and the potential formation of new collaborations among attendees, the atmosphere was kept informal and preceded by an organized group visit to the VIGAMUS (Video-Games Museum) in Rome. Also, two interactive and gamified sessions were carried out during the conference day, one focusing on group brainstorming for the design of innovative game solutions and the other focusing on discussing their deployment and exploitation challenges.

Contributions to the conference were solicited in the form of full and short research papers. After a thorough review process of the papers received, for which we thank the Technical Program Committee, nine were accepted for presentation at the conference.

On behalf of the Organizing Committee of PERGAMES 2014, we would like to thank EAI and CREATE-NET for technical sponsorship of the event. A special thank also to the volunteer students from the Faculty of Architecture, University of Rome La Sapienza, and to Prof. Ivan Paduano, in particular, for their local support and endless patience.

Last but not least, we would like to thank all the authors who submitted papers, making the conference possible, and the authors of accepted papers for their valuable contribution.

Edna Pasher
Gabriel Bendersky
Silvia Gabrielli

First International Conference on IoT Technologies for HealthCare
HealthyIoT 2014
Rome, Italy, October 27–28, 2014

Preface

In this dedicated Internet of Things technologies for healthcare section of the publication, it is our pleasure to introduce to you a wide selection of innovative and insightful research papers that were presented at the First International Conference on IoT Technologies for Healthcare. The HealthyIoT 2014 conference was an IoT co-located event which took place in Rome, Italy, during October 27–29, 2014, forming one of the main conferences in the IoT360 Summit.

HealthyIoT 2014 was the first one of an international scientific event series dedicated to the IoT and healthcare. The IoT, as a set of existing and emerging technologies, notions, and services, can provide many solutions to delivery of electronic healthcare, patient care, and medical data management. The event brought together technology experts, researchers, industry and international authorities contributing toward the assessment, development, and deployment of healthcare solutions based on IoT technologies, standards, and procedures.

The conference was organized by CREATE-NET in collaboration with the European Alliance for Innovation in Slovakia, and its partner, the European Alliance for Innovation, in Trento, Italy.

A total of 15 research papers are featured in this publication, with contributions by researchers from across Europe and around the world. The publication includes manuscripts written and presented by authors from different countries, including China, Germany, Greece, Italy, Portugal, Romania, Sweden, and the UK. Topics including healthcare support for the elderly, real-time monitoring systems, wearables, and healthcare security systems are covered.

In conclusion, we would like to once again express our sincere thanks to all the authors and attendees of the conference in Rome, Italy, and also the authors who contributed to the creation of this HealhthyIoT publication.

Antonio J. Jara

International Conference IoT as a Service
IoTaaS 2014
October 27–28, 2014, Rome, Italy

Preface

These are the proceedings of the First Internet of Things as a Service (IoTaaS) Conference. IoTaaS is an international venue for publishing innovative and cutting-edge results on the convergence of next-generation technologies and methodologies reshaping our way of living. This conference focuses on the Internet of Things (IoT) in general and in particular on providing innovative and enabling capabilities "as a service." The cloud serves as the central focal point for consumption and delivery of such technologies and applications.

The IoT era is widely seen as looming just around the corner, expected to have a significant impact on most aspects of entities of all kinds, from citizens through enterprises small and large to government bodies. The amount of smart devices is huge and grows at a staggering rate, while connectivity gets a wider coverage. Smart objects are immersed in everyday life and the amount and variety of contextual data they can produce, or the actions they can take on their immediate environment, is enormous. At the same time smart objects are becoming more capable and sophisticated by having stronger processing power, larger amounts of storage, and longer battery life.

For this trend to have a big impact, be successful, and be widely adopted and useful it needs to be tightly integrated with the most advanced operational technology trend of cloud-based "Everything as a Service." IoT poses various specific challenges that are not yet covered by existing cloud offerings, chief among these are the heterogeneity, security, and scalability issues. In addition, developing and deploying IoT-based applications should be made as accessible as possible such that the entry barrier for new innovations in this area is lowered. Thus, an appropriate cloud should support a high level of "as a service" paradigm. This deployment paradigm will enable the easy adoption of IoT-based services and applications by end users, while calling for smart object providers as well as platform middleware providers to architect their solutions accordingly. Moreover, the same rule of thumb applies also for the ingestion and exposure of smart objects via the platform. The supporting business model would support a pay-as-you-go paradigm, enabling small to large entities to participate and contribute.

We received many good papers. These papers went through a rigorous review process that selected the papers in the program. The selected papers cover a wide spectrum of topics belonging to IoTaaS. We have papers on networking considerations for IoT, platforms for IoTaaS, adapting to the IoT environment, modeling IoTaaS, machine-to-machine support in IoT, as well as composite applications. We also have a position paper on the third phase FI-PPP (Future Internet – Private Public Partnership) project encouraging SMEs to start experimenting in this challenging new area. To top all these interesting topics, we have two keynote talks. One by Aleardo Furlani from INNOVA, who discusses enabling IoT business opportunities. The other by Peter Niblett from IBM, with an industry view. We believe that this strong program laid a concrete foundation for this conference for years to come.

Eliezer Dekel
Benjamin Mandler

First International Conference on Cognitive Internet of Things Technologies – COIOTE 2014
Rome – October 27, 2014

Organization

General Co-chairs

Imrich Chlamtac	Create-Net, Trento, Italy
Frederik Santens	Imtech ICT, Belgium
Liviu Goraş	Gheorghe Asachi University, Iaşi, Romania
Ramanathan Subramanian	ADSC, Singapore
Athanasios V. Vasilakos	University of Western Macedonia, Greece
Radu-Laurenţiu Vieriu	University of Trento, Italy

Technical Program Chair

Artur Arsénio	Beira Interior University/YDreams Robotics, Portugal

Technical Program Co-chair

Erik Mannens	MMLab/iMinds-UGent, Belgium

Web Chair

Stanislau Semeniuta	University of Trento, Italy

Techincal Program Committee

Frederik Santens	Imtech ICT, Belgium
Ramanathan Subramanian	ADSC, Singapore
Radu-Laurenţiu Vieriu	University of Trento, Italy
Abdur Rahim Biswas	Create-Net, Italy
Nenad Stojanovic	iCEP, Germany
Mohan Kankanhalli	National University of Singapore, Singapore
Vassilios Vonikakis	ADSC, Singapore
Nuno Garcia	Beira Interior University, Portugal
Neeli R. Prasad	Aalborg University, Denmark

Nik Bessis	University of Derby, UK
Wesley De Neve	MMLab/iMinds-UGent, Belgium
Ruben Verborgh	MMLab/iMinds-UGent, Belgium
Simon Mayer	ETH Zürich, Switzerland

"Affordances in IoT" Special Session Organizers

Alice Ruggeri	University of Turin, Italy
Alessio Antonini	University of Turin, Italy
Luigi Di Caro	University of Turin, Italy
Livio Robaldo	University of Turin, Italy

International Conference on Pervasive Games
PERGAMES 2014
Rome, Italy, 26 October 2014

Organization

General Chair

Edna Pasher   Founder & CEO - EPA Management Consultants, Israel

General Co-chair

Gabriel Bendersky   Edna Pasher PhD & Associates, Israel

Steering Committee Chair

Imrich Chlamtac   CREATE-NET, Italy

Technical Program Committee Chair

Silvia Gabrielli   CREATE-NET, Italy

Publication Chair

Irit Luft Madar   Methodica Ltd., Israel

First International Conference on IoT Technologies for HealthCare
HealthyIoT 2014
Rome, Italy, October 27–28, 2014

Organization

Steering Committee Chair

Imrich Chlamtac   President of Create-Net, President of European Alliance for Innovation, Italy

Steering Committee Members

Joel J.P.C. Rodrigues   Instituto de Telecomunicações, University of Beira Interior, Portugal

Antonio J. Jara   Institute of Information Systems, University of Applied Sciences Western Switzerland (HES-SO), Switzerland

Shoumen Palit Austin Datta   School of Engineering Massachusetts Institute of Technology; Industrial Internet Consortium, USA

General Chairs

Joel J.P.C. Rodrigues   Instituto de Telecomunicações, University of Beira Interior, Portugal

Antonio J. Jara   Institute of Information Systems, University of Applied Sciences Western Switzerland (HES-SO), Switzerland

Publication Chair

Codrina Lauth   Copenhagen Business School, Embedded Software Lab. and Grundfos Holding A/S, Corporate R&T Dept., Denmark

Publicity Chair

Andrej Kos   University of Ljubljana, Faculty of Electrical Engineering, Slovenia

Local Chair

Raffaele Giaffreda   CREATE-NET, Italy

Technical Program Members

Gerald Bieber	Fraunhofer Institute for Computer Graphics, Germany
Dimitrios Kosmopoulos	Technical Educational Institute of Crete Estavromenos, Greece
Ilias Maglogiannis	University of Piraeus, Greece
Matt Bishop	University of California, Davis, USA
Venet Osmani	CREATE-NET, Italy
Jun Suzuki	University of Massachusetts, Boston, USA
Silvia Gabrielli	CREATE-NET, Italy
Abdelmajid Khelil	Huawei European Research Center, Germany
Emad Felemban	Umm Al-Qura University, Saudi Arabia
Faisal Karim	Mehran University, Pakistan
Kunal Mankodiya	Carnegie Mellon University, USA
Manish Mahajan	Software Lead, Osterhout Design Group, USA

International Conference IoT as a Service
IoTaaS 2014
October 27–28, 2014, Rome, Italy

Preface

General Chairs

Eliezer Dekel   IBM Research - Haifa, Israel
Benny Mandler   IBM Research - Haifa, Israel

Program Chair

Benny Mandler   IBM Research - Haifa, Israel

Program Committee Members

Gari Singh   IBM
Vivi Fragopoulou   FORTH, Greece
Dana Petcu   West University of Timisoara, Romania
Stephan Steglich   Fraunhofer FOKUS, Germany
Beniamino Di Martino   Second University of Naples, Italy
Kostas Magoutis   University of Ioannina and ICS-FORTH, Greece
Sotiris Ioannidis   FORTH, Greece
Joachim Posegga   Institute for IT Security and Security Law (ISL),
                         University of Passau, Germany
Dimosthenis Kyriazis   National Technical University of Athens, Greece
Iacopo Carreras   U-Hopper, Italy
Marios Dikaiakos   University of Cyprus, Cyprus

Contents – Part I

PERGAMES 2014

HealthyIoT 2014

IoTaaS 2014

Contents – Part II

SaSeIoT 2014

COIOTE 2014

PowerOnt: An Ontology-Based Approach for Power Consumption Estimation in Smart Homes

Dario Bonino, Fulvio Corno, and Luigi De Russis[✉]

Dipartimento di Automatica e Informatica, Politecnico di Torino,
Corso Duca Degli Abruzzi 24, 10129 Torino, Italy
{dario.bonino,fulvio.corno,luigi.derussis}@polito.it

Abstract. The impact of electricity consumption in buildings on the overall energy budget of European and North-American states is steadily growing and requires solutions for achieving a more sustainable development. Smart metering and energy management system can be hardly afforded by residential homes, for their cost and the required granularity. Empowering smart homes with suitable power consumption models allows to estimate, in real-time, the current home consumption on the basis of currently active devices. In this paper we introduce an ontology based power consumption model (PowerOnt) for smart homes, and we discuss some application use cases where the proposed approach may successfully be exploited. Results show that the modeling approach has the potential to support energy efficiency measures into residential homes with few or no metering devices.

Keywords: Power consumption · Ontology · Smart home · Electricity

1 Introduction

According to statistics from both the US Department of Energy and the European Union Energy Commission, electricity consumption will increase in the next years, with residential and commercial buildings raising their aggregate figure up to 73 % of the total yearly consumption. Smart homes can play a pivotal role by enabling users to better organize their daily activities in order to reduce the global home consumption, by suggesting and promoting new, more efficient behaviors and by preventing or postponing the activation of energy greedy appliances, possibly coordinating with local power sources. Fine grained metering is one of the key factor for these "energy positive" innovations in the homes although implied costs still prevent its application inside home environments. As a consequence, homes are still "locked" into a stale condition where only one meter (if any) is installed and almost no policy can be applied. To overcome this issue and start improving energy efficiency of residential habitations we propose to enrich smart homes with explicit, machine understandable information, in form of appliance-level power consumption data, either nominal or measured on

© Institute for Computer Sciences, Social Informatics and Telecommunications Engineering 2015
R. Giaffreda et al. (Eds.): IoT360 2014, Part I, LNICST 150, pp. 3–8, 2015.
DOI: 10.1007/978-3-319-19656-5_1

the specific device. Such a detailed modeling allows to estimate the total power absorbed by a smart home by knowing device activations, only. If such a capability is complemented by the availability of one, or more, real meters, estimation can be improved and results may increase their accuracy scaling gracefully to the full metering case, where every device is connected to a dedicated meter. The PowerOnt ontology model presented in this paper is specifically designed to model nominal, typical and real power consumption of each device in a home and its modular design allows to plug the same model into different ontology-based modeling frameworks for smart homes.

2   Use Cases

To better exemplify how a relatively simple and abstract model of energy consumption such as PowerOnt can positively impact the energy consumption in habitations, we depict two different use cases, of increasing complexity, where power modeling assumes a crucial role for sustaining better consumption policies.

Meterless monitoring Many research contributions, in literature, show that householders can decrease their electricity absorption by 5 %-15 % by just being informed about their current energy consumption habits [1]. To make home inhabitants aware of their current energy habits, most approaches exploit In-Home energy Displays (IHDs) [2,3] showing the amount of power currently consumed, the energy absorbed since a given start time and information to promote positive changes in the householders lifestyle. Metering is a functional requirement for IHDs, if no metering information is available in the home, no feedback can be given and no improvement can be achieved. By simply plugging PowerOnt device descriptions into an existing smart home, i.e., by inserting a proper software module into the existing smart home gateway, it is possible to estimate the current home consumption from the activation states of the connected devices, even if no meter is installed.

Better Practices Suggestion Given a smart home with one or more meters installed, PowerOnt may be used by the home gateway to implement advanced suggestion policies, stimulating positive changes of the home inhabitants behaviors. At every device activation, e.g., by means of a button, the home gateway intelligence may, in fact, check the alternative ways for achieving the same final state, and suggest to activate the one having the lowest impact on the home energy consumption. For example, imagine that the bathroom illumination can be obtained by either switching on the bathroom ceiling lamp, or by raising up the bathroom shutter. Every solution can be profiled under the electrical consumption point of view, using information encoded in PowerOnt, and the less consuming one can be identified. If the user does not select the best activation (energetically speaking), the smart home can exploit IHDs to inform the inhabitant of the existence of a better habit, e.g., raising the shutter instead of lighting the lamp.

3   PowerOnt

PowerOnt is a light-weight ontology designed to model power consumption of electrical devices and appliances in smart homes (see Fig. 1), supporting the previously depicted use cases. A minimal approach is adopted, reducing

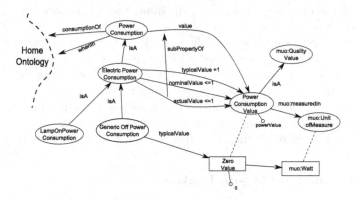

Fig. 1. PowerOnt, class hierarchy

modeling primitives (classes and relations) to those strictly needed to support power consumption modeling. Relations to described devices and appliances are left "open," i.e., their descriptions shall be completely formalized depending on the ontology-based home/device model to which PowerOnt is connected.

3.1   Structure

Two main classes compose the ontology, namely `poweront:PowerConsumption` and `poweront:PowerConsumptionValue`. They respectively model the kind of power absorbed by a given device or appliance, e.g., electric power, and the amount (value) of consumed power in terms of International System units, e.g., Watt. The `poweront:PowerConsumption` concept is specialized into `poweront:ElectricPowerConsumption`, modeling electric power typically absorbed by home devices and appliances. Devices can be described by either instantiating the type of power they absorb or by further specializing the electric power consumption class and by instantiating the corresponding descendants, e.g., `poweront:LampOnPowerConsumption` that models power absorbed by switched-on lamps. Power values are referred to their unit of measure by means of the `muo:measuredIn` relation, defined in the standard MUO ontology[1], that relates a `poweront:PowerConsumptionValue` instance to a `muo:UnitOfMeasure` instance. Power consumption classes are related to (at least) one power consumption value by means of the `poweront:value` relation. Such a relation is further specialized to allow specifying typical, nominal and actual consumption values.

---

[1] http://idi.fundacionctic.org/muo/.

Given an instance of a class descending from `poweront:PowerConsumption`, e.g., of `LampOnPowerConsumption`, such an instance can be connected to: (a) a *typical* power value derived from the consumption of a generic device of the same type, e.g., lamps in a home typically consume around 60/90 W; (b) an optional *nominal* power value declared by the device manufacturer, e.g., the living room lamp has a nominal power consumption of 30 W; (c) an optional *actual* power value measured on the real device, e.g., the living room lamp actually consumes 28,92 W.

Two "open" relations, respectively named `poweront:consumptionOf` and `dogP:whenIn`, model the power absorbed by a given device in a given operating condition. The former relates a device, expressed in whatever ontology (range unspecified) with its corresponding power consumption described in PowerOnt. The latter further specializes this relation by associating the power consumption with a specific device operating condition, e.g., state; also in this case the relation is left open to achieve maximum modeling flexibility (range unspecified).

3.2 Sample Integration with DogOnt

To better clarify power consumption modeling through PowerOnt we consider a specific integration sample, where PowerOnt is integrated with the DogOnt[2] ontology model for Smart Environments [4]. Integrating PowerOnt and DogOnt means exploiting DogOnt concepts as the ranges of `poweront:consumptionOf` and of `poweront:whenIn`. In DogOnt, devices that can be connected to a smart gateway, i.e., controlled, are modeled by the concept `dogont:Controllable`. Therefore, PowerOnt in DogOnt will specialize the `poweront:consumptionOf` range to `dogont:Controllable`. Moreover, since in DogOnt different device operating conditions are explicitly modeled by means of concepts belonging to the `dogont:StateValue` hierarchy, the PowerOnt `poweront:whenIn` relation range will be set at `dogont:StateValue`.

The resulting integration is reported in Fig. 2 where DogOnt concepts are reported in bold while PowerOnt concepts are reported in italic font. The PowerOnt ontology integrated with DogOnt is available at http://elite.polito.it/ontologies/poweront.owl.

4   Example Application

We can use the first use case presented in Sect. 2 (*Meterless energy monitoring*) as a practical example to exploit some PowerOnt functionalites. We can consider the devices present in a bathroom: a lamp on the top of the bathroom mirror, a shutter and the ceiling lamp. Only the shutter is metered. If we want to obtain the consumption of such home appliances (metered or not), in order to promote energy saving, we could use a SPARQL query, thus reporting either the typical, nominal, or measured value. As shown in Fig. 3, SPARQL querying

---

[2] Available at http://elite.polito.it/ontologies/dogont.owl.

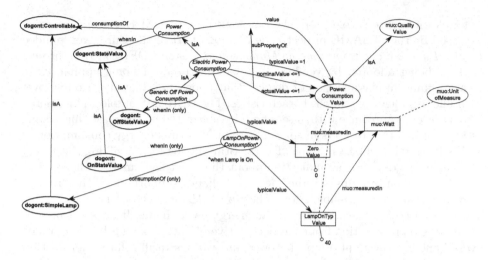

Fig. 2. Integration of PowerOnt and DogOnt

is exploited to extract, for each controlled device `?device` located in the bath-room, the list of its state values `?stateValue` and to further retrieve the power consumption values `?consumption` for each state value. Then, the typical con-sumption value (`?typicalConsumption`), the nominal (`?nominalConsumption`) and the measured one (`?actualConsumption`) are extracted, if available, from `?consumption`.

```
SELECT ?device, ?typicalConsumption, ?nominalConsumption, ?measuredConsumption
WHERE
{
?device a dogOnt:Controllable.
?device dogOnt:isIn <http://elite.polito.it/ontologies/samples/samplePower.owl#Bathroom>.
?consumption a powerOnt:ElectricPowerConsumption.
?device dogOnt:hasState ?state.
?state dogOnt:hasStateValue ?stateValue.
?consumption powerOnt:consumptionOf ?device.
?consumption powerOnt:whenIn ?stateValue.
OPTIONAL{?consumption powerOnt:typicalValue ?typicalConsumption}.
OPTIONAL{?consumption powerOnt:nominalValue ?nominalConsumption}.
OPTIONAL{?consumption powerOnt:actualValue ?measuredConsumption}
}
```

Fig. 3. SPARQL query for the "Monitoring" case

5   Related Works

Several ontologies for energy management in smart homes have been proposed in the literature. Most of them, differently from PowerOnt, are not modular and they do not use standard ontologies (such as MUO) to define units of measure.

Example of such ontologies are the ontology part of DEHEMS, or the ontology used by the SESAME project. The ontology part of the European founded *Digital Environment Home Energy Management System* (DEHEMS) [5] project aims at being adopted by vendors and manufacturers of home appliances to create a uniform classification of devices that allows automated reasoning over their energy efficiency related characteristics. The DEHEMS ontology, in general, associates each appliance with: a set of advice generated by the reasoning system as recommendation to users in specific case of abnormal energy consumption; b a "EU Energy Label Class" and a "Energy Star" rating for classifying the energy efficient of the device; c an indication about the "Wattage" used; d the value of the "Wattage on Standby" (if the specific appliance supports it); e the "Energy Consumed" in every possible state. The *SESAME* project [6], instead, uses an ontology-based approach to describe an energy-aware home. It does not provide appliances representation from the perspective of energy saving but it relies on overall energy consumption, peak power and various tariff information as they are provided by smart meter supplier.

6   Conclusions and Future Works

In this paper we introduce PowerOnt, an ontology based power consumption model for intelligent environments, able to provide, for each controlled home appliance, either a typical power consumption, a nominal or a measured consumption. Future work includes the usage of PowerOnt in the open source Dog gateway[3] and the realization of the proposed use cases.

References

1. Darby, S.: The Effectiveness of Feedback on Energy Consumption. Technical report, Environmental Change Institute, University of Oxford (2006)
2. He, H.A., Greenberg, S.: Motivating Sustainable Energy Consumption in the Home. In: ACM CHI Workshop on Defining the Role of HCI in the challenges of Sustainability (2009)
3. Riche, Y., Dodge, J., Metoyer, R.A.: Studying always-on electricity feedback in the home. In: Proceedings of the 28th international conference on Human factors in computing systems, CHI 2010, pp. 1995–1998. ACM, New York (2010)
4. Bonino, D., Corno, F.: DogOnt - ontology modeling for intelligent domotic environments. In: Sheth, A.P., Staab, S., Dean, M., Paolucci, M., Maynard, D., Finin, T., Thirunarayan, K. (eds.) ISWC 2008. LNCS, vol. 5318, pp. 790–803. Springer, Heidelberg (2008)
5. Shah, N., Chao, K.-M.: Ontology for Home Energy Management Domain. Technical report, University of Coventry (2011)
6. Tomic, S., Fensel, A., Pellegrini, T.: Sesame demonstrator: ontologies, services and policies for energy efficiency. In: Proceedings of the 6th International Conference on Semantic Systems. ACM, New York (2010)

---

[3] See http://dog-gateway.github.io for further information.

A Learning Approach for Energy Efficiency Optimization by Occupancy Detection

Vitor Mansur[1(✉)], Paulo Carreira[1,2], and Artur Arsenio[3,4]

[1] Department of Computer Science and Engineering,
Universidade de Lisboa, Lisbon, Portugal
{vitor.mansur,paulo.carreira}@ist.utl.pt
[2] INESC-ID Lisboa, Lisbon, Portugal
[3] Department of Computer Science, Universidade da Beira Interior,
Covilhã, Portugal
arsenio@alum.mit.edu
[4] YDreams Robotics, Lisbon, Portugal

Abstract. Building Automation Systems control HVAC systems aiming at optimizing energy efficiency and comfort. However, these systems use pre-set configurations, which usually do not correspond to occupants' preferences. Although existing systems take into account the number of occupants and the energy consumption, individual occupant preferences are disregarded. Indeed, there is no way for occupants to specify their preferences to HVAC system. This paper proposes an innovation in the management of HVAC systems: a system that tracks the occupants preferences, and manages automatically the ventilation and heating levels accordingly to their preferences, allowing the system to pool its resources to saving energy while maintaining user comfort levels. A prototype solution implementation is described and evaluated by simulation using occupants' votes. Our findings indicate that one of the algorithms is able to successfully maintain the appropriate comfort levels while also reducing energy consumption by comparing with a standard scenario.

Keywords: Energy savings · Users preferences · Occupancy detection · HVAC system · Thermal comfort

1 Introduction

Heating, Ventilation and Air Conditioning (HVAC) systems account for up to 60 % of the total energy consumption of commercial buildings [1]. In modern buildings, HVAC system settings are configured centrally on the management console of the Building Automation System (BAS). Despite the fact that BASs aim at saving energy while maintaining occupant comfort [2], HVAC settings are only reviewed seasonly to account for large climate and occupancy variations. Indeed, settings are not adjusted in real-time to take into account fast dynamics of occupant preferences leading to overcooling or overheating. In practice, since occupants cannot control the HVAC thermal settings, they may experience discomfort while the system is probably cooling or heating above what is required and wasting energy. If occupants were given the

© Institute for Computer Sciences, Social Informatics and Telecommunications Engineering 2015
R. Giaffreda et al. (Eds.): IoT360 2014, Part I, LNICST 150, pp. 9–15, 2015.
DOI: 10.1007/978-3-319-19656-5_2

opportunity to control the system, situations of excessive service delivery that energy expenditure would be less frequent.

Energy management systems (EMS) are concerned with finding sources of waste and acting to improve energy savings. EMSs corrective action also typically targets HVAC systems in order to reduce energy waste. However, if occupants are not in the loop, these improvements are under-optimal. An intelligent climate control solution that takes into account occupant opinions regarding comfort is potentially capable of minimizing the energy consumption while maintaining the occupants comfort.

Studies show that the use of occupancy detection techniques with light and HVAC systems is beneficial to energy optimization, reaching savings values from 10 % up to 50 % [3–5]. However occupancy detection does not always have an acceptable accuracy rate. A promising approach is to use Radio Frequency Identification (RFID) systems to detect occupants with reliable accuracy, and retrieve occupants' information such as their comfort preferences. This can lead to a higher occupancy detection accuracy and energy management control.

Maximizing occupant comfort from individual preferences is challenging because preferences can be contradictory. Even if possible for occupants to change HVAC system settings, it still may difficult to reach a consensual set-point value so that every single occupant feel comfortable. To date, there is no platform that maximizes comfort by collecting information on the occupant preferences and (i) compute a setpoint which will control the temperature based on their feedback, (ii) encourage occupants to save energy by presenting them information on the other occupant votes, (iii) takes into account occupants preference history to improve decision making, and (iv) makes automatic decisions to configure the HVAC subsystem automatically.

This paper describes an approach that enables occupants of a given room to give their opinion on HVAC system configuration. A machine learning algorithm calculates a setpoint temperature that best fits their suggestions and find the most appropriate actuation to minimize energy consumption while at the same time maximize comfort. The proposed system incorporates dynamic user feedback control loops in order to optimize the energy/comfort trade-off.

2 Solution Architecture

The proposed solution tracks occupant through RFID card-reading, interacts with occupants on a web-front displayed on their mobile devices, computes set-points and sends commands to the HVAC sub-system through an OPC gateway. The system architecture is depicted in Fig. 1. The system consists of the following modules [6]:

RFID Module that retrieves the users information from the RFID tag on a student card. RFID card readers were mounted and two doors entrances and wired to two Arduino systems (Arduino Board plus RFID and LCD shields), coupled to another system, a Raspberry Pi, to aggregate the information of these systems and send it to the Storage Module. An entrance acknowledge feedback is presented to the user on the (LCD) screen (it could also be sent to a smartphone).

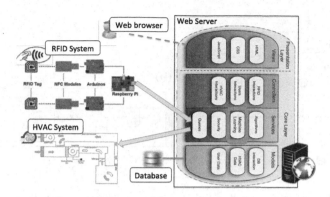

Fig. 1. Solution architecture and modules. On the left, the occupancy detection and HVAC modules (the peripheral modules) on the right, the application core modules.

Backend Application Interface consists of the presentation layer running on the web server to abstract the access to the database.

Storage Module uses a PostgreSQL Database to store and manage user information.

Application Core acts as the brain of the system, performing all computation including the simulation and the learning algorithm. Some of the main functions are:

- Occupancy detection: Knowing and deciding if a user is on the room or not, based on information received from the RFID System.
- User voting & feedback handling: Collecting user's votes and send users feedback regarding ambient variables.
- Setpoint calculation: Collecting the occupant's votes, validate them and calculate a new setpoint which minimizes discomfort.
- Learning algorithm: Learn information about occupant's behaviour and predict a best decision to make [7].
- Interaction with HVAC System: Send information about the new set-point and receive information about the ambient variables.

2.1 Occupancy Detection Using RFID

In order to adjust automatically to occupant preferences, the system must know the identities of the occupants. The main algorithm works in three stages: the first one is to detect the RFID tag (or student card), the second one is to route this information through a Raspberry Pi and add a simple security layer to the information. Finally, in the last stage, receives the information through a web service, adds a presence flag on the user database, saves the date, time and hour that the user entered the room and return the response to the Arduino's LCD and the entrance. Figure 2 depicts the flow of interactions that are triggered when a tag is read.

(a)

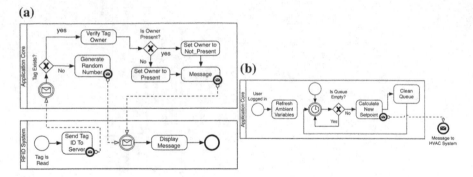

Fig. 2. (a) RFID System's interaction with the Main Application. It starts by sending the read tag ID to the Core, which verifies if the owner exists and defines it as present or abscent. (b) Main functions of the Application Core: Refresh ambient variables, calculates the setpoint periodically and cleans queue.

2.2 Setpoint Calculation

The setpoint calculation algorithm is responsible for gathering the occupants' votes and calculating a setpoint, which tries to minimize the probability of negative voting, thus maximizing overall comfort for users in the room.

After a user votes, the Application Core starts by verifying if the user is in the room; if not, the process ends with an error message. Next, it verifies if the user has already voted; if so, it automatically overwrites the last request, adds it to a queue and stores it on the database with all the relevant information of the status of the room.

The system verifies the voting queue at specific intervals. If the queue is not empty, it calculates the new setpoint, cleans the queued requests and sends the new setpoint to the HVAC system. Then, it returns to waiting on the queue. Figure 2b illustrates the process. Setpoint computations are based always on the direction of the majority of votes. Therefore, the temperature settings will converge to an average value where most occupants feel comfortable. This algorithm assumes that a vote is correlated with the dissatisfaction of the occupant regarding current temperature settings, so the occupant wants to change it by voting to increase or decrease the temperature. The vote calculation starts by collecting all the queued votes and calculating the number of people in the room. It compares the percentage of votes relatively to the number of people in the room. The difference between the votes to increase and decrease the temperature should be greater than 10 %; if its not the case, the algorithm only cleans the queue and does not change the setpoint. The calculation decides if the setpoint should increase or decrease the temperature considering the majority of the votes changing it from 1°C.

2.3 Learning Algorithm

By having users configuring the HVAC System with votes, the overall performance can be improved enabling the system to automatically configure itself. First it is necessary to gather all the votes, identify patterns into it and learn them to take decisions in the future. Many learning algorithms are able to identify patterns on input data with a large number of examples. In this particular case, the system will not have a large amount of data to identify patterns. The analysed input consists of a stream of users votes who want to raise, maintain, or decrease the temperature. After collecting these votes, a learning algorithm is applied to separate this data into clusters according to data similarity. This way, it becomes possible à-posteriori the auto configuration of the room's setpoint without further needing the occupants to vote.

We employ an unsupervised learning algorithm to configure the setpoint according to a prediction based on the actual status of the room. The application core achieves this by loading the information about the room and comparing it to a set of previously calculated scenarios. Then it decides which setpoint is most appropriate. The algorithm retrieves the information on each vote made and saves it on the database during the submission of a user request. The users vote will not interfere with the set-point estimation, it is solely used for the purpose of training the Learning Algorithm. The k-means algorithm [8] used is a method of cluster analysis that divides into k clusters a set of n observations, each cluster S being associated with a centroid C. Each observation should belong to the cluster with the nearest mean. First, the algorithm starts by mapping the clusters by choosing k random values and define them as the new centroids, then it iterates and calculate a new centroid [9]. Each centroid is related to a system decision. The algorithm calculates once per day the new centroids, updating all the new requests and labeling each one of them, based on all previous votes, and new ones made on the previous day. This method makes it possible to calculate the setpoint, and simultaneously using data to train the algorithm to achieve better results. Once the system has the clusters calculated, it takes the information on current variables such as the indoor temperature, hour of day, number of occupants and calculates the cluster that fits better these variables. Then verifies which is the decision (for temperature setpoint definition) associated with the cluster.

3   Experimental Evaluation

The proposed algorithms were evaluated on a simulation of a real life environment using EnergyPlus package. The simulation environment consists of a room where occupants are able to cast a vote with the intent of setting the temperature, which best fits their comfort [6]. The system computes the new setpoint and adjusts the HVAC system accordingly. The data collected in order to evaluate the system corresponds to the overall daily comfort value, the daily mean energy consumption in KWh and the mean daily setpoint. Two scenarios were considered.

In the baseline scenario, the temperature within the room did not vary throughout the day, independently on the occupant's votes. Simulations were made using fixed setpoints from 20-22°C. According to Fig. 3a and Table 1, the mean energy consumption is 67,89 KWh, standard deviation of 9,37 KWh, and the mean confort value is 75,7 with standard deviation of 1,58.

In the other scenario, the system adjusts the room temperature based on the learning algorithm and occupants votes. The Learning Algorithm scenario was tested in two experiments, one using k-means algorithm during 10 days of simulations to train it employing 9 centroids (k = 9), and the other employing 3 centroids (k = 3). It is shown that a larger number of clusters decrease energy consumption at a cost of a smaller confort level. Such trade-off is also seen in both learning experiments compared to the baseline scenario, as shown in Table 1 and Fig. 3b.

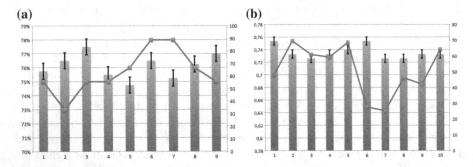

Fig. 3. The red line shows the percentage of the computed comfort (left axis scale), and the blue bars shows the energy consumption in KWh of each simulation (right axis scale); (a) Baseline simulations results; (b) k-means simulation results, with k = 3.

Table 1. Simulations experimental results (Energy Use in KWh, Comfort in %, and Setpoint in °C).

	Baseline Scenario		k = 9 and Days = 10			k = 3, Days = 10		
	Energy Use	Comfort	Energy Use	Comfort	Setpoint	Energy Use	Comfort	Setpoint
Mean	67,89	75,67	52,49	66,44	20,24	62,22	70,78	21,67
Std Deviation	9,37	1,58	39,74	2,38	4,45	4,18	4,01	0,41
Superior CV	74,25	76,7	77,12	67,91	22,99	64,81	73,26	21,93
Inferior CV	61,54	64,96	27,85	64,96	17,48	59,63	68,29	64,96

4   Conclusions

The use of BAS and EMS systems is becoming evermore common and sophisticated and seeking to promote energy savings by integrating new sources of data, such as user preferences, in real-time. Our hypothesis was that developing a learning system based on occupants input could allow controlling a HVAC system, to minimize the energy consumption while maximizing average user comfort. The results using the k-means algorithm suggest that it is possible to allow a room to configure the HVAC system based on a machine learning technique. Despite the comfort rate, which is approximately 5 % lower than the baseline, the energy consumption had a decrease of 5–KWh on the mean consume. This suggests there was a reduction on the energy consumption while abstaining from a higher occupant comfort rate.

Acknowledgments. Work developed in the scope of SMARTCAMPUS Project and supported by EU funds (http://greensmartcampus.eu). P. Carreira was supported by Fundação para a Ciência e a Tecnologia, under project PEst-OE/EEI/LA0021/2013.

References

1. Yang, R., Wang, L.: Development of multi-agent system for building energy and comfort management based on occupant behaviors. Energy Build. **56**, 1–7 (2013)
2. Soucek, S., Zucker, G.: Current developments and challenges in building automation. e & i Elektrotech. und Informationstechnik **129**(4), 278–285 (2012)
3. Boman, M., Davidsson, P.: Energy saving and added customer value in intelligent buildings. In: International Conference on the Practical Application of Intelligent Agents and Multi-Agent Technology, vol. 1, pp. 505–516 (1998)
4. Klein, L., Kwak, J., Kavulya, G., Jazizadeh, F., Becerik-Gerber, B., Varakantham, P., Tambe, M.: Coordinating occupant behavior for building energy and comfort management using multi-agent systems. Autom. Constr. **22**, 525–536 (2012)
5. Padmanabh, K., Adi Malikarjuna, V.: iSense: a wireless sensor network based conference room management system. In: Proceedings of the First ACM Workshop on Embedded Sensing Systems for Energy-Efficiency in Buildings, pp. 37–42 (2009)
6. Mansur, V.: Energy Efficiency Optimization Through Occupancy Detection and User Preferences. Instituto Superior Tecnico, MsC Thesis (2014)
7. Arsenio, A.: Development of neural mechanisms for machine learning. Int. J. Neural Syst. **15** (1–2), 41–54 (2011)
8. MacKay, D.: Information Theory, Inference and Learning Algorithms, pp. 316–322. Cambridge University Press, New York (2003)
9. Sun, Z., Wun, Y.: Multispectral image compression based on fractal and K-Means clustering. In: 1st International Conference on Information Science and Engineering, (1), pp. 1341–1344 (2009)

Intelligent Multi-platform Middleware
for Wireless Sensor and Actuator Networks

Rui Francisco[1,3] and Artur Arsenio[2,3(✉)]

[1] Computer Science Department, Universidade de Lisboa, Lisbon, Portugal
rui.francisco@ydreamsrobotics.com
[2] Computer Science Department, Universidade da Beira Interior,
Covilhã, Portugal
artur.arsenio@ydreamsrobotics.com
[3] YDreams Robotics, Lisbon, SA, Portugal

Abstract. Wireless Sensor and Actuator Networks (WSAN), composed by small sensing nodes for acquisition, collection and analysis of data, are often employed for communication between Internet objects. However the WSAN have some problems such as sensors' energetic consumption and CPU load. The massive storage capacity, large processing speeds and the rapid elasticity makes Cloud Computing a very good solution to these problems. To efficiently manage devices' resources, and achieve efficient communication with various platforms (cloud, mobile), this paper proposes a middleware that allows flows of AI applications' execution to be transferred between a device and the cloud.

Keywords: Internet of things · Wireless sensor and actuator networks · Cloud computing · Middleware · State machines

1 Introduction

It is expect that in a few years our lives become more dependent of internet objects connected by WSAN in areas such as environmental, medical, transportation, entertainment and city management. Although there has been an evolution of the nodes in WSAN, these continue to have limited battery, limited computation power, etc. Due to these problems, the network node can crash due to lack of sufficient resources to perform, and jeopardize the smooth operation of the infrastructure. So, especially for demanding AI applications, internet objects using sensors and actuators require specific middleware for integrated operation with networked resources [1, 2].

Cloud computing provides attractive solutions for these issues [3]. Indeed, it allows the reduction of the initial costs associated with the computational infrastructure. Another relevant aspect is that the cloud computing resources are easily and automatically adjustable according to the real infrastructure needs. This way, the computational resources are easily scalable following the growth of the infrastructure. Another important point is related with the fact that the customer only pays for the cloud resources that he actually uses. Mostly important, cloud computing resources provide almost unlimited battery, storage, and computing power.

So, we need an efficient solution that monitors the WSAN node capability to execute operations, and communicates transparently with the cloud infrastructure.

© Institute for Computer Sciences, Social Informatics and Telecommunications Engineering 2015
R. Giaffreda et al. (Eds.): IoT360 2014, Part I, LNICST 150, pp. 16–22, 2015.
DOI: 10.1007/978-3-319-19656-5_3

2 Solution Architecture

The system consists of devices running applications (egg clients: cell phones, tablets, and computers, as shown in Fig. 1a) and the cloud that makes data processing and saves data. The communication protocols are TCP, UDP, SSH and HTTP Rest, and a publish/subscribe model for internal communications in the device. Devices run applications developed by programmers, having constraints such as limited memory and battery (contrary to the cloud). These applications will run the management and cloud client side modules for programmers to use our middleware. The former monitors hardware components, and communicates to the cloud client whenever a component reaches a critical condition. The cloud client interchanges application's control messages and data to the cloud server module (see Fig. 1b).

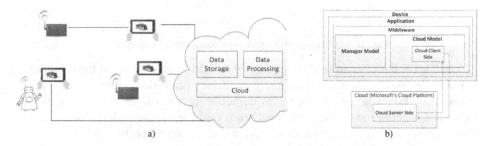

Fig. 1. (a) System Architecture and (b) its Components.

2.1 Manager Module

The management module aims to determine hardware components state (battery, CPU and memory), as well as the Wi-Fi connection state. The programmer defines each component's critical state on a configuration file, before the middleware starts to be used. Whenever one of these components achieves a value above a critical value (and WiFi signal is strong) a certain execution will no longer be run on the device, being transferred to the cloud. Figure 2a shows the management model's state machine.

The management model is initialized in the "Middleware" state when the "Application" state sends an initialization command. The "Middleware" state contains the monitored component conditions, which are updated by the "Monitoring" state through a shared queue between the two states. The "Middleware" state is always checking the conditions of the Wi-Fi signal quality and the conditions of the battery, CPU and memory, through calls to device hardware that runs the middleware. The values obtained are compared with the critical values stipulated by the application programmer. The load CPU analysis is a bit different from the other checks, because a notification is only sent if the read values are superior to the critical value for three times in a row (to avoid reactions to sporadic peaks). If the signal quality of the wireless network is below the critical value stipulated by the programmer the remaining monitoring tests will not be performed. After each monitoring cycle of the hardware components, the "Monitoring" state goes into sleep mode for one minute.

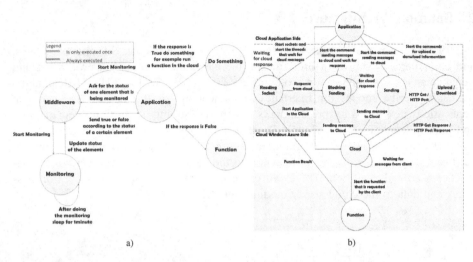

Fig. 2. (a) Management, and (b) Cloud, state machines.

The "Application" state sends requests to the "Middleware" state on the conditions of a component (e.g. battery). If the reply is "False" (transition between the "Application" and "Function" states), it means no action is needed, since the state of the component is below the critical status (and hence running with enough resources on the device). This way the programmer's application can continue to run without any changes, and no event is initiated. In case of a "True" response sent by the "Application" state, the machine transits to the "Do Something" state, meaning the component exceeds the critical value. In this case the programmer chooses the actions to take after receiving the message. One possible option is to use cloud platform provided services for performing certain actions. This way it is removed some load on the device that is running the application, releasing resources (e.g. memory).

2.2   Cloud Model - Client

The cloud module state machine is shown in Fig. 2b. The communication between the application and the cloud is initialized when the programmer application makes an initialization call to the middleware. The first step is for the client to boot the server in the cloud via an SSH command and to create TCP and UDP sockets. The access settings of Post and Get commands of HTTP Rest protocol are also configured, so that whenever the programmer intends an application to perform an upload or download of information in the cloud, it is sent a Post or Get command to the cloud.

The middleware in the cloud responds (transitions between "Application", "Upload/Download" and "Cloud") states either: (i) with a confirmation that the information was successfully saved; or (ii) there was an error while performing the operation of storage; or (iii) the information as requested by the get command; or (iv) error due to failure on obtaining the requested information.

In a blocking call connection, a message is sent to the cloud with the following information: the function ID and its arguments. After the message is sent the state

"Blocking Socket" enters in a blocking state and waits for the result of the function that is going to be executed in the cloud, delivered by the state "Reading Socket". In the non-blocking case, the state is not blocked after the message is sent (the program continues to run). Once the cloud returns the response, this is saved in the device memory until the program needs to access it. The state "Reading Socket" after being initialized enters in block mode waiting for new entries in the socket that arrive from the state "Cloud". A new message on the socket will be processed differently depending on the information of one message field. If the message is from a blocking function, the result is sent to the state "Sending Blocking", otherwise the function ID and its result will be stored in the device memory until the program needs the result.

2.3   Cloud Model - Server

The Cloud Server side module is initialized at the application server once it receives an SSH connection with the start command, locking the "Cloud" state, and waiting to receive messages from the client. Upon receipt of the message and its decoding, it is possible to identify the function ID that is intended to be performed and its arguments (going from state "Cloud" to "Function" state). The "Function" state consists of the execution of the functions that were chosen by the programmer to run in the cloud. At the end of the execution of a function a message is sent to the client (state "Reading Socket) with the function ID and its result. It is also sent a small packet to identify if the response is to the blocking or the non-blocking function.

3   Experimental Results Assessment

The metrics were the Percentage of Energy consumed and CPU Load. It was used 1 BQ Edison with Android OS, and one virtual machine with one core and 1,75 GB of RAM. We applied OpenCV to build a face detection and tracking application, heavy in terms of CPU processing power, battery consumption and generated traffic, since it makes significant image processing. Two experimental setups were implemented:

1. The baseline: the application that detects/tracks the human face is the only running on the Android OS (no middleware).
2. Integration with the middleware: the same application only sends messages composed with frames, getting these from the camera, and sending these to the cloud, being the frames' analysis made in the cloud.

3.1   Energy Consumed

The experiments on the 2 aforementioned scenarios lasted 40 min and were repeated 5 times. As shown in Fig. 3. and Table 1, there is no evidence of gains by transferring some application execution flows to the cloud. Results are even slightly better when the middleware was not used (difference never exceeded 8 %).

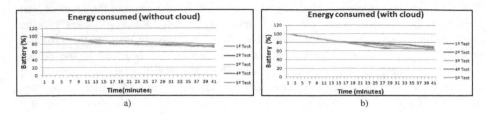

Fig. 3. Energy Consumed (a) without using the cloud; and (b) using the cloud.

Table 1. Energy Consumed (as percentage of battery charge) and CPU Load

Experimental setup	Without Cloud	With Cloud
Average working battery charge (at the end)	73,6%	66,4%
Standard Deviation	2,70	3,04
Average of battery spent by the five tests	25,2%	32,6%
Standard Deviation	3,11	3,04
Average Of the CPU Load	68,98%	45,84%
Standard Deviation	3,53	1,15

This similarity may be due to excessive use of the video camera, which consumes a lot of battery power, although this component is also used extensively without the middleware. The constant access to the wireless network should be the largest impact on the results, since the higher transmission rate implies higher energy spending [4].

3.2   CPU Load

To check potential middleware advantages in relation to CPU load, the "Face Detect/ Tracking" application was subjected to tests lasting 20 m and repeated five times. In Table 1 and Fig. 4, there is a significant gain with the migration of the detection and tracking algorithms to the cloud. This gain is due to the heavier work done now in the cloud, which alleviates the processing needs of the device's CPU running the application (just grabs image frames on the device and sends them).

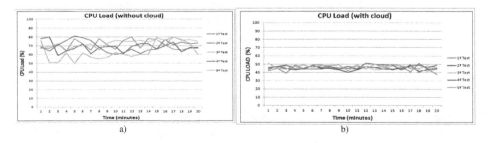

Fig. 4. CPU Load (a) without, and (b) with, the presence of the middleware

Hence, in situations where applications compete for CPU time in processing constrained devices, this solution can bring very interesting benefits. The image processing algorithms requires a lot of CPU load to be executed, which may prevent simultaneously other applications to run properly. The same also happens with image processing application that ceases to have the CPU just for itself, competing for resources such as CPU processing time, and this competition may create difficulties to its execution, such as a smaller frame rate, getting this way less frames per second.

To check if the middleware solution can solve this competition problem for limited resources, the following test scenarios were performed: checking the CPU status whenever an exhaustive analysis of 100 frames needs to be made, and checking the time consumed for both processing these set of images in the tablet or in the cloud.

According to Table 2, CPU load reaches saturation values for single tablet processing. But usage of cloud processing originates a significantly lower CPU load at the tablet. Hence the integration of the middleware may be beneficial to run reliably multiple applications on a device of limited resources, because with the transferring of execution flows to the cloud much of the processing is done outside the device, thus freeing some of the CPU load, so that other device applications can also be executed.

Table 2. CPU Comparative load in exhaustive case.

	Without Cloud	With Cloud
CPU Load average (%)	98,69	25,53
CPU Load standard deviation (%)	1,20	2,28
Average (execution time)(ms)	1292	1100
Standard deviation (ms)	5,60	4,80

4 Conclusions

This paper proposed a state machine based middleware to manage the transferring of execution flows between terminal devices and the cloud. The main goal was, using cloud technology, to address the problem of a device's lack of resources such as limited memory and battery. Experimental evaluation showed that offloading the execution flows into the cloud does not necessarily reduces energy consumption (or increases battery lifetime), because more battery energy may be required for wireless communications. Experiments indicate however that using the cloud to solve the lack of device resources is quite advantageous, because it allows reducing the CPU load. This may lead to battery with extended autonomy. But most importantly, it avoids applications entering in blocking states due to lack of memory, and allows running more applications in a simple device that otherwise would exceed the available resources. The decision whether to run an application locally or remotely is done dynamically, according to the status of available resources, as checked through active monitoring. More recently [5], we have successfully integrated the proposed middleware with a WSAN platform, OpenHAB, for smart home automation.

This middleware will be most beneficial for programmers who want to make the most of the hardware resources available on the devices.

Acknowledgments. Work developed in the scope of the Monarch project: Multi-Robot Cognitive Systems Operating in Hospitals, FP7-ICT-2011-9-601033, supported by EU funds. Artur Arsenio was also supported by CMU-Portuguese program through Fundação para Ciência e Tecnologia, under Augmented Human Assistance project CMUP-ERI/HCI/0046/2013.

References

1. Kranz, M., Rusu, R., Maldonado, A., Beetz, M., Schmidth, A.: A player/stage system for context-aware intelligent environments. In: Proceedings of the System Support for Ubiquitous Computing Workshop (UbiSys), September 2006
2. Quigley, M., Gerkey, B., Conley, K., Faust, J., Foote, T., Leibs, J., Berger, E., Wheeler, R., Ng, A.: ROS: an open-source robot operating system. In: ICRA Workshop on Open Source Software, vol. 3. No. 3.2 (2009)
3. Hunziker, D., Gajamohan, M., Waibel, M., D'Andrea, R.: Rapyuta: The roboearth cloud engine. In: IEEE International Conference on Robotics and Automation (ICRA) (2013)
4. Balasubramanian, N., Balasubramanian, A., Venkataramani, A.: Energy consumption in mobile phones: a measurement study and implications for network applications. In: Proceedings 9th ACM SIGCOMM Conference on Internet Measurement Conference (2009)
5. Francisco, R.: Flexible, Multi-platform Middleware for Wireless Sensor and Actuator Networks. MsC Thesis, IST (2014)

Sense-Deliberate-Act Cognitive Agents for Sense-Compute-Control Applications in the Internet of Things and Services

Amir H. Moin[✉]

fortiss, An-Institut Technische Universität München,
Munich, Germany
moin@fortiss.org

Abstract. In this paper, we advocate Agent-Oriented Software Engineering (AOSE) through employing Belief-Desire-Intention (BDI) intelligent agents for developing Sense-Compute-Control (SCC) applications in the Internet of Things and Services (IoTS). We argue that not only the agent paradigm, in general, but also cognitive BDI agents with sense-deliberate-act cycle, in particular, fit very well to the nature of SCC applications in the IoTS. However, considering the highly constrained heterogeneous devices that are prevalent in the IoTS, existing BDI agent frameworks, even those especially created for Wireless Sensor Networks (WSNs), do not work. We elaborate on the challenges and propose possible approaches to address them.

Keywords: Internet of things and services · Agent oriented software engineering · Intelligent agents · Cognitive agents · BDI · Constrained devices

1 Introduction

The Internet of Things and Services (IoTS) is an expanded version of the Internet containing not only the components of the Internet such as Web 2.0, but also constrained embedded devices such as sensors and actuators. As a crucial infrastructure for Cyber Physical Systems (CPS), in which the physical world merges with the virtual world of cyberspace [1], the IoTS is believed to have sufficient power to trigger the next (i.e., fourth) industrial revolution. However, it turns out that with this great power an enormous degree of complexity in software systems is inevitable. This is due to a number of reasons such as the tremendously large number of "things" (i.e., devices), heterogeneity of things and services as well as the variety of communication protocols.

Sense-Compute-Control (SCC) applications [2] are a typical group of applications in the IoTS. A SCC application senses the environment (e.g., temperature, humidity, light, UV radiation, etc.) through sensors, performs some computation (often decentralized, i.e., distributed) and finally prompts to take one or more actions through actuators (very often sort of control) in the environment.

© Institute for Computer Sciences, Social Informatics and Telecommunications Engineering 2015
R. Giaffreda et al. (Eds.): IoT360 2014, Part I, LNICST 150, pp. 23–28, 2015.
DOI: 10.1007/978-3-319-19656-5_4

There exist two main differences between these applications in the IoTS and the similar ones in the field of Wireless Sensor and Actuator Networks (WSAN), a predecessor of the field of the IoTS. First, the scale of the network is quite different. While WSANs typically have several hundreds or thousands of nodes, SCC applications in the IoTS may have several millions or billions of nodes. Second, the majority of nodes in a WSAN are more or less similar to each other. However, here in the IoTS we have a wide spectrum of heterogeneous devices, ranging from tiny sensor motes with critical computational, memory and energy consumption constraints to highly capable servers for cloud computing. Heterogeneity is a property inherited from another predecessor field, known as Pervasive (Ubiquitous) computing [3].

One of the recent paradigms in software engineering that helps in dealing with complexity is Agent-Oriented Software Engineering (AOSE). In fact, it is the intersection of the field of Multi-Agent Systems (MAS), the successor of Distributed Artificial Intelligence (DAI), with software engineering. Although the research field of MAS is only about two decades old, many methodologies have been proposed in this area. They could be mainly categorized into two groups [4,5]: software engineering (e.g., Gaia, Prometheus and O-MaSE) and knowledge engineering (e.g., CoMoMAS, MAS-CommonKADS and Tropos). Our focus here is on the former category, a field that is known as Agent-Oriented Software Engineering (AOSE).

AOSE helps in dealing with complexity in software development through raising the level of abstraction via the higher level concepts of agents, roles, organizations, collaboration, interaction protocols, etc. Yet, cognitive agents (e.g., BDI agents) raise the level of abstraction beyond that level. Moreover, MASes are intrinsically peer-to-peer distributed systems with asynchronous communication often based on message-passing with unicast, multicast and broadcast possibilities. This is a model which fits perfectly fine to the nature of SCC systems in the IoTS. Because, unlike web applications in the Internet, where the client/server model is prevalent, in the IoTS the peer-to-peer network topology (either pure or hybrid) makes more sense. Also, the asynchronous communication based on message-passing is much more scalable and efficient comparing other alternatives for distributed systems such as synchronous Remote Procedure Calls (RPC), in which the client should block (i.e., busy-wait) until the server finishes the processing of its request.

There exist several research works that have proposed BDI MAS approaches for the IoTS, WSANs, etc. However, considering the fact that the majority of heterogeneous things in the IoTS are highly constrained devices in terms of computational power, memory space, energy consumption, etc., to our knowledge, none of the proposed BDI-based approaches could work in practice for the SCC applications in the IoTS. Therefore, as the main contribution, we propose possible approaches for addressing this problem.

The paper is structured as follows. In Sect. 2, we explain the idea of employing BDI agents for SCC applications in the IoTS, elaborate on the practical technical challenges and propose two possible approaches for addressing those challenges.

This is followed by a brief review of the related work in this area in Sect. 3. Finally, we conclude and mention our future work in Sect. 4.

2   BDI Agents for SCC Applications

Intelligent agents have a number of key properties which distinguish them from other software paradigms. Some of them are listed below [4].

1. *Autonomy:* An agent can perform its task without any supervision.
2. *Reactiveness:* An agent reacts in a timely manner to the changes in its environment.
3. *Proactiveness:* An agent is not only reactive, but also proactive in the sense that it is goal-oriented and pursues its own goals.
4. *Sociality:* An agent interacts with other agents often through message-passing. A group of agents collaborating with each other in order to achieve a common goal form a society known as organization.

In a broad sense, the AOSE research area can be divided into two groups [6]. The first group is more concentrated on the MAS paradigm as middleware (e.g., Java Agent DEvelopment Framework (JADE) [7]), while the second one is about reasoning-oriented agent frameworks (e.g., the Jadex BDI system [6]). Our discussion here is more related to the latter category, i.e., reasoning.

As mentioned in the previous section, cognitive agents provide a very high level of abstraction for hiding complexity in AOSE. A number of cognitive architectures for agents have been proposed in the literature. One of the well-known software models for cognitive intelligent agents is Belief-Desire-Intention (BDI). BDI is not only simple to implement, but also corresponds nicely to the way that people talk about the human behavior in psychology [6].

As depicted in Fig. 1, a BDI agent has a set of beliefs, a set of desires, a set of intentions and a set of plans. Beliefs are informational attitudes about the

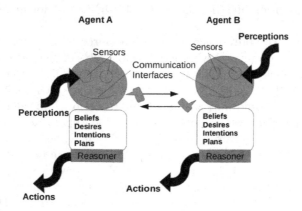

Fig. 1. Belief-Desire-Intention (BDI) agents, figure inspired by [8]

surrounding environment (i.e., the local personal view of the agent from the world that it perceives through its sensors) as well as the internal state of the agent itself. Desires are motivational attitudes that represent the wishes of the agent. These wishes may even be conflicting with each other. A consistent subset of desires is called goals. Goals can have different types such as achieve-goals (for achieving a state) or maintain-goals (for maintaining a state over a period of time). Another important component, is the set of plans. Each plan consists of a sequence of actions for achieving a goal and can even contain subgoals. Hence, other plans are needed to achieve the subgoals of one plan. This way, a hierarchy of plans is formed. Moreover, intentions are those goals that the agent is currently committed to achieve them based on its plans [6].

The BDI model is implemented in a number of MAS frameworks, namely PRS, dMARS, JACK Intelligent Agents^{TM}, JAM, AgentSpeak, 3APL, Dribble, Coo-BDI, Brahms, and Jadex. So far, BDI agents have proven to be very useful in various areas such as industrial automation, simulation, air traffic control systems, e-commerce systems, virtual environments, online multi-player games, etc. Among the customers of only one of the BDI frameworks, called dMARS (a predecessor of Jadex), are NASA (space shuttle malfunction handling), AirServices, Thomson Airsys (air traffic control), Daimler Chrysler (supply chain management, resource and logistics management) and Hazelwood Power (process control) [9].

From the above explanation, it is clear that the BDI model fits very well to the logic of SCC applications in the IoTS. Moreover, as mentioned in Sect. 1, MASes are intrinsically very close to the nature of the IoTS. Therefore, for our application domain, i.e., SCC applications in the IoTS, we advocate the BDI model for MASes. State-of-the-art BDI systems such as the free open source Jadex BDI agents framework [6] are much more mature and advanced comparing the initial BDI frameworks. Moreover, Jadex, which supports both stationary and mobile agents, can be deployed on different middleware such as JADE. JADE is a free open source FIPA[1]-compliant middleware for the development and runtime execution of peer-to-peer applications based on the MAS paradigm [7]. Furthermore, there exist an extension of JADE known as JADE-LEAP, for mobile platforms (e.g., Android).

However, given the prevalence of highly resource-constrained things in the IoTS, such as tiny sensor motes with only few kilobytes of memory and extremely limited computational (i.e., CPU) as well as power (i.e., electrical energy) resources, neither Jadex nor any other state-of-the-art BDI agent framework, that we are aware of, could work for such limited platforms in the IoTS. In order to address this problem, we propose three possible approaches. First, one may tailor JADE to work atop very compact and efficient virtual machines of Java-like byte-code languages that are especially designed for motes such as the IBM Mote Runner. Second, an existing C/C++ BDI framework such as the classic BDI reasoner called PRS (e.g., OpenPRS) may be evolved in order to work for this purpose. Finally, the more feasible solution is to develop a BDI framework

---

[1] http://www.fipa.org/.

from scratch, especially for SCC applications in the IoTS that works for constrained devices too, similar to the non-BDI Mobile-C, a mobile agent platform for mobile C/C++ agents on constrained embedded devices, or Agila [10] and actorNet [11] which both run on TinyOS for Wireless Sensor Network (WSN) applications.

Last but not least, one drawback of the BDI model is that its reasoning power often comes at the cost of increased computational overhead. However, by using the BDI model more judiciously and making correct design choices, one can overcome this problem. For a nice practical example on this issue for using BDI with Brahms language based on efficient design choices in contrast to inefficient ones at NASA Ames Research Center, please refer to [12].

3   Related Work

MASes are widely used in the field of Wireless Sensor and Actuator Networks (WSAN). ActorNet [11] is an agent-based platform with an extremely lightweight interpreter that can operate on low-power sensor nodes with as little as 4KB RAM. The programming language for agents is functional and very similar to the Scheme programming language in terms of its syntax. The communication model is based on message passing. ActorNet is specifically designed for mobile agents on Mica2 sensor motes running TinyOS. Moreover, Agila [10] is an agent-based middleware for mobile agents on Mica2, MicaZ, and Tmote Sky motes running TinyOS. It has an assembly-like programming language with proprietary ISA for agents [13].

In contrast, MAPS (Mobile Agent Platform for Sun SPOT) [14] and AFME (Agent Factory Micro Edition) [15] are Java-based frameworks. The agent model in the former is Finite-State-Machines (FSM), while the latter is based on the BDI model. However, they can only run on Sun SPOT (Sun Small Programmable Object Technology), but not on the more constrained tiny sensor motes that are much more prevalent in the IoTS.

4   Conclusion and Future Work

Although there exist overlapping areas in the two young research fields of the IoTS and Multi-Agent Systems, where the latter is only about one decade older than the former, the research and development communities are still isolated from each other. We believe that the R&D work in the field of the IoTS could benefit a lot from the advances in MASes. Similarly, the IoTS could become an interesting testbed for MASes.

In this paper, we advocated Agent Oriented Software Engineering (AOSE), in particular Belief-Desire-Intention (BDI) cognitive intelligent agents, for Sense-Compute-Control (SCC) applications in the Internet of Things and Services (IoTS). Considering the specific requirements and the constrained devices which are prevalent in the IoTS, we elaborated on challenges for pursuing this aim and proposed possible approaches for addressing them. The implementation and validation of the proposed approaches remained as future work.

References

1. Broy, M.: Cyber physical systems (Part 1). it-Inf. Technol. **54**(6), 255–256 (2012)
2. Patel, P., Morin, B., Chaudhary, S.: A model-driven development framework for developing sense-compute-control applications. In: Proceedings of the 1st International Workshop on Modern Software Engineering Methods for Industrial Automation, MoSEMInA 2014, New York, NY, USA, pp. 52–61. ACM (2014)
3. Patel, P., Pathak, A., Teixeira, T., Issarny, V.: Towards application development for the internet of things. In: Proceedings of the 8th Middleware Doctoral Symposium, MDS 2011, New York, NY, USA, pp. 5:1–5:6. ACM (2011)
4. Sturm, A., Shehory, O., Dori, D.: Evaluation of Agent-Oriented Methodologies (2004)
5. Weiß, G.: Agent orientation in software engineering. Knowl. Eng. Rev. **16**(4), 349–373 (2001)
6. Braubach, L., Pokahr, A., Lamersdorf, W.: Jadex: A BDI-agent system combining middleware and reasoning. In: Unland, R., Calisti, M., Klusch, M. (eds.) Software Agent-Based Applications, Platforms and Development Kits, Whitestein Series in Software Agent Technologies, Birkhäuser Basel, pp. 143–168 (2005). http://dx.doi.org/10.1007/3-7643-7348-2_7
7. Bellifemine, F., Caire, G., Poggi, A., Rimassa, G.: JADE, A White Paper (2003)
8. Huhns, M.N., Singh, M.P.: Cognitive agents. IEEE Internet Comput. **2**(6), 87–89 (1998). doi:10.1109/4236.735992
9. Mascardi, V., Demergasso, D., Ancona, D.: Languages for Programming BDI-style Agents: an Overview (2005)
10. Fok, C.-L., Roman, G., Lu, C.: Rapid development and flexible deployment of adaptive wireless sensor network applications. In: Proceedings of the 25th IEEE International Conference on Distributed Computing Systems, ICDCS 2005, pp. 653–662, June 2005
11. Kwon, Y., Sundresh, S., Mechitov, K., Agha, G.: Actornet: an actor platform for wireless sensor networks. In: Proceedings of the Fifth International Joint Conference on Autonomous Agents and Multiagent Systems, AAMAS 2006, New York, NY, USA, pp. 1297–1300. ACM (2006)
12. Wolfe, S.R., Sierhuis, M., Jarvis, P.A.: To BDI, or Not to BDI: design choices in an agent-based traffic flow management simulation. In: Proceedings of the 2008 Spring Simulation Multiconference, SpringSim 2008, Society for Computer Simulation International, San Diego, CA, USA, pp. 63–70 (2008)
13. Aiello, F., Carbone, A., Fortino, G., Galzarano, S.L:Java-based mobile agent platforms for wireless sensor networks. In: Proceedings of the 2010 International Multiconference on Computer Science and Information Technology (IMCSIT), pp. 165–172, Oct 2010
14. Aiello, F., Fortino, G., Gravina, R., Guerrieri, A.: A Java-based agent platform for programming wireless sensor networks. Comput. J. **54**(3), 439–454 (2011)
15. Muldoon, C., O'Hare, G.M.P., Collier, R., O'Grady, M.J.: Agent factory micro edition: a framework for ambient applications. In: Alexandrov, V.N., van Albada, G.D., Sloot, P.M.A., Dongarra, J. (eds.) ICCS 2006. LNCS, vol. 3993, pp. 727–734. Springer, Heidelberg (2006)

A Novel Term-Term Similarity Score Based Information Foraging Assessment

Ilyes Khennak[✉], Habiba Drias, and Hadia Mosteghanemi

Laboratory for Research in Artificial Intelligence,
USTHB, Algiers, Algeria
{ikhennak,hdrias,hmosteghanemi}@usthb.dz

Abstract. The dramatic proliferation of information on the web and the tremendous growth in the number of files published and uploaded online each day have led to the appearance of new words in the Internet. Due to the difficulty of reaching the meanings of these new terms, which play a central role in retrieving the desired information, it becomes necessary to give more importance to the sites and topics where these new words appear, or rather, to give value to the words that occur frequently with them. For this aim, in this paper, we propose a novel term-term similarity score based on the co-occurrence and closeness of words for retrieval performance improvement. A novel efficiency/effectiveness measure based on the principle of optimal information forager is also proposed in order to assess the quality of the obtained results. Our experiments were performed using the OHSUMED test collection and show significant effectiveness enhancement over the state-of-the-art.

Keywords: Information retrieval · Information foraging theory · Query expansion · Term proximity · Term co-occurrence

1 Introduction

The experimentation and evaluation phase is the main phase to judge the success and failure of the implemented systems and achieved programs. The performance and quality of a retrieval system is measured on the basis of effectiveness and efficiency [2]. From the theoretical standpoint, the effectiveness is indicated by returning only what user needs and efficiency is indicated by returning the results to the user as quickly as possible [3,9]. From the practical standpoint the effectiveness, or relevance, is determined by measuring the precision, recall, etc., and efficiency is determined by measuring the search time [7]. The Reliance on these two measures varies from one community to another. The information retrieval community, for example, is focusing too much on the quality of the top ranked results while the artificial intelligence community, which started paying attention to information retrieval, ontologies and the Semantic Web [16], is focusing on the retrieval process cost. Accordingly, and in order to establish consensus between communities and adopt both effectiveness and efficiency measures, the Information Foraging Theory has been proposed to do so. The information foraging is a

© Institute for Computer Sciences, Social Informatics and Telecommunications Engineering 2015
R. Giaffreda et al. (Eds.): IoT360 2014, Part I, LNICST 150, pp. 29–41, 2015.
DOI: 10.1007/978-3-319-19656-5_5

theory that describes information retrieval behavior [13,14]. It is derived from a food foraging theory called optimal foraging theory that helps biologists understand the factors determining an animal's food preference and feeding strategies. The basis of foraging theory is a cost and benefit assessment of achieving a goal.

We introduce in the early part of this study the basic principles and concepts of information foraging theory which is employed later in the experimental section to evaluate the retrieval systems. The second part is devoted to presenting and discussing our suggested approach for improving retrieval performance. The major purpose of this proposed approach is to provide an effective similarity measurement for query expansion based on the co-occurrence and closeness of terms. This approach assigns importance, during the retrieval process, to words that frequently occur in the same context. For instance, the term *'COIOTE'* is often recurred in the same sites where the words *'Conference'*, *'Italy'*, and *'2014'* are clustered. the reliance on this principle was not a coincidence but was the result of studies carried out recently regarding the evolution and growth of the Web. All of these studies have shown an exponential growth of the Web and rapid increase in the number of new pages created. In his study [15], Ranganathan estimated that the amount of online data indexed by Google had increased from 5 exabytes in 2002 to 280 exabytes in 2009. According to [22], this amount is expected to be double in size every 18 months. Ntoulas et al. [12] read these statistics in terms of the number of new pages created and demonstrated that their number is increasing by 8 % a week. The work of Bharat and Broder [1] went further and estimated that the World Wide Web pages are growing at the rate of 7.5 pages every second. This revolution, which the Web is witnessing, has led to the appearance of two points:

- The first point is the entry of new words into the Web which is estimated, according to [21], at about one new word in every two hundred words. Studies by [8,20] have shown that this invasion is mainly due to: neologisms, first occurrences of rare personal names and place names, abbreviations, acronyms, emoticons, URLs and typographical errors.
- The second point is that the users employ these new words during the search. Chen et al. [5] indicated in their study that more than 17 % of query words are out of vocabulary (Non dictionary words), 45 % of them are E-speak (lol), 18 % are companies and products (Google), 16 % are proper names, 15 % are misspellings and foreign words (womens) [19].

Out of these two points which the web is witnessing and due to the difficulty, or better, the impossibility to use the meanings of these words, we proposed a method based on finding the locations and topics where these words appear, and then trying to use the terms which neighbor and occur with the latter in the search process. We will use the best-known instantiation of the Probabilistic Relevance Framework system: Okapi BM25, and the Blind Relevance Feedback: Robertson/Sparck Jones' term-ranking function as the baseline for comparison, and evaluate our approach using OHSUMED test collection. The main contributions of our work in this paper are the following:

– The adoption of an external correlation measure in order to evaluate the co-occurrence of words with respect to the query features.
– The determination of an internal correlation measure in order to assess the proximity and closeness of words relative to the terms of the query.

In the next section, we will introduce the information foraging theory. The BM25 model and the Blind Feedback approach are presented in Sect. 3. In Sect. 4 we will explain our proposed approach and finally we will describe our experiments and results.

2   Information Foraging Theory

The information foraging is a theory proposed by [14]. It is becoming a popular theory for characterizing and understanding web browsing behavior [6]. The theory is based on the behavior of an animal deciding what to eat, where it can be found, the best way to obtain it and how much energy the meal will provide.

For example, imagine a predator that faces the recurrent problem of deciding what to eat. Energy flows into the environment and comes to be stored in different forms. Different types of habitat and prey will yield different amounts of net energy. By analogy, imagine an academic researcher that faces the recurrent problems of finding relevant information. Information flows into the environment to be represented in different types of external media. The different information sources will have different profitabilities in terms of the amount of valuable information.

The basis of foraging theory is a *cost* and *benefit* assessment of achieving a goal where cost is the amount of resources consumed when performing a chosen activity and the benefit is what is gained from engaging in that activity.

Conceptually, the *optimal forager* finds the best solution to the problem of maximizing the rate of benefit returned by effort expended given the energetic profitabilities of different habitats and prey, and the costs of finding and pursuing them. By analogy, the *optimal information forager* finds the best solution to the problem of maximizing the rate of valuable information gained per unit cost.

Reference [14] expressed the rate of valuable information gained per unit cost, by the following formula:

$$R = \frac{G}{T} \tag{1}$$

where:

R, is the rate of gain of valuable information per unit cost,
G, is the ratio of the total amount of valuable information gained,
T, is the total amount of time spent.

In order to adopt both effectiveness and efficiency measures during the experimentation phase, we suggest considering the parameters G and T in representing the effectiveness and efficiency measures, respectively.

Accordingly, we propose to evaluate and compare the quality of the results obtained by our suggested approach relying on the principle of optimal information forager and using the basis of the rate R, where G and T represent respectively the total number of relevant documents returned by the retrieval system, and the total amount of search time.

3   Probabilistic Relevance Framework

The probabilistic Relevance framework is a formal framework for document retrieval which led to the development of one of the most successful text-retrieval algorithms, Okapi BM25. The classic version of Okapi BM25 term-weighting function, in which the weight w_i^{BM25} is attributed to a given term t_i in a document d, is obtained using the following formula:

$$w_i^{BM25} = \frac{tf}{k_1((1-b) + b\dfrac{dl}{avdl}) + tf} w_i^{RSJ} \tag{2}$$

where:
tf, is the frequency of the term t_i in a document d;
k_1, is a constant;
b, is a constant;
dl, is the document length;
$avdl$, is the average of document length;
w_i^{RSJ}, is the well-know Robertson/Sparck Jones weight [17]:

$$w_i^{RSJ} = \log \frac{(r_i + 0.5)(N - R - n_i + r_i + 0.5)}{(n_i - r_i + 0.5)(R - r_i + 0.5)} \tag{3}$$

where:
N, is the number of documents in the whole collection;
n_i, is the number of documents in the collection containing t_i;
R, is the number of documents judged relevant;
r_i, is the number of judged relevant documents containing t_i.

The RSJ weight can be used with or without relevance information. In the absence of relevance information (the more usual scenario), the weight is reduced to a form of classical idf:

$$w_i^{IDF} = \log \frac{N - n_i + 0.5}{n_i + 0.5} \tag{4}$$

The final BM25 term-weighting function is therefore given by:

$$w_i^{BM25} = \frac{tf}{k_1((1-b) + b\dfrac{dl}{avdl}) + tf} \log \frac{N - n_i + 0.5}{n_i + 0.5} \tag{5}$$

Concerning the internal parameters, a considerable number of experiments have been done, and suggest that in general values such as $1.2 < k_1 < 2$ and

$0.5 < b < 0.8$ are reasonably good in many cases. Robertson and Zaragoza [18] have indicated that published versions of Okapi BM25 are based on specific values assigned to k_1 and b: $k_1 = 2, b = 0.5$ As part of the indexing process, an inverted file is created containing the weight w_i^{BM25} of each term t_i in each document d.

The similarity score between the document d and a query q is then computed as follows:

$$Score_{BM25}(d, q) = \sum_{t_i \in q} w_i^{BM25} \qquad (6)$$

During the interrogation process, the relevant documents are selected and ranked using this similarity score.

3.1   Blind Relevance Feedback for Query Expansion

One of the most successful techniques to improve the retrieval effectiveness of document ranking is to expand the original query with additional terms that best capture the actual user intent. Many approaches have been proposed to generate and extract these additional terms. The Blind Relevance Feedback (or the Pseudo-Relevance Feedback) is one of the suggested approaches. It uses the pseudo-relevant documents, i.e. the first documents retrieved in response to the initial query, to select the most important terms to be used as expansion features.

In its simplest version, the approach starts by performing an initial search on the original query using the BM25 term-weighting and the previous document-scoring function (formula 6), suppose the best ranked documents to be relevant, assign a score to each term in the top retrieved documents using a term-scoring function, and then sort them on the basis of their scores. One of the best-known functions for term-scoring is the *Robertson/Sparck Jones* term-ranking function, defined by formula 3. The original query is then expanded by adding the top ranked terms, and re-interrogated by using the BM25 similarity score (formula 6), in order to get more relevant results.

In addition to the BM25 Model, we will use the Robertson/Sparck Jones term-scoring function for Relevance Feedback as a baseline to compare the results of our proposed approach.

4   The Closeness and Co-occurrence of Terms for Effectiveness Improvement

The main goals of our proposed method is to return only the relevant documents. For that purpose, we have introduced the concept of co-occurrence and closeness, during the search process. This concept is based, at first, on finding for each query term the locations where it appears and then selecting, from these locations, the terms which frequently neighbor and co-occur with that query term. To put it simply, we recover for each query term the documents where it appears, and then assess the relevance of the terms contained in these documents to the query term on the basis of:

1. The co-occurrence, which gives value to words that appear in the largest possible number of those documents.
2. The proximity and closeness, which gives value to words in which the distance separating them and the query term within a document, with respect to the number of words, is small.

These words are then ranked on the basis of their relevance to the whole query and the top ranked ones are added to that query in order to repeat the search process.

we started our work by reducing the search space through giving importance to documents which contain at least two words of the initial query. This means that the terms, which will be added to the original query, will depend only on this set of documents. The following formula allows us to select the documents that contain at least two words of the query, i.e. to pick out any document d whose $Score_{Bigram}$ to a query q is greater than zero:

$$Score_{Bigram}(q, d) = \sum_{\substack{(t_i, t_j) \in q}}^{i \neq j} (w_i^{BM25} + w_j^{BM25}) \tag{7}$$

As we previously mentioned, we will find, in the first step, the terms which often appear together with the query terms. Finding these words is done by assigning more importance to words that occur in the largest number of documents where each term of the query appears. We interpret this importance via the measurement of the external distance of each term t_i of the R_c' vocabulary to each term $t_{j_{(q)}}$ of the query q (R_c, is the set of documents returned by using the formula (7)). This distance, which does not take in consideration the content of documents, computes the rate of appearance of t_i with $t_{j_{(q)}}$ in the collection of documents R_c. In the case where t_i appears in all the documents in which $t_{j_{(q)}}$ occurs, the value of the external distance will be 1.0; and in the case where t_i does not appear in any of the documents in which $t_{j_{(q)}}$ occurs, the value of the external distance will be 0.0. Based on this interpretation, the external distance $ExtDist$ of t_i to $t_{j_{(q)}}$ is calculated as follows:

$$ExtDist(t_i, t_{j_{(q)}}) = \frac{\sum_{d_k \in R_c} x_{(i,k)} * x_{(j,k)}}{\sum_{d_k \in R_c} x_{(j,k)}} \tag{8}$$

where:
$$x_{(i,k)} = \begin{cases} 1 \text{ if } t_i \in d_k, \\ 0 \text{ else.} \end{cases}$$
d_k, is a document that belongs to R_c.
The total external distance between a given term t_i and the query q is estimated as follows:

$$ExtDist(t_i, q) = \sum_{t_{j_{(q)}} \in q} ExtDist(t_i, t_{j_{(q)}}) \tag{9}$$

Our dependence on this distance came as a result of the remarkable outcomes achieved in [10,11]. The distance was used during the indexing process to compute the external distance between each pair of terms of the dictionary which appear in at least one document. After that and during the search process, the original query was expanded by adding, for each term t of the initial query, the term whose external distance to t is the highest.

In the second step, we will find the terms which are often neighbors to the query terms. Therefore, we attribute more importance to terms having a short correlation with the query keywords. We interpret this importance via the measurement of the internal correlation between each term t_i of V_R and each term $t_{j_{(q)}}$ of the query q. This correlation, which takes into consideration the content of documents, computes the correlation between t_i and $t_{j_{(q)}}$ within a given document d in terms of the number of words separating them. The more t_i is close to $t_{j_{(q)}}$, the greater is its internal correlation. For this purpose, we used the well-known Gaussian kernel function to measure the internal correlation $IntDist$ between t_i and $t_{j_{(q)}}$ within a given document d:

$$IntDist_{(d)}(t_i, t_{j_{(q)}}) = exp\left[\frac{-(i-j)^2}{2\sigma^2}\right] \tag{10}$$

where:
i (resp. j), is the position of the term t_i (resp. $t_{j_{(q)}}$) in d;
σ, is a parameter to be tuned.

The terms t_i and $t_{j_{(q)}}$ may appear more than once in a document d. Therefore, the internal distance between the term pair $(t_i, t_{j_{(q)}})$ is estimated by summing all possible $IntDist_{(d)}$ between t_i and $t_{j_{(q)}}$. Thus, the preceding formula becomes:

$$IntDist_{(d)}(t_i, t_{j_{(q)}}) = \sum_{occ(t_i, t_{j_{(q)}})} exp\left[\frac{-(i-j)^2}{2\sigma^2}\right] \tag{11}$$

where:
$occ(t_i, t_{j_{(q)}})$, is the number of appearance of the term pair $(t_i, t_{j_{(q)}})$ in the document d.

The average internal correlation between t_i and $t_{j_{(q)}}$ in the whole R is then determined as follows:

$$IntDist(t_i, t_{j_{(q)}}) = \frac{\sum_{d_k \in R} IntDist_{(d_k)}(t_i, t_j)}{C(t_{j_{(q)}})} \tag{12}$$

The following formula calculates the total internal correlation between a given term t_i and the query q :

$$IntDist(t_i, q) = \sum_{t_{j_{(q)}} \in q} IntDist(t_i, t_{j_{(q)}}) \tag{13}$$

Finally, in order to compute the total correlation $(Dist)$, the values of $ExtDist$ and $IntDist$ were normalized between 0 and 1. The overall correlation between t_i and q is obtained using the following formula:

$$Dist(t_i, q) = \lambda ExtDist(t_i, q) + (1 - \lambda)IntDist(t_i, q) \tag{14}$$

where:
λ, is a parameter to adjust the balance between the external and internal correlations ($\lambda \in [0, 1]$).
Using formula (14), we evaluate the relevance of each term $t \in V_R$ with respect to the query q. Then we rank the terms on the basis of their relevance and add the top ranked ones to the original query q. Based on the BM25 similarity score, presented in Sect. 3, we retrieve the relevant documents, as follows:

$$Score_{BM25}(d, q') = \sum_{t_i \in q'} w_i^{BM25} * \beta \tag{15}$$

where:
q', is the expanded query;
$\beta = \begin{cases} 1 \text{ if } t_i \in q, \\ Dist(t_i, q) \text{ else.} \end{cases}$

5   Experiments

In order to evaluate the effectiveness of the proposed approach, we carried out a set of experiments. First, we describe the dataset, the software, and the effectiveness measures used. Then, we present the experimental results.

5.1   Dataset

Extensive experiments were performed on OHSUMED test collection. The collection consists of 348 566 references from MEDLINE, the on-line medical information database, consisting of titles and/or abstracts from 270 medical journals over a five-year period (1987-1991). In addition, the OHSUMED collection contains a set of queries, and relevance judgments (a list of which documents are relevant to each query).

In order that the results be more accurate and credible, we divided the OHSUMED collection into 6 sub-collections. Each sub-collection has been defined by a set of documents, queries, and a list of relevance documents. Table 1 summarizes the characteristics of each sub-collection in terms of the number of documents it contains, the size of the sub-collection, and the number of terms in the vocabulary (dictionary).

Regarding the queries, the OHSUMED collection includes 106 queries. Each query is accompanied by a set of relevance judgments chosen from the whole collection of documents. Partitioning the collection of documents into sub-collections leads inevitably to a decrease in the number of relevant documents

Table 1. Characteristics of the sub-collections used for evaluating the proposed approach.

Size of the collection:	(#documents)	50000	100000	150000	200000	250000	300000
	(Mb)	26.39	52.36	80.72	107.58	135.05	164.31
Number of terms in the dictionary		81937	120825	156009	184514	211504	237889

for each query. In other words, if we have n documents relevant to a given query q with respect to the entire collection, then surely we will have m documents relevant to the same query with respect to one of the sub-collections, where the value of n is certainly greater or equal to the value of m and, the probability of non-existence of any relevant document for a given query could be possible. In this case, in which the value of m is equal to 0, we have removed, for each sub-collection c, every query does not include any relevant document in c. Table 2 shows the number of queries (Nb $Queries$) for each sub-collection, the average query length in terms of number of words (Avr $Query$ Len), the average number of relevant documents (Avr Rel Doc).

Table 2. Some statistics on the OHSUMED sub-collections queries.

#documents	50000	100000	150000	200000	250000	300000
Nb Queries	82	91	95	97	99	101
Avr Rel Doc	4.23	7	10.94	13.78	15.5	19.24
Avr Query Len	6.79	6.12	5.68	5.74	5.62	5.51

5.2   Software, Effectiveness Measures

The BM25 model, the Relevance Feedback technique presented in Sect. 3, and the proposed approach have been implemented in Python. All the experiments have been performed on a Sony-Vaio workstation having an Intel i3-2330M/2.20GHz processor, 4GB RAM and running Ubuntu GNU/Linux 12.04. The precision and the Mean Average Precision (MAP) have been used as measures to evaluate the effectiveness of the systems and to compare the different approaches. As indicated is Sect. 2, the principle of optimal information forager has been employed to assess the performance of the search methods.

5.3   Results

Before proceeding to compare the quality of the suggested approach with the BM25 and the Pseudo-Relevance Feedback methods, we fixed the parameter σ of the internal correlation (formula (10)). For this aim, we considered the internal correlation as the total correlation ($Dist$), i.e. $\lambda = 0$, and systematically tested a set of fixed σ values from 1 to 40 in increments of 5. Table 3 presents the precision

Table 3. The best performance of the proposed approach for different σ.

PSD	10		20		50	
σ	P@10	MAP	P@10	MAP	P@10	MAP
1	0.1060	0.2110	0.1048	0.2208	0.1073	0.2193
5	0.1109	**0.2265**	0.1121	0.2252	0.1146	**0.2241**
10	0.1109	0.2253	0.1121	**0.2255**	0.1146	0.2231
15	0.1109	0.2231	0.1121	0.2245	0.1146	0.2228
20	0.1109	0.2230	0.1121	0.2245	0.1146	0.2235
25	0.1109	0.2230	0.1121	0.2245	0.1146	0.2233
30	0.1109	0.2230	0.1121	0.2245	0.1146	0.2233
35	0.1109	0.2230	0.1121	0.2245	0.1146	0.2233
40	0.1109	0.2230	0.1121	0.2245	0.1146	0.2233

values after retrieving 10 documents ($P@10$) and the Mean Average Precision (MAP) reached by the proposed approach, while using the sub-collection of 50000 documents. The number of pseudo-relevant documents (denoted by PSD) was tuned at 10, 20 and 50.

From Table 3, we can conclude that the appropriate values of σ, which bring the best performance, are 5 and 10.

For all the following experiments, the parameters σ and λ were set to 5 and 0.5, respectively. Moreover, the number of expansion terms added to the initial query for the proposed system and the Pseudo-Relevance Feedback approaches was set to 10, which is a typical choice [4].

In the first stage of testing, we evaluated and compared the results of the suggested approach (EXT/INT), which use both the external and internal correlations, with those of BM25 and RSJ (Robertson/Sparck Jones algorithm for Relevance Feedback); where we computed the precision values after retrieving 10 documents ($P@10$). Figure 1 shows the precision values for the EXT/INT, the BM25 and the RSJ techniques.

In the second stage of testing, we computed the Mean Average Precision (MAP) score to evaluate the retrieval performance of the EXT/INT, the BM25, and the Relevance Feedback method.

From Fig. 1a and b, we note an obvious superiority of the suggested approach EXT/INT compared with the BM25, and this superiority was more significant in comparison to the RSJ technique. Despite the superiority shown in Fig. 1c, the result was not similar to that observed in Fig. 1a and b, however, the precision values of the proposed approach were the best in all the sub-collections.

Through Fig. 1 we can conclude that the proposed method EXT/INT, compared with the rest of the search techniques, succeeded to improve the ranking of the relevant documents and made them in the first place. The precision values of the suggested system, after retrieving 10 documents, show a clear and significant superiority in front of each of BM25 and RSJ techniques, and this confirms the effectiveness of the EXT/INT approach.

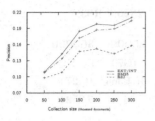 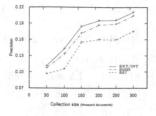 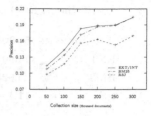

(a) Precision after retrieving 10 documents (P@10),
(PSD=10).

(b) Precision after retrieving 10 documents (P@10),
(PSD=20).

(c) Precision after retrieving 10 documents (P@10),
(PSD=50).

Fig. 1. Effectiveness comparison of the EXT/INT approach to the state-of-the-art.

Figure 2 shows a clear advantage of the EXT/INT approach compared to the RSJ in all the sub-collections. It also shows a slight superiority over the BM25 results.

As previously explained in Sect. 2, we propose to use the principle of optimal information forager in order to adopt both effectiveness and efficiency measures in evaluating the quality of the obtained results. For this purpose, we calculate for each query the rate R, illustrated in formula 1, where the parameter G was taken as the number of relevant documents retrieved and the parameter T as the total amount of search time. The different rates, each of which is linked to a query, are then summed and divided by the total number of queries. As a result, we obtain an average rate $R(Q)$ defined as follows:

$$R(Q) = \frac{1}{|Q|} \sum_{i=1}^{|Q|} \frac{G_{q_i}}{T_{q_i}} \tag{16}$$

where:
$|Q|$, is the total number of queries,
G_{q_i}, is the number of relevant documents retrieved for query q_i,
T_{q_i}, is the total time spent in processing q_i.

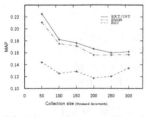 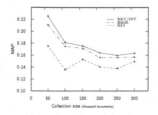 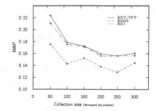

(a) Mean Average Preci-
sion (MAP), (PSD=10).

(b) Mean Average Preci-
sion (MAP), (PSD=20).

(c) Mean Average Preci-
sion (MAP), (PSD=50).

Fig. 2. Mean Average Precision (MAP) results of the EXT/INT approach, the BM25 and the RSJ methods.

Table 4. R(Q)-score achieved by EXT/INT, BM25 and RSJ.

#documents	50000	100000	150000	200000	250000	300000
EXT/INT	14.9049	10.7110	10.1994	9.9643	9.0079	9.2276
BM25	16.0251	11.7612	11.2681	10.9097	10.0364	10.2747
RSJ	11.1365	7.3431	7.0448	6.6212	5.7615	5.9524

It can be seen from Table 4 that the BM25 overcame the EXT/INT approach in terms of $R(Q)$ values. This superiority is mainly due to the short time taken by BM25 during the search process as it used only the original query words. However, it is clear that the proposed method produces the best results over the RSJ in all cases.

6 Conclusion

In this paper, we proposed a novel term-term similarity score based on the co-occurrence and closeness of words for retrieval performance improvement. We have introduced in this work, the concept of the External/Internal similarity of terms.

We thoroughly tested our approach using the OHSUMED test collection. The experimental results show that the proposed approach EXT/INT achieved a significant improvement in effectiveness.

Although the main purpose of relying on the principle of optimal information forager, and in particular the $R(Q)$ Score, in assessing the quality of retrieval systems was not to get better results compared to BM25 and RSJ methods, but rather to introduce a new measure in order to compare the performance of retrieval systems, taking into account both effectiveness and efficiency measures.

Even though our methods perform quite well, there are some remaining issues that need to be investigated further. One limitation of this work is the use of a single test collection. The other one is that the semantic aspect of terms was not exploited in order to improve the search effectiveness.

References

1. Bharat, K., Broder, A.: A technique for measuring the relative size and overlap of public web search engines. Comput. Netw. ISDN Syst. **30**(1), 379–388 (1998)
2. Cambazoglu, B.B., Aykanat, C.: Performance of query processing implementations in ranking-based text retrieval systems using inverted indices. Inf. Process. Manage. **42**(4), 875–898 (2006)
3. Cambazoglu, B.B., Baeza-Yates, R.: Scalability Challenges in Web Search Engines. In: Melucci, M., Baeza-Yates, R. (eds.) Advanced Topics in Information Retrieval. The Information Retrieval Series, vol. 33, pp. 27–50. Springer, Heidelberg (2011)
4. Carpineto, C., Romano, G.: A survey of automatic query expansion in information retrieval. ACM Comput. Surv. **44**(1), 1–50 (2012)

5. Chen, Q., Li, M., Zhou, M.: Improving query spelling correction using web search results. In: EMNLP-CoNLL 2007: Proceedings of the 2007 Joint Conference on Empirical Methods in Natural Language Processing and Computational Natural Language Learning, pp. 181–189. ACL, Stroudsburg (2007)
6. Dix, A., Howes, A., Payne, S.: Post-web cognition: evolving knowledge strategies for global information environments. Int. J. Web Eng. Technol. 1(1), 112–126 (2003)
7. Dominich, S.: The Modern Algebra of Information Retrieval. Springer, Heidelberg (2008)
8. Eisenstein, J., OConnor, B., Smith, N.A., Xing, E.P.: Mapping the geographical diffusion of new words. In: NIPS 2012: Workshop on Social Network and Social Media Analysis: Methods, Models and Applications (2012)
9. Frøkjær, E., Hertzum, M., Hornbæk, K.: Measuring usability: are effectiveness, efficiency, and satisfaction really correlated? In: CHI 2000: Proceedings of the SIGCHI Conference on Human Factors in Computing Systems, pp. 345–352. ACM, New York (2000)
10. Khennak, I.: Classification non supervisée floue des termes basée sur la proximité pour les systèmes de recherche d'information. In: CORIA 2013: Proceedings of the 10th French Information Retrieval Conference, pp. 341–346. Unine, Neuchâtel (2013)
11. Khennak, I., Drias, H.: Term proximity and data mining techniques for information retrieval systems. In: Rocha, Á., Correia, A.M., Wilson, T., Stroetmann, K.A. (eds.) Advances in Information Systems and Technologies. AISC, vol. 206, pp. 477–486. Springer, Heidelberg (2013)
12. Ntoulas, A., Cho, J., C. Olston.: What's new on the web?: the evolution of the web from a search engine perspective. In: WWW 2004: Proceedings of the 13th International Conference on World Wide Web, pp. 1–12. ACM, New York (2004)
13. Pirolli, P.: Information Foraging Theory: Adaptive Interaction with Information. Oxford University Press, Oxford (2007)
14. Pirolli, P., Card, S.: Information foraging. Psychol. Rev. 106(4), 643–675 (1999)
15. Ranganathan, P.: From microprocessors to nanostores: rethinking data centric systems. IEEE Comput. 44(1), 39–48 (2011)
16. Ramos, C., Augusto, J.C., Shapiro, D.: Ambient intelligence the next step for artificial intelligence. IEEE Intell. Syst. 23(2), 15–18 (2008)
17. Robertson, S.E., Jones, K.S.: Relevance weighting of search terms. J. Am. Soc. Inform. Sci. 27(3), 129–146 (1976)
18. Robertson, S., Zaragoza, H.: The probabilistic relevance framework: BM25 and beyond. Found. Trends Inf. Retrieval 3(4), 333–389 (2009)
19. Subramaniam, L.V., Roy, S., Faruquie, T.A., Negi, S.: A survey of types of text noise and techniques to handle noisy text. In: AND 2009: Proceedings of The Third Workshop on Analytics for Noisy Unstructured Text Data, pp. 115–122. ACM, New York (2009)
20. Sun, H.M.: A study of the features of internet english from the linguistic perspective. Studies in Literature and Language 1(7), 9–103 (2010)
21. Williams, H.E., Zobel, J.: Searchable words on the web. Int. J. Digit. Libr. 5(2), 99–105 (2005)
22. Zhu, Y., Zhong, N., Xiong, Y.: Data explosion, data nature and dataology. In: Zhong, N., Li, K., Lu, S., Chen, L. (eds.) BI 2009. LNCS, vol. 5819, pp. 147–158. Springer, Heidelberg (2009)

A Cloud-Based Bayesian Smart Agent Architecture for Internet-of-Things Applications

Veselin Pizurica$^{(\boxtimes)}$ and Piet Vandaele

Waylay, Gaston Crommenlaan 8, 9050 Ghent, Belgium
{veselin,piet}@waylay.io

Abstract. The Internet-of-Things (IoT) connects devices with embedded sensors to the Internet and is expected to grow at a spectacular rate. IoT will drive increased quality of life for individual as well as spur business growth and efficiency gains in industry. Actions based on real-time information, better decision making and remote diagnostics are some key areas where IoT can make a difference. This paper presents a smart agent architecture for the Internet-of-Things based on Bayesian Network technology that can be used for automation, notification, diagnostics and troubleshooting use cases.

Keywords: Bayesian networks · Internet-of-Things · Decision making · Artificial intelligence

1 Introduction

The Internet-of-Things provides us with lots of sensor data. However, the data by themselves do not provide value unless we can turn them into actionable, contextualized information. Big data and data visualization techniques allow us to gain new insights by batch-processing and off-line analysis of sensor data. Real-time sensor data analysis and decision-making is often done manually but to make it scalable, it is preferably automated. Artificial Intelligence provides us the framework and tools to go beyond trivial real-time decision and automation use cases for IoT.

In this paper, we present a cloud-based smart agent architecture for real-time decision taking in IoT applications. Section 2 reviews the concept of a rational agent. Section 3 describes the architecture of an agent suited for IoT applications. Section 4 explains why Bayesian technology is a good choice as agent logic for IoT applications. Section 5 explains how the agent can be embedded in an overall IoT solution. Finally, Sect. 6 summarizes and concludes the paper.

2 Rational Agent

The rational agent is a central concept in artificial intelligence [1]. An agent is something that perceives its environment through sensors and acts upon that environment via actuators. For example, a robot may rely on cameras as sensors and act on its environment via motors.

© Institute for Computer Sciences, Social Informatics and Telecommunications Engineering 2015
R. Giaffreda et al. (Eds.): IoT360 2014, Part I, LNICST 150, pp. 42–47, 2015.
DOI: 10.1007/978-3-319-19656-5_6

A rational agent is an agent that does 'the right thing'. The right thing obviously depends on the performance criterion set for the agent, but also on an agent's prior knowledge of the environment, the sequence of observations the agent has made in the past and the choice of actions that an agent can perform (Fig. 1).

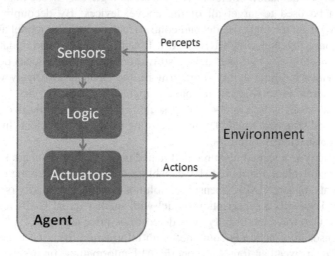

Fig. 1. Rational agent architecture [1].

An agent consists of an architecture and logic. The architecture of an agent typically consists of a computing device with physical sensors and actuators. The architecture allows ingesting sensor data, running logic on the data and acting upon the outcome. The logic itself is the heart of the agent and is the agent program that maps percepts of the environment to actions on that environment. It computes and reasons based on the available data and its knowledge of the environment.

3 Agent Architecture for IoT Applications

As described above, an agent is composed of an architecture and logic. Each poses specific challenges in the context of IoT. This section describes architectural considerations for the smart agent. Section 4 discusses the choice of logic.

3.1 Agent Location

In an IoT context, the agent can be located at different places:

- Close to the sensors and actuators, e.g. on a home gateway, a smartphone or on onsite server or private cloud infrastructure in an industrial environment.
- In a (public) cloud.
- Somewhere in between, such as switches and routers at the network edge. For the latter, Cisco coined the term fog computing [2].

In many respects, a cloud-based architecture is the preferred solution for a smart agent.

A cloud solution is device-agnostic and decouples logic from the presentation layer. So whether logic gets presented on an Android Smartphone, an iPhone, a tablet or as a web app (or any combination of the above), the cloud logic only needs to be developed once and can be used to target all of the above devices. By decoupling the user interface (view) from the logic (model and control), an architectural model arises where logic is built once together with a REST API. It can be changed and updated without necessarily impacting any end-user device software. This model reduces development time and increases business agility. Furthermore, the cloud brings many well-known advantages in terms of software maintenance, upgrades, roll-backs, etc.

Cloud logic scales well: cloud-capacity scales horizontally, while distributed HW often needs to be swapped when HW resources are no longer sufficient. In that sense, cloud logic is also more future-proof.

Cloud capacity is a shared resource and hence per-customer costs are substantially lower than for equivalent distributed HW capabilities. This can make a big difference in market segments that are CAPEX-sensitive. Solutions that rely primarily on cloud may be better suited towards a subscription model with smaller initial CAPEX investment for customers. Gateways are usually considered to be price-sensitive.

In case sensor information is combined with information from the Internet such as social media data, weather forecast, generic API information, or user profile information (which is by definition not bound to any particular device), the cloud is the natural place for these things to come together.

Similarly when integrating multiple IoT vertical solutions, e.g. the integration of an alarm system from vendor A with a home automation system of vendor B, that integration is likely to happen via APIs exposed in the back-end, rather than via direct integration between devices in the home. Using battery-powered devices to retrieve all this information from the cloud for local execution of the logic may drain battery resources.

Finally, cloud intelligence also allows easy generation of analytics regarding the usage of the logic itself. Which rules fired and why? How often?

However, in some application domains a cloud-based model is not optimal. In some cases, bandwidth is expensive or the amount of data is so large that connectivity and bandwidth are the bottleneck, i.e. data does not get easily into the cloud. You can think of applications relying on camera video feeds or certain industrial applications, e.g. Virgin Atlantic reported that Boeing 787 s will create half a terabyte of data per flight [3].

In those cases, local, on-premise processing or preprocessing, compression or buffering of data conserves bandwidth and associated costs. In a multi-tiered architecture, local preprocessing complements core logic that still resides in the cloud.

In other use cases, availability and latency are crucial aspects of a service, e.g. in process control in industry. For time-critical applications that require response times in the order of milliseconds, cloud-based logic can be replaced by fog or onsite logic.

In sum, there are compelling arguments for a cloud-based architecture but some verticals have boundary conditions that do not allow doing that.

3.2 Software-Defined Sensors and Actuators

Besides the location of the agent, the agent architecture also specifies how the agent interacts with sensors and actuators in its environment. In the context of IoT, applications can benefit from enriching sensor data with other types of information such as location, social media data, wearables, big data, open data, data from the API economy etc. The usage of additional sources of information leads to increased precision, personalization and contextualization of IoT applications, see e.g. [4].

Therefore, a smart agent architecture requires a generalized sensor and actuator concept that allows not only accepting raw sensor data but also other types of information. We call this concept a 'software-defined-sensor' and 'software-defined-actuators'.

4 Rational Agent Logic for IoT

The choice for a particular type of agent logic is influenced by the characteristics of the environment in which an agent needs to operate [1].

The simplest agent relies on 'if-then-else' constructs that are available in any programming language or rules engine. These agent implementations belong to the class of simple reflex agents. Their advantage is simplicity and familiarity; the main drawback is that they are only applicable if the action to be taken depends only on the current observation.

A second option is flowchart models such as used in business process modeling systems. These agents belong to the class of model-based reflex agents. They can maintain state of past observations, but can become very complex when the number of inputs and states rises. Moreover, when uncertainty is involved, flowchart based models may not come to satisfactory conclusions.

A third option is to use graph modeling technology, such as Bayesian networks, which is an implementation of goal- or utility-based agents. Below we illustrate why Bayesian networks match IoT environment characteristics.

Bayesian logic is the technology of choice when working in environments that cannot be completely observed, i.e. when not all aspects that could impact a choice of action are observable. In IoT, due to the complexity of the environment or due to cost constraints on the number of sensors, the environment may not be fully observable.

Bayesian logic is suited for applications with unreliable, noisy or incomplete data or when domain knowledge is incomplete such that probabilistic reasoning is required. In IoT, sensors may not be responding, out-of-service or quality of sensor data may be low or inaccurate. In all these cases, Bayesian technology is the best choice.

Bayesian logic is suited for use cases where the number of causes for a particular observation is so large, that it is nearly impossible to enumerate them explicitly. For example, when a door pressure sensor observes that a door is open, somebody may have forgotten to close the door, somebody may still be standing at the door while having a conversation, somebody may have briefly left open the door but will return soon, etc. Bayesian networks allow you to pick the most relevant options and model all others as 'other causes' via so-called leaky nodes.

Bayesian networks are well suited to model expert-knowledge together with knowledge that is retrieved from accumulated data [5]. In a data-driven approach, humans can specify the main attributes of Bayesian logic while the exact (conditional) probabilities can be learned in an automatic way from the available data.

From an implementation perspective, Bayesian networks allow more compact modelling in case the number of variables and states rises. The modeling of the logic and as-well-as the ongoing maintenance and updates to the logic will be simpler than for alternative technologies.

Finally, Bayesian networks are more amenable to use cases where there are asynchronous information flows, i.e. when not all information streams are synchronized, since the inference (i.e. the computation of posterior probability given observations on other variables) can be executed as new evidence comes in, for any node. As noted above, contextualized IoT applications will require the combination of many input sources, and therefore Bayesian networks may also be a good choice.

A couple of authors have suggested the usage of Bayesian Network technology as a valuable technology for IoT [6–10], however without implementation architecture as defined in this paper.

5   Embedding the Smart Agent in an IoT Solution

In many cases, the Bayesian logic will form part of a larger IoT application that has other components such as dedicated user interfaces, device management, big data analysis etc. Therefore, it is required that the Bayesian logic can be integrated in an overall solution. This can be done by exposing the architecture as a REST service, which means the agent, sensors and actuators can be controlled from the outside, and the intelligent agent can be integrated as part of a bigger solution. Figure 2 summarizes the cloud-based smart agent architecture proposed in this paper.

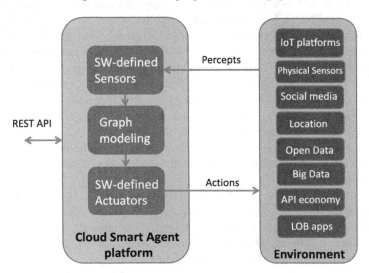

Fig. 2. A cloud-based Bayesian smart agent architecture for IoT applications.

6   Conclusion

This paper has presented a smart agent architecture for real-time decision making in IoT applications. It is based on a cloud architecture with flexible, generalized sensor and actuator capabilities via a software-defined-sensor and software-defined-actuator layer. At its core it uses Bayesian network technology. This paper has demonstrated that Bayesian technology matches challenges and environmental conditions of IoT. Its API-driven architecture makes it compatible with modern SaaS development practices and allows integration in broader IoT solutions.

References

1. Russell, S., Norvig, P.: Artificial Intelligence: A Modern Approach, 3rd edn. Pearson, London (2014)
2. Cisco: Fog Computing, Ecosystem, Architecture and Applications. http://www.cisco.com/web/about/ac50/ac207/crc_new/university/RFP/rfp13078.html
3. Finnegan, M.: Boeing 787 s to create half a terabyte of data per flight, says Virgin Atlantic, ComputerWorldUK (2013). http://www.computerworlduk.com/news/infrastructure/3433595/boeing-787s-create-half-terabyte-of-data-per-flight-says-virgin-atlantic/
4. Scoble, R., Israel, S.: Age of Context: Mobile, Sensors, Data and the Future of Privacy. CreateSpace Independent Publishing Platform, Seattle (2013)
5. Koller, D., Friedman, N.: Probabilistic Graphical Models Principles and Techniques. Massachusetts Institute of Technology, Cambridge (2009)
6. Ko, K.-E., Sim, K.-B.: Development of context aware system based on Bayesian network driven context reasoning method and ontology context modeling. In: International Conference on Control, Automation and Systems, 2008, ICCAS 2008, pp. 2309–2313, October 2008
7. Park, H.-S., Oh, K., Cho, S.-B.: Bayesian network-based high-level context recognition for mobile context sharing in cyber-physical system. Int. J. Distrib. Sens. Netw. **2011**, 10 (2011)
8. Perera, C., Zaslavsky, A., Christen, P., Georgakopoulos, D.: Context aware computing for the internet of things: a survey. http://arxiv.org/pdf/1305.0982.pdf
9. Renninger, H., von Hasseln, H.: Object-Oriented Dynamic Bayesian Network-Templates for Modelling Mechatronic Systems. http://www.dbai.tuwien.ac.at/user/dx2002/proceedings/dx02final21.pdf
10. Carner, P.: Beyond home automation: designing more effective smart home systems. In: 9th IT & T Conference School of Computing, 1 October 2009

Design and Implementation of IoT-Based Intelligent Condition Management System for the Industrial Facilities

Jaekeun Lee, Soono Seo, Myeong-in Choi, Yongkwen Hwang,
Tacklim Lee, and Sehyun Park[(⊠)]

School of Electrical and Electronics Engineering, Chung-Ang University,
84 Heuseok-Ro, Dongjak-Gu, Seoul, Korea
{li0825, ssoabc, auddlscjswo, dydrms06, tacklim34,
shpark}@cau.ac.kr

Abstract. A condensation phenomenon occurs when the water vapor in the air turn into water droplets. Many industrial facilities are damaged by the condensation phenomenon. An ammunition storage is one of the facilities that are damaged by this phenomenon. Therefore, this paper proposes an IoT-based intelligent condition management system (ICMS) in for the industrial facilities. The proposed system prevents a condensation phenomenon by measuring the temperature and humidity and provides alerting service about intrusion and gas exposure through a smartphone application. Therefore, it has become possible to manage the ammunition efficiently.

Keywords: Environmental monitoring system · Condensation phenomenon · Ammunition storage · Zigbee communication · Internet of things

1 Introduction

A condensation phenomenon is easily shown in our daily lives. This phenomenon is caused by difference between internal temperature and external temperature. Generally, when the air temperature gets high, the amount of saturated water vapor is increased. However, if warm air suddenly becomes cold, the amount of saturated water vapor is also reduced [1]. For this reason, water vapor changes to water droplets. The condensation phenomenon easily occurs during the summer when temperature and humidity are especially high. This phenomenon causes a lot of problems. For example, water droplets corrode metals and woods and promote the growth of mold. The army ammunition storage facility is also one of the facilities damaged by condensation. Because most ammunition is expensive, scale of damage is greater than the other problems. Therefore, many studies have been conducted in order to prevent this problem. However, most studies have presented a solution of the problem with architectural approaches. And, this solution can only be applicable to the initial construction of ammunition storage and requires high cost. Currently, most of ammunition storages were built in the form of igloo for the purpose of protection and camouflage. The igloo type ammunition storage has bad air circulation between inside and outside.

© Institute for Computer Sciences, Social Informatics and Telecommunications Engineering 2015
R. Giaffreda et al. (Eds.): IoT360 2014, Part I, LNICST 150, pp. 48–53, 2015.
DOI: 10.1007/978-3-319-19656-5_7

Thus, it is particularly vulnerable to condensation. Nowadays, in order to prevent the condensation phenomenon, an administrator opens the door of ammunition storage and directly checks the value of temperature hygrometer which is installed internally. If it is the condensation conditions, the administrator should turn on the fan using the internal switch of ammunition storage. This management system is an inconvenient for managing temperature and humidity.

Recently, with the changes in the IoT paradigm, many studies on IoT based temperature and humidity monitoring system have been conducted [2, 3]. Devices shown in these studies consist of a sensor module, a communication module, and a micro controller unit (MCU). The sensor module measures ambient temperature and humidity. The communication module sends the information, which is collected through the sensor module, to users via WiFi, Bluetooth, ZigBee communication. The MCU analyzes the information of temperature and humidity and creates services for the users. By controlling the appliances in the room through this monitoring system, user can be provided optimal air control service in the space [4]. However, these studies have mostly focused on home and building as application target areas.

Therefore, this paper proposes an IoT-based intelligent condition management system (ICMS) for the industrial facilities. The ICMS measures the temperature and humidity and determines whether the condition phenomenon occurred based on these collected information. If it is condensation condition, ICMS turns on the fan installed inside the ammunition storage. The operating fan reduces the difference between internal temperature and external temperature by letting outside air in. This method is capable of automatically preventing condensation according to the condition of the ammunition storage and improves the conventional method which has been managed manually. The ICMS also includes a motion sensor and a gas sensor. Therefore, if an intruder enters the ammunition storage or gas is detected in the space, an administrator can be provided alerting service through a smartphone application.

2 System Architecture

The architecture of the proposed system is shown in Fig. 1. The ICMS is installed in each of the ammunition storages. It collects the information of temperature, humidity, movement, and gas in the internal ammunition storage. A server is located in the center of ammunition storages. It plays a role in storing the information which has been measured by the ICMS and transmitting these information to administrator. The ICMSs adjacent to the server are named header node, the others are named general node. The general nodes transmit the measured information to header nodes. And, the header nodes transmit these information to the server. This method helps to prevent server overload. The ICMS and server are connected via ZigBee communication, and the server is connected to administrator's smartphone via military's intranet. The two key functions that the proposed system has are as follows.

2.1 Preventing the Condensation Using an ICMS

Figure 2 describes the process of preventing the condensation phenomenon in the proposed system. The possibility that the condensation will occur is deeply related to

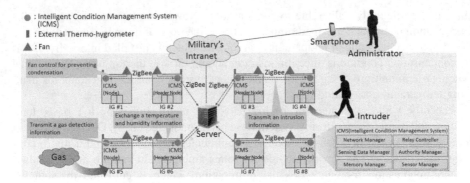

Fig. 1. Overview of the proposed system architecture.

the difference between indoor and outdoor temperature. Thus, in this Fig. 2, the high possibility that the condensation will occur means the temperature difference between indoor and outdoor ammunition storage is over one degree or the humidity is over 80 %. Moreover, ICMS has an ability to control the fan by comparing the internal and external temperature information collected from the sensor manager. The process of the comparison process is performed by the sensing data manager in ICMS. In the scenario 1, when ICMS detects a high possibility that the condensation will occur, the network manager of ICMS forwards a control packet to the fan and an information packet to the server. Then, the fan is activated by the relay controller and the server

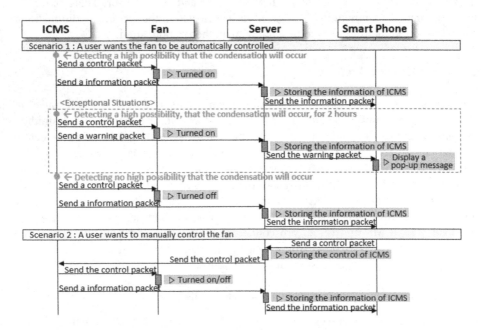

Fig. 2. Sequence diagram for preventing the condensation using an ICMS.

stores the information packet. After storing the information of ICMS, the server sends the information packet to the smart phone. Similarly, when ICMS does not detect the high possibility that the condensation will occur, ICMS forwards a control packet to the fan and an information packet to the server. After receiving the control packet, the fan is deactivated and the server stores the information of ICMS. Then, the server transfers the information packet to the smart phone.

In Fig. 2, the exceptional situation means that the environmental condition has not be improved for 1 h after the fan is turned on. For example, the exceptional situation is can occur due to the fan's breakdown. If ICMS detects the exceptional situation, ICMS will transfer the control packet to the fan again and the warning packet to the server. Then, the server stores the information of ICMS and sends the warning packet to the smart phone. After the smart phone receives the warning packet, the smart phone shows a pop-up message that alarms the administrator through the mobile phone application. Due to this pop-up message, the administrator can immediately recognize the problem of the ammunition and quickly handle the problem.

Furthermore, the administrator is able to remotely control the power supply of fan by using the smart phone. The scenario 2 in Fig. 1 shows the process of the remote control. When an administrator sends a control packet to the ICMS through the server, the authority manager of ICMS first identifies the administrator for the security, and then the control packet is sent to the fan. For this purpose, the authority manager has an ability to entitle specific administrators to access the ICMS. If an administrator has access authority, ICMS will forward the control packet to the fan to activate or deactivate the fan. After the fan is turned on or off, the ICMS sends an information packet to the server. Then, the server stores the information of ICMS and transfers the information packet to the administrator's smart phone.

2.2 Providing an Alerting Service Through Smartphone Application

Figure 3 describes the process of warning the administrator of an intruder's movement or a gas leak in the ammunition storage. When ICMS detects the motion of human or gas exposure, ICMS forwards a warning packet to the server. The server, then, stores the information of ICMS and transfers the warning packet to the smart phone. After receiving the warning packet, the smart phone immediately warns the administrator of detecting the motion of a human or a gas leak with a pop-up message of the mobile phone application.

3 Implementation and Test

Figure 4(a) shows the prototype of ICMS. It consists of a micro controller unit (MCU), a power module, an environmental monitoring sensor module, a ZigBee (IEEE 802.15.4) module, and a buzzer. The environmental monitoring sensor module is divided into 3 parts: a temperature and humidity sensor, a gas sensor, and a motion sensor. A smartphone application is shown in Fig. 4(b). Using the mobile application, an administrator is able to both observe the condition of the ammunition storage and

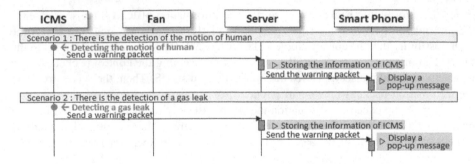

Fig. 3. Sequence diagram for alerting service.

remotely control the fan to decrease a gap between indoor temperature and outdoor temperature. Moreover, the mobile application displays pop-up messages and warns an administrator of urgent problems such as detecting an intruder and the air condition that has not been improved for 1 h. We implemented the proposed system in the test bed shown in Fig. 4(c). It was made as a model analogous to the environment of an ammunition storage. The test bed consists of ICMS, an external thermometer, and a fan. Figure 4(d) shows temperature changes in the test bed. When the temperature difference became over one degree between inside and outside, the fan was activated.

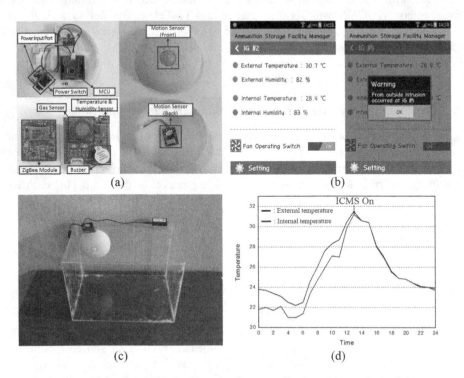

Fig. 4. (a) Prototype of the ICMS, (b) smartphone application, (c) test bed of the proposed system, (d) experimental result.

And then, the temperature difference was decreased. Owing to this process of the proposed system, the condensation phenomenon could be prevented.

4 Conclusion

For the efficient ammunition storage management, an intelligent condition management system (ICMS) is proposed. The ICMS measures temperature and humidity in real time and turns on an installed fan by analyzing these measured values. Therefore, it prevents condensation phenomenon automatically. The ICMS also provides alerting service for security and safety. An administrator can receive the message about intrusion or gas exposure via smartphone application. We implemented the proposed system in a test bed to verify efficiency. The proposed system prevented the condensation phenomenon by controlling a fan.

Acknowledgments. This work was supported by the MSIP (Ministry of Science, ICT and Future Planning), Korea, under the ITRC (Information Technology Research Center) support program (NIPA-2014-H0301-14-1044) supervised by the NIPA(National IT Industry Promotion Agency), and by the Human Resources Development (No. 20124030200060) and the Energy Efficiency & Resources (No. 20132010101850) of the Korea Institute of Energy Technology Evaluation and Planning (KETEP) grant funded by the Korea government Ministry of Trade, Industry and Energy.

References

1. Jia, L., Peng, X.: Heat transfer in flue gas with vapor condensation. Tsinghua Sci. Technol. **7**, 177–181 (2002)
2. Lazarescu, M.T.: Design of a WSN platform for long-term environmental monitoring for IoT applications. IEEE Trans. Sel. Top. Circuits Syst. **3**, 45–54 (2013)
3. Chi, Q., Yan, H., Zhang, C., Pang, Z., Xu, L.D.: A reconfigurable smart sensor interface for industrial WSN in IoT environment. IEEE Trans. Ind. Informat. **10**, 1417–1425 (2014)
4. Perera, C., Zaslavsky, A., Christen, P., Georgakopoulos, D.: Context aware computing for the Internet of things: a survey. Commun. Surv. Tuts. **16**, 414–454 (2014)

A Cognitive Approach to Affordance Learning in Robotic Ecologies

Mauro Dragone[✉]

Trinity College Dublin, College Green, Dublin 2, Ireland
dragonem@tcd.ie
https://www.scss.tcd.ie/~dragonem/

Abstract. The Robotic Ecology vision shares many similarities with the one pursued by the IoT community: The ideal aim on both fronts is that arbitrary combinations of devices should be able to be deployed in unstructured environments, such as those exemplified in a typical household, and there efficiently cooperate to the achievement of complex tasks. While this has the potential to deliver a range of modular and disruptive applications, a pressing and open research question is how to reduce the amount of pre-programming required for their deployment in real world applications. In order to inspire similar advancements within the IoT community, this extended abstract discusses how this goal has been addressed by pioneering the concept of a self-learning robotic ecology within the EU project RUBICON (Robotic UBIquitous Cognitive Network); how such an approach relates to the concept of Affordances at the basis of Gibsons' theory of ecological psychology; and how it can be used to drive the gradual adaptation of a robotic ecology to changing contexts and evolving requirements.

Keywords: Robotic ecology · Affordances · Cognitive systems

1 Robotic Ecologies

In [1], Saffiotti and Broxvall discuss the implications of their PEIS-Ecology instantiation of the Robotic Ecology approach from an ecological (Gibsonian) point of view, by conceiving the interaction between each device and its environment in terms of mutuality and reciprocity. An ecology of simple devices can achieve complex tasks by performing several steps in a coordinated fashion while also exchanging sensor data and other useful information in the process. Note how such a viewpoint falls into the framing assumption of ecological psychology, which, as Greeno notes [2] "...*involves a shift of the level of primary focus of cognitive analysis from processes that can be attributed to individual agents to interactive processes in which agents participate, cooperatively, with other agents and with their physical systems that they interact with*".

Saffiotti and Broxvall emphasise how its embodied nature is what makes confronting an ecological view in a robotic ecology characteristically different from what is usually done in pure software systems, e.g., for the orchestration

© Institute for Computer Sciences, Social Informatics and Telecommunications Engineering 2015
R. Giaffreda et al. (Eds.): IoT360 2014, Part I, LNICST 150, pp. 54–57, 2015.
DOI: 10.1007/978-3-319-19656-5_8

of web-services. Noticeably, the semantic of services (the function that they can provide) is usually advertised to the network irrespective of the components that may actually come to use them. On the contrary, just as with Affordances [3], intended as behavioural possibilities, a robotic ecology must be described in terms of relations (configurations) between its components. For instance, a ceiling camera can track and inform a mobile robot about its location in the environment (thus *affording localization* to the robot). However, this can be done as long as the robot in question (i) is not too small, (ii) is inside the field of view of the camera, and (iii) its color can be distinguished from the one of the floor.

A PEIS Ecology adopts temporal constraints to represent the possible relations between PEIS components, e.g., stating that navigation must occur while location information is available, or that a class of robots is able to push a given object. These relations are then shared and resolved into global configurations, by using either a centralized constraint satisfaction solver or a multi-agent, reactive approach. However, both methods lack learning capabilities and rely instead on pre-programmed, static and brittle domain knowledge. The inability of modelling other (unforeseen at design time) information in the domain, including possible synergies, conflicts and other inter-dependencies between their many components, is what breaks the modularity of the development of these systems, and ultimately impacts on their ability to pro-actively and smoothly adapt to changing contexts and evolving requirements. These are the key issues addressed in RUBICON [4], as outlined in the next section.

2   The RUBICON Approach

The most appealing aspects of the concept of affordances as a source of inspiration in Robotics are (i) its implicit emphasis on the relationship between an agent and the environment, and (ii) its grounding in the paradigm of direct perception. The central question for Gibson was whether affordances can be directly perceived. In their stride to build physically embodied agents, roboticists have thus sought to enable robots with the ability to learn to recognize affordances, thus ultimately reducing the complexity of representation and reasoning.

A common approach has been the utilization of an exploratory stage, in which the robot tries out different action primitives and observes their consequences. To this end, roboticists have usually based their works on more formal, e.g., functional elaboration of affordances seen as opportunities for action and inherently suited to be used as pre-conditions in a planning context by virtue of their predictive quality (see [5] for a survey). A service robot may thus learn how to poke, push, pull, rotate and lift objects, and also for what objects and in what situations its actions can more successfully achieve given results. A mobile robot may learn to infer the traversability of its surroundings by mapping from the space of the features extracted from its range sensors, to the effects (success/fail) of a number of basic manoeuvres. Techniques supporting online learning usually exploit curiosity measures to guide the robot's exploration process, by reducing unnecessary interaction with the environment when the robot is confident that it will not bring about new information.

Equipping robotic ecologies with similar learning abilities poses a formidable number of issues: from the computational constraints and the number of the devices involved, to the difficulty of identifying suitable and reliable teaching information to drive system's adaptation. RUBICON [4] addressed these problems by supporting a self-sustaining dynamic between cognitive capabilities realized in a modular architecture, shown in Fig. 1.

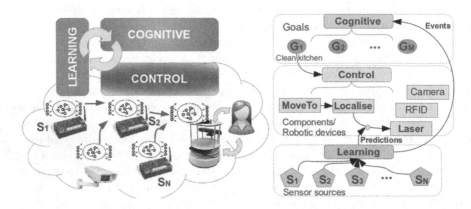

Fig. 1. High-level, hierarchical RUBICON architecture: Sensor data is processed as much as possible locally on computational constrained and robotic devices. Information is extracted and exploited by the higher layers.

The central component of the RUBICON architecture is a plan-based Control Layer (an evolution of the system employed in PEIS, as described in Sect. 1), which is able to decide which components (e.g. robot behaviours) and/or devices need to collaborate to achieve given service goals. The key approach to enabling system adaptation is to (i) improve its ability to extract meaning from noisy and imprecise sensed data, and (ii) learn what goals to pursue, and (iii) how to pursue them, from experience, rather than by relying on pre-programmed goal-deliberation strategies and plan pre-conditions.

The first and the last of these challenges are met by the Learning Layer, a distributed and adaptable learning infrastructure based on echo state networks, and which is used to process time series of data gathered by the sensors in the ecology. Its outputs are used to recognize events concerning the state of the environment and of the users, and predict the success/fail rate in using given devices and/or other components in the ecology. This information is used by the Control Layer to inform its configuration of the ecology. The second challenge is the responsibility of the Cognitive Layer, which uses Self-Organising Fuzzy Neural Networks to reason over the events recognized by the Learning Layer in order to predict the user's activation of appliances and robotic services.

In our reports [4], we have described how our system, equipped with some initial knowledge and supervised information, can be trained to provide some basic services. The system can use this as a starting point and self-adapt to the preferences of the user and to modification to the environment in a number of ways: firstly, the Cognitive Layer can learn to predict the user's routines. For instance, by observing past instances in which the user has summoned her cleaner robot to the kitchen after eating her meal, the system learns to send the robot without waiting for the user's request. Secondly, the Control Layer can monitor the performances and the outcomes of its own plans, and feed them (as teaching signals) to the Learning Layer in order to learn previously un-modelled plan pre-conditions. For instance, in [6], we have shown how a robot can learn to use the information it receives from itw own sensors and the sensors embedded in the environment (e.g. infrared sensors signalling the movements of the user and/or the robot) to predict (i) what are the best situations in which cleaning a certain room will be less likely to annoy the user, and (ii) when is best to use the RFID-based localization component in place of its own laser (e.g., after the user installs a new mirror that disturbs the robot's laser). Finally, the Cognitive Layer can "explore" (in a manner similar to the one adopted in curiosity-driven, robot manipulators) by trying out new goals in different situations in order to gather further experience and/or feedback from the user.

Our approach allows robotic ecologies to be driven by easily identifiable (albeit rough) rules, while delegating, over time, symbolic reasoning to data-driven inference for the purpose of learning to recognize the affordances of their environment, directly from sensor features. This is a clear improvement over past solutions, which demanded for all goal rules and plan pre-conditions to be specified a priori. What makes it a practical approach, which limits the computational cost of our learning solutions and enables us to use fully automatic feature selection algorithms, is (i) the existence of a finite set of pre-defined and simple goals, (ii) their clear distinction to the plans to achieve them, and (iii) the reduced number of sensor sources included in current smart homes. Future research should increase the scalability of these systems, and address the challenging problem of autonomously learning what goals are achievable to the ecology.

References

1. Saffiotti, A., Broxvall, M.: Affordances in an ecology of physically embedded intelligent systems. In: Rome, E., Hertzberg, J., Dorffner, G. (eds.) Towards Affordance-Based Robot Control. LNCS (LNAI), vol. 4760, pp. 106–121. Springer, Heidelberg (2008)
2. Greeno, J.G.: Gibson's affordances. Psychol. Rev. **1012**, 336–342 (1994)
3. Gibson, J.J.: The Theory of Affordances. Lawrence Erlbaum (1977)
4. Robotic ubiquitous cognitive network (rubicon) website (2014). http://www.fp7rubicon.eu/
5. Horton, T.E., Chakraborty, A., Amant, R.S.: Affordances for robots: A brief survey. Avant **3**(2), 70–84 (2012)
6. Bacciu, D., Gallicchio, C., Micheli, A., Di Rocco, M., Saffiotti, A.: Learning context-aware mobile robot navigation in home environments. In: The 5th International Conference on Information, Intelligence, Systems and Applications, IISA 2014, pp. 57–62, July 2014

High-Level Programming and Symbolic Reasoning on IoT Resource Constrained Devices

Salvatore Gaglio[1,2], Giuseppe Lo Re[1], Gloria Martorella[1],
and Daniele Peri[1(✉)]

[1] DICGIM University of Palermo,
Viale Delle Scienze, Ed. 6, 90128 Palermo, Italy
{salvatore.gaglio,giuseppe.lore,gloria.martorella,
daniele.peri}@unipa.it
[2] ICAR CNR,
Viale delle Scienze, Ed. 9, 90128 Palermo, Italy

Abstract. While the vision of Internet of Things (IoT) is rather inspiring, its practical implementation remains challenging. Conventional programming approaches prove unsuitable to provide IoT resource constrained devices with the distributed processing capabilities required to implement intelligent, autonomic, and self-organizing behaviors. In our previous work, we had already proposed an alternative programming methodology for such systems that is characterized by high-level programming and symbolic expressions evaluation, and developed a lightweight middleware to support it. Our approach allows for interactive programming of deployed nodes, and it is based on the simple but effective paradigm of executable code exchange among nodes. In this paper, we show how our methodology can be used to provide IoT resource constrained devices with reasoning abilities by implementing a Fuzzy Logic symbolic extension on deployed nodes at runtime.

Keywords: High-level programming · Resource constrained devices · Knowledge representation · Fuzzy Logic

1 Introduction

According to the Internet of Thing (IoT) vision [1], all kinds of devices, although computationally limited, might be used to interact with people or to manage information concerning the individuals themselves [6]. Besides reactive responses on input changes, the whole network may exhibit more advanced behaviors resulting from reasoning processes carried out on the individual nodes or emerging from local interactions. However, nodes' constraints leave the system designers many challenges to face, especially when distributed applications are considered [9]. Conventional programming methodologies often prove inappropriate on resource constrained IoT devices, especially when knowledge must be treated with a high level representation or changes of the application goals may be required after the network has been deployed [8]. Moreover, the implementation of intelligent mechanisms, as well as symbolic reasoning, through rigid

© Institute for Computer Sciences, Social Informatics and Telecommunications Engineering 2015
R. Giaffreda et al. (Eds.): IoT360 2014, Part I, LNICST 150, pp. 58–63, 2015.
DOI: 10.1007/978-3-319-19656-5_9

layered architectures, reveals impracticable on resource constrained devices such
as those commonly used in Wireless Sensor Networks (WSNs). Often this issue is
faced through the adoption of an intelligent centralized system that uses WSNs as
static sensory tools [3]. Indeed, integration of WSN devices in the IoT seems quite
natural and desirable, provided that the aforementioned issues be addressed. In
our previous work [4,5], we introduced an alternative programming methodology, along with a lightweight middleware, based on high-level programming and
executable code exchange among WSN nodes. The contribution of this paper
consists in the extension of the methodology to include symbolic reasoning even
on IoT resource constrained devices. The remainder of the paper is organized
as follows. In Sect. 2 we describe the key concepts of our methodology and the
symbolic model we adopted. In Sect. 3, we extend the symbolic approach characterizing our programming environment with Fuzzy Logic, and in Sect. 4 we show
an application to make the nodes reason about their position with respect to
thermal zones of the deployment area. Finally, Sect. 5 reports our conclusions.

2   Key Concepts of the Development Methodology

Mainstream praxis to program embedded devices consists in cross-compilation of
specialized application code together with a general purpose operating system.
The resulting object code is then uploaded to the on-board permanent storage. Instead, our methodology is based on high-level executable code exchange
between nodes. This mechanism, while abstracted, is implemented at a very low
level avoiding the burden of a complex and thick software layer between the
hardware and the application code. Indeed, a Forth environment runs on the
hardware providing the core functionalities of an operating system, including
a command line interface (CLI). This also allows for interactive development,
which is a peculiar feature of our methodology that can be used even to repro-
gram deployed nodes. This way, nodes can be made expand their capabilities by
exchanging pieces of code among themselves in realtime. The CLI is accessible
through either a microcontroller's UART or the on-board radio [4]. The Forth
environment is inherently provided with an interpreter and a compiler. Both can
be easily extended by defining new *words* stored in the *dictionary*. Being Forth a
stack-based language, words use the stack for parameters passing. A command,
or an entire program, is thus just a sequence words. The description of a task
in natural language and its implementation can be thus made very similar. Our
programming environment is composed of some nodes wirelessly deployed and a
wired node that behaves as a bridge to send user inputs to the network. In previous work [5], we introduced the syntactic construct that implements executable
code exchange among nodes:

$$\texttt{tell: } \langle code \rangle \texttt{ :tell}$$

in which ⟨*code*⟩ is a sequence of words, sent as character strings, to be remotely
interpreted by the receiver node. The address of the destination node is left
on the top of the stack. A numeric as well as a string value, can be taken at

runtime from the top of the stack and inserted in the outgoing packet when special markers, such as ~ for numbers and ~s for strings are encountered.

3   Distributed Processing and Symbolic Reasoning

In our programming environment, purely reactive behaviors can be easily implemented on the remote nodes by sending them the sequence of words to be executed if certain conditions are met. Let us consider the following command given through the CLI of the bridge node:

```
bcst tell: close-to-window? [if] red led on [then] :tell ;
```

This command broadcasts (bcst is the reserved address for the purpose) the code between the tell: and :tell words. Once received, each node executes the word close-to-window? to evaluate if it is close to the window and, if so turns the red LED on. The word close-to-window?, already in the dictionary, performs temperature and luminosity measurements and checks if both sensory readings are above a predefined threshold. As it can be noticed, the code is quite understandable, although all the words operate just above the hardware level by setting ports or enabling the ADCs to read temperature and light exposure. This code, as well as those in the rest of the paper, has been used on Iris Mote nodes equipped with the MTS400 sensor board to acquire data about temperature and light exposure. For the sake of showing how it is possible to incorporate in our middleware new abstractions to support intelligent applications here we introduce a Fuzzy Logic extension. Fuzzy Logic has the peculiarity to be appropriate to implement approximate reasoning in several contexts as well as for machine learning purposes [10]. We adopted a classic Forth Fuzzy Logic implementation [11] that we enriched with the possibility to exchange definitions and evaluation among nodes. Moving on with the above example, in place of two crisp variables, the fuzzy variables temp and lightexp can be easily defined on deployed nodes, using the word fvar to define the related membership functions (Fig. 1) placed between tell: and :tell. A node can be made measure light exposure, and fuzzify it with the code:

```
lightexp measure apply
```

while the code:

```
lightexp.low @
```

pushes onto the stack the truth value by using the built-in word @ (*fetch*). Rather than through a thresholding process, a device can establish if it is close to the window through the evaluation of fuzzy rules in the form:

```
temp.high @ lightexp.high @ & => close-to-window
```

where temp.high and lightexp.high are membership functions of the fuzzy input variable temp and lightexp respectively, and close-to-window is one of the linguistic labels associated to the output variable. Similarly to the case of the thresholding process, if both the temperature and the light exposure levels are high a node can infer to be under sunlight, and thus close to the window.

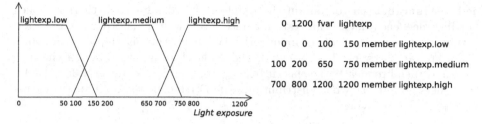

Fig. 1. Fuzzy set associated with the fuzzy variable `lightexp`. On the right side, the code to define the fuzzy variable `lightexp` and its membership functions. The definition domain, corresponding to the raw readings values interval [0,1200], is given before the word `fvar`, while the word `member` defines each of the three trapezoidal membership functions by using four control points (bottom-left, top-left, top-right, and bottom-right).

4 Inferring Nodes' Distribution According to Thermal Zones

Let us suppose we intend to make the deployed nodes able to discover their distribution with respect to thermal zones of an environment lighted by some windows exposed to direct sunlight, and lamps. Each node assesses in turn the thermal zone it belongs to, and makes the others aware of this information. We defined the syntactic construct `classification` to make the nodes able to classify according to an arbitrary number of fuzzy variables. With the previously defined input variables `temp` and `lightexp` the code:

```
temp lightexp 2 classification thermal-zone
```

creates the new word `thermal-zone`, which is bound to the two fuzzy variables `temp` and `lightexp`. The new word `thermal-zone` measures the temperature and luminosity, fuzzifies the crisp inputs and evaluates the rules by storing the firing strength for each rule, indicating the degree to which the rule matches the inputs. The rule generation process considers all the possible combinations of all the membership functions, -i.e. in this case, the set of all ordered pairs (a,b) where a and b are linguistic terms associated respectively with `temp` and `lightexp`. When handling few variables, this does not cause excessive memory occupation. It offers instead the advantage of considering a fine-grained classification based on all the n-tuples, that in this case, are all valid. However, optimization methods for the reduction of a large scale rule base may be required in real-time fuzzy systems [2,7,12]. When needed, the table is traversed to compute the membership grade of the output by aggregating all rules. The rule with the maximum strength is taken as the output membership class. This way, each node is able to classify itself into one of the thermal zones. To support more sophisticated behaviors, it is possible to exploit the mechanism of code exchange among nodes to trigger the process of neighbor discovery in order to keep track of their classification into thermal-zones. For this purpose, it is necessary to define the table `nodes-distribution` to contain the number of nodes for each thermal zone. For instance, each device can transmit once, after waiting (word `on-timer`) for a time that is function of its unique ID. When its time is elapsed, the word `classification-spread` is executed, the node classifies itself into a thermal zone and then broadcasts the class it belongs to, together with the code to make the others update the whole distribution. The Forth code required for the entire process is the following:

```
: local-update nodes-distribution update ;
: spread dup local-update bcst [tell:] ~ local-update [:tell] ;
: classification-spread thermal-zone spread ;
  on-timer ' classification-spread
```

in which the word **spread** creates a message with the code to make the other devices update locally the `nodes-distribution`. At the end of the **update** process, each node holds the current nodes distribution in terms of thermal zones, as such:

```
Class 1 2 3 4 5 6 7 8 9
   # 5 1 0 0 0 0 0 1 1
```

Five nodes belongs to class 1, one node to class 2 and so on. Each node knows the number of nodes in the network and their position, without any centralized computation. Once some nodes are moved from their position to another, and the process is triggered again, each node is able to detect the new distribution. Moreover, the analysis of the nodes distribution may lead a node to classify itself as an outlier, to trigger self-diagnosis operations, and even to take specific actions, by reasoning about the whole network configuration and its membership thermal zone. The interactivity granted by our approach permits the programmer to communicate with the network through the serial shell of the bridge node. For instance, the programmer can tell the nodes belonging to class 8 to turn their red LED on:

```
bcst tell: thermal-zone 8 class? [if] red led on [then] :tell ;
```

5   Conclusions

In this paper, we showed how distributed symbolic reasoning can be implemented on resource constrained IoT devices by exploiting executable code exchange. Our contribution aims to fill the lack in the absence of programming paradigms enabling a vast adoption of IoT in everyday life. The possibility to exchange executable code makes the system adaptive and autonomous, since each node can evolve on the basis of realtime inputs, in terms of both data and executable code, from other nodes and from the user. We showed how abstractions and symbolic expression evaluation can be efficiently incorporated into a programming model for such networks by exploiting both interpretation and compilation of code. As an example, we described the syntactic constructs that can be defined to make the nodes aware of their position with respect to a subdivision of the environment into thermal zones. Our methodology reveals suitable for implementing more advanced behaviors on IoT devices since symbolic reasoning is performed even on inexpensive and resource constrained microcontrollers.

References

1. Atzori, L., Iera, A., Morabito, G.: The internet of things: a survey. Comput. Netw. **54**(15), 2787–2805 (2010)
2. De Paola, A., Lo Re, G., Pellegrino, A.: A fuzzy adaptive controller for an ambient intelligence scenario. In: Gaglio, S., Lo Re, G. (eds.) Advances onto the Internet of Things. AISC, pp. 47–59. Springer, Heidelberg (2014)
3. De Paola, A., Ortolani, M., Lo Re, G., Anastasi, G., Das, S.K.: Intelligent management systems for energy efficiency in buildings: a survey. ACM Comput. Surv **47**(1), 13:1–13:38 (2014)
4. Gaglio, S., Lo Re, G., Martorella, G., Peri, D.: A fast and interactive approach to application development on wireless sensor and actuator networks. In: Accepted at the 19th IEEE International Conference on Emerging Technologies and Factory Automation (ETFA 2014) (2014)
5. Gaglio, S., Re, G.L., Martorella, G., Peri, D.: A lightweight middleware platform for distributed computing on wireless sensor networks. Procedia Comput. Sci. **32**, 908–913 (2014). http://www.sciencedirect.com/science/article/pii/S1877050914007108, The 5th International Conference on Ambient Systems, Networks and Technologies (ANT-2014), The 4th International Conference on Sustainable Energy Information Technology (SEIT-2014)
6. Guo, B., Zhang, D., Yu, Z., Liang, Y., Wang, Z., Zhou, X.: From the Internet of things to embedded intelligence. World Wide Web **16**(4), 399–420 (2013)
7. Jin, Y.: Fuzzy modeling of high-dimensional systems: complexity reduction and interpretability improvement. IEEE Trans. Fuzzy Syst. **8**(2), 212–221 (2000)
8. Kortuem, G., Kawsar, F., Fitton, D., Sundramoorthy, V.: Smart objects as building blocks for the internet of things. IEEE Internet Comput. **14**(1), 44–51 (2010)
9. Martorella, G., Peri, D., Toscano, E.: Hardware and software platforms for distributed computing on resource constrained devices. In: Gaglio, S., Lo Re, G. (eds.) Advances onto the Internet of Things. Advances in Intelligent Systems and Computing, vol. 260, pp. 121–133. Springer International Publishing, Switzerland (2014)
10. Navara, M., Peri, D.: Automatic generation of fuzzy rules and its applications in medical diagnosis. In: Proceedings of the 10th International Conference on Information Processing and Management of Uncertainty, Perugia, Italy, vol. 1, pp. 657–663 (2004)
11. VanNorman, R.: Fuzzy Forth. Forth Dimensions **18**, 6–13 (1997)
12. Yam, Y., Baranyi, P., Yang, C.T.: Reduction of fuzzy rule base via singular value decomposition. IEEE Trans. Fuzzy Syst. **7**(2), 120–132 (1999)

BlockMagic, A Hybrid Educational Environment Based on RFID Technology and Internet of Things Concepts

Orazio Miglino[1], Raffaele Di Fuccio[1(✉)], Andrea Di Ferdinando[2],
and Carlo Ricci[3]

[1] Università di Napoli "Federico II", Naples, Italy
raffaele.difuccio@unina.it
[2] Consiglio Nazionale delle Ricerche, Istituto di Scienze e Tecnologie della
Cognizione, Rome, Italy
[3] Fondazione Lega del Filo D'Oro, Osimo, Italy

Abstract. The new improvements of ICT technologies allow the opportunity to use these tools in the learning context and create smart environments for children and teachers in schools. In this paper, we present Block Magic (BM), a tool that exploits the Internet of Things theory using RFID technology. This tool allows the children to play traditionally with well-known didactic materials, the traditional Logic Blocks, but in connection with a PC and a dedicated software that increase the interaction. BM stimulates different learning activities for specific skills as mathematics, logic, language, problem solving and creativity. This low-cost and user-friendly technology allows enhancing the learning/ teaching session due to the software feedbacks and the session tracker. The software is able to track the sessions of each child, and supporting the learner with a hidden Adaptive Tutoring System (ATS) that presents to the children the right exercises, based on the learners' replies. BM was tested in four different countries (Germany, Spain, Italy and Greece) in the kindergartens and the primary schools, the target groups were in the range 3–7 years old. The tool was tested in a larger scale evaluation that involved 22 teachers and 495 children. The results shows a high degree of acceptability; that appreciated the concept and the innovation features. The trials showed some issues to be fixed, as the usability. BM was a research developed in the framework of a funded by the EU Commission.

Keywords: Internet of things · Innovation · Augmented Reality System · Research projects · RFID technologies · Assistive learning

1 Introduction

The Internet of Things theory was the drive of the research of Block Magic. The project, funded by the European Commission and ended in the November 2013, aimed to start from the Radio Frequency Identification Technology (RFID) creating a sort of interactive net between the children in schools, the learning materials and the teachers. This hybrid environment [1, 2] was based on traditional psycho-pedagogical activities

© Institute for Computer Sciences, Social Informatics and Telecommunications Engineering 2015
R. Giaffreda et al. (Eds.): IoT360 2014, Part I, LNICST 150, pp. 64–69, 2015.
DOI: 10.1007/978-3-319-19656-5_10

well-know from the teachers. These activities exploited the structured materials used in rehabilitation centers, baby-parks, children's hospitals and the homes. The structured materials are materials that have a fixed numbers of "n" elements and "m" categories. The structure is represented by the rules that connect the single parts. Typical examples of structured materials are logic blocks, cards, teaching tiles, etc. These materials allow analytical thought, using the isolation of a single quality (e.g. dimension, shape, color, etc.) and allowing the focalization of attention on a single part of the object, and then, with a gradual analytical process, the ability for clustering and serialization, in order to understand the object.

The Logic Blocks was the didactic materials chosen in the Block Magic project for their wide adoption by the schools. These are different pieces or blocks that differ each other for different attributes as color, thickness, geometric shape and dimension. (see Fig. 1).

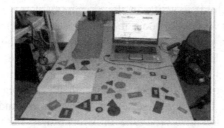

Fig. 1. The Block Magic system

Traditionally these materials aim at empowering the proactive function of learning processes and cooperative dynamics between the pairs (children in our case). It is fundamental underline, that these Logic Blocks, in the traditional uses, propose an important hurdle. It allows the active participation of pupils, but is extremely expensive because of the continue supervision of the teachers/parents and the needs of personalized educational interventions that are impossible in this context.

The research project Block Magic, ended in November 2013 and funded in the framework of the programme LLP-Comenius by the European Commission, worked in order to overcome this limit, and connect the smart learning environment exploiting the strength of the manipulation. These interactions seem to be determinant in the human knowledge cognitive representation as showed by the theoretical perspective of the Internet of Things [3, 4] and the Embodiment Cognition [5]. It demonstrated using experiments, empirical studies, clinical observations and computational modelling [6] that it is captured in our neurocognitive structures as a holistic space-based sensory-motor representation.

1.1   Technology

The technology becomes important for an increase of the satisfaction of the users and the Internet of Things rules require an interconnection between the things in a smart configuration enhanced by the technology.

In this point of view, the technology that matches with these purposes is the RFID (Radio Frequency Identification/Near Field Communication).

RFID systems consists of an antenna and a transceiver, which is able to read the radio frequency and transfer the information to a device, and a small and low cost tag, which is an integrated circuit containing the RF circuitry and information to be transmitted.

The aim of the project Block Magic was to create hybrid platforms matching two different contexts, from one side the digital world usual for the new digital natives interconnecting more tools in a traditional environment (school or home, etc.), for the other side the physical world with strong and well-consolidated psych-pedagogical practices.

These hybrid systems propose some improvements respect the state of art of the physical and the digital world. The strength points are the ability: (i) to overcome the limits of the excessive orientation of the screen, typical of the digital applications, because the user (the child) is active in the execution of the task, playing with the device and with the environment tools in the same time; (ii) to assess the session performed by a learner, giving a supporting tool for the teachers; (iii) to reduce the costs of the traditional lesson that use the structured material, because they need a continue support of the teacher; (iv) to permit an highly individualized learning path; (v) to connect the elements in a traditional environment, creating a smart environment.

On these bases, an international research Consortium funded by the European Commission produced the first prototype of BlockMagic based on STELT (Smart Technology to Enhance Learning and Teaching) a developing tools to build-up educational games with RFID sensors [7].

From a more general point of view, the ambition of BlockMagic project is to redefine the learning-teaching Logic Block materials through the use of a cheap Smart Technology creating hybrid smart environments. In this prospective BlockMagic aims to reinforce the traditional teaching methods for kindergarten and primary school.

2 The Block Magic Framework

2.1 Block Magic Platform

Block Magic is a hardware-software prototype that uses RFID sensors and an Artificial Tutoring System in order to connect different tools in an environment like school or home. The general objective is to reduce the presence of an adult that supervises the activities (teacher or parent). The hardware is based on RFID-TAG (tiny stickers) are on traditional logic block pieces that can be recognized by an active reader connected to a Tablet/PC. The PC/tablet is equipped with the Block Magic software that simulate the actions of teachers, proposing exercises, giving feedbacks and maintaining a record of an individual learning history (Fig. 2).

Operatively, when a user places one or more blocks on the active reader of BlockMagic, in connection via Bluetooth or cable to a PC/tablet, the system recognizes the blocks and gives some opportune aural and sound feedbacks to the learner. These feedbacks support the pupil in order to solve different exercises regarding different skill

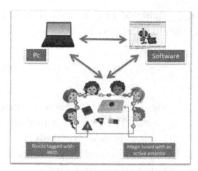

Fig. 2. The framework of the Block Magic system

(mathematics, logic, problem solving, creativity, etc.). The "smart" software engine, developed during the project, receives input from the board and generates an "action" directly on the screen.

2.2 Scenarios/Learning Activities

The methodology defined in the project has three main scenarios: (1) Individual Game Scenario and (2) Social Game Scenario, (3) Special Needs Scenario. In the Individual Game Scenario, the learner has to solve a task autonomously using life skills (mathematical, logical, strategic, and creative or language skills). In the Social Game Scenario, the group plays/learns with Block Magic and the "social skill" can emerge in this context. In the Special Needs Scenario, special games were proposed to children having severe disabilities.

The teacher has the role to set the classroom and introduces the blocks and the magic board to the children, leaving the kids free to play these materials. The BlockMagic software allows to the educators to personalize the training for every child, choosing the exercises proposed for the children in order to seek defined educational objectives. The teacher acts differently in the Individual Game Scenario and in the Social Game scenario. In the first case, the educator represents an observer and in case of request of help, he/she could support the kids. In the second case, the teacher interacts with the children, providing support, observing, creating obstacle, based on the characteristics of the specific exercises.

2.3 Trials

The methods, exercises and technologies developed by BlockMagic Consortium were tested in kindergartens and primary schools with selected children and teachers in Greece, Italy and Spain between 3 to 7 years old. The trials involved 10 teachers, 257 students, and 2 children with special needs in 4 schools. In Italy, in the structures of LegaDelFiloD'Oro were performed trial for children with special needs.

During the trails, the researchers of the project supervised the sessions reporting observations and comments. After the sessions, the researchers made some face-to-face interview with teachers that participated in the trials. The interview were focused on three aspects (ergonomics, usefulness and satisfaction) for the three scenarios.

3 Results

The observations and the interview with the experts collected about the Individual Scenario shows an encouraging view. The hidden nature of the tools permits a high degree of acceptance from the teachers and the kids in the schools. Their main approaches was positive and they considered it as a normal tool for the schools, underlining some positive points and some weaknesses.

Regarding the usefulness, the teachers considered Block Magic an important tool that could be added in the daily school routines, with some improvements that will allow an easier use. The exercises provided in BlockMagic are considered balanced for children in that range of ages. In their opinion BlockMagic stimulates mainly mathematical and logical skills and with a minor degree also creativity, strategic and language. In particular, the creativity is stimulated but the children prefer to build picture using the blocks out of the BlockMagic platform. The feature that the teachers mainly appreciate was the direct feedback. The teachers considered that Block Magic stimulates the children to learn, in particular the children with problems in concentrations.

Regarding the ergonomics, the teachers referred that the prototype has some features to be improved, some exercises contain some obstacles for a correct performing. For example: the repetition of a same action, the need of place a block in order to start a game, etc. However, the observations showed that the children after a little time of understanding were highly confident with the tool. The pupils learned quickly the functionalities of BlockMagic and there was few requests of support from teacher. The learners asked for helps only when lacked the exercise information. However, a problem emerged with the children between the 3 and 4 years old for the difficulty in distinguishing the thickness of magic blocks.

Regarding the satisfaction, the children appreciated the whole tool, with a strong preference for the aural feedback (the BlockMagic software is set to call the user by own name). This feature surprises the children and allows a quick interaction. All children looked forward to play again with the BlockMagic tool. The teachers appreciated this element, because the children enjoyed "to learn" because they considered they were playing a game.

4 Conclusions

The BlockMagic project funded by the EU Commission, developed a structured methodology that take from the experience of well consolidated psycho-pedagogical approaches and a functional platform (hardware/software) using the RFID technology and the Internet of Things (IoT) approach. The BlockMagic kits were tested it with selected children and teachers in Greece, Italy, Germany and Spain in kindergartens and primary schools. The results achieved during this experimentation were very encouraging for all the three real cases: individual scenario, social scenario and special needs scenario. The observations performed by the researchers and the interviews collected with the teachers involved demonstrates that the BlockMagic prototype is a tool that could be easily introduced in the daily routines of real classrooms. The children are very attracted and excited during the BlockMagic session and they consider it as a game. The system allows a good interaction in social contexts and supports the group activities. In addition, BlockMagic reduced the negative feedbacks for children with special needs during the execution of the sessions in comparison with traditional methods.

It is necessary to underline some limits reported by the teachers in particular regarding the ergonomics. This element will represent the direction that the authors will seek in order to improve the features of this hybrid system.

Acknowledgments. The BlockMagic project (517936-LLP-1-IT-COMENIUS-CMP) has been funded with support from the European Commission. This publication reflects the views only of the author, and the Commission cannot be held responsible for any use which may be made of the information contained therein.

References

1. Dienes, Z.P.: The Elements of Mathematics. Herder and Herder, Inc., New York (1971)
2. Dienes, Z.P.: Large Plastic Set, and Learning Logic, Logical Games. Herder & Herder, New York (1972)
3. Kranz, M., Holleis, P., Schmidt, A.: Embedded interaction: interacting with the internet of things. IEEE Internet Comput. **14**(2), 46–53 (2010)
4. De La Guía, E., Lozano, M.D., Penichet, V.M.: Interacting with Objects in Games Through RFID Technology (2013)
5. Borghi, A.M., Cimatti, F.: Embodied cognition and beyond: acting and sensing the body. Neuropsychologia **48**, 763–773 (2010)
6. Ponticorvo, M., Miglino, O.: Encoding geometric and non-geometric information: a study with evolved agents. Anim. Cognit. **13**(1), 157–174 (2010)
7. Miglino, O., Di Fuccio, R., Barajas, M., Belafi, M., Ceccarani, P., Dimitrakopoulou, D., Ricci, C., Trifonova, A., Zoakou, A.: Enhancing manipulative learning with smart object. In: Learning Innovations and Quality: The Future of Digital Resources, pp. 112–119 (2013)

A Reputation-Based Distributed District Scheduling Algorithm for Smart Grids

D. Borra[1]([✉]), M. Iori[2], C. Borean[2], and F. Fagnani[1]

[1] Dipartimento di Scienze Matematiche, Politecnico di Torino, Turin, Italy
domenica.borra@polito.it
[2] Swarm Joint Open Lab, Telecom Italia, Lazio, Italy

Abstract. In this paper we develop and test a distributed algorithm providing Energy Consumption Schedules (ECS) in smart grids for a residential district. The goal is to achieve a given aggregate load profile. The NP-hard constrained optimization problem reduces to a distributed unconstrained formulation by means of Lagrangian Relaxation technique, and a meta-heuristic algorithm based on a Quantum inspired Particle Swarm with Lévy flights. A centralized iterative reputation-reward mechanism is proposed for end-users to cooperate to avoid power peaks and reduce global overload, based on random distributions simulating human behaviors and penalties on the effective ECS differing from the suggested ECS. Numerical results show the protocols effectiveness.

Keywords: Distributed algorithms · Autonomous demand response management · Energy consumption scheduling · Smart power grids · Reputation algorithm

1 Introduction

The balance between demand and supply plays a leading role in smart grids applications and modern technologies aim to develop energy optimization algorithms able to provide efficient residential district dispatchment. A large literature has been devoted to decentralized versions of optimization algorithms applied to power systems, see, e.g., [15], due to distributed energy generation and demand, renewables such as photovoltaic resources, storage devices, with changes in real time. Multi-agent planning, as in [11], is often formulated as a combinatorial optimization problem: each agent has its own objectives, resources, constraints, and at the same time it has to share and compete for global resources and constraints. Moreover, new roles in the energy market are emerging, such as energy aggregators as intermediate between energy utilities and home users, managing uncertainties due to variable customer actions, metereology and electricity prices. Given the huge number of agents, the optimization problem is often computationally intractable in a centralized fashion, and given the time-varying cost and constraints in energy demand-response (DR) problems, a fast single-agent planning algorithm is appealing. In this paper, as in [6], customers

© Institute for Computer Sciences, Social Informatics and Telecommunications Engineering 2015
R. Giaffreda et al. (Eds.): IoT360 2014, Part I, LNICST 150, pp. 70–76, 2015.
DOI: 10.1007/978-3-319-19656-5_11

are incentivized to move their loads in off-peak hours despite their individual needs through marginal costs, using reputation scores as feedback. In [6] a cooperative game reduces peak-to-average ratio of the aggregate load and the Nash equilibria are reached using centralized information, whereas our approach is completely distributed. Evolutionary Game theory and Reinforcement Learning techniques have been applied to swarm intelligence problems, as in [1,5,12,14].

Our focus is on energy distribution to a residential district, according to the European Project INTrEPID [9]. In this scenery, the district global load is sensed by power meters, and using non-intrusive load-monitoring techniques (NILM, as in [8]) or smart plugs, the disaggregated data are available, turning the "blind" system to a decentralized smart grid [2]. A centralized unit senses local loads, and communicates with agents through smart-phone app or similar devices proposing day-ahead optimal Energy Consumption Schedules (ECS). Agents may accept the suggested ECS or not, according to individual needs.

Our contribution is twofold. First, we provide a mathematical formalization of the optimization problem, decoupling the global constraint through Lagrangian relaxation as in [10], see Sect. 2. Second, in Sect. 3 we design optimal ECS in a distributed fashion at two levels: at the agent level applying meta heuristic optimization techniques as QPSOL (Quantum Particle Swarm with Levy's Flights) described in [3], in order to get feasible optimal suggested ECS; at the district level a reputation-reward mechanism provides incentives for users leading to an emerging cooperative behavior. Section 4 describes the numerical results, and we draw the conclusions of our study in Sect. 5.

2   Model Description

Consider a district with N users, each i-th agent has n_i appliances that are schedulable, like washing machine (WM), dish washer (DW) and tumbler dryer (TD). Refrigerator load is also included as background profile. The state of the multi-agent system is given by $x = (x_1, \ldots, x_N)$, i.e., a vector of schedules that each user has to execute in a given time slot, and x_i is defined by the start times of all the n_i appliances of user i and their type (WM, DW, TD) with well-known load profiles. Due to energy and time constraints, the goal to find a global optimum of the constrained optimization problem, called *primal problem*:

$$\min_{x=(x_1,\ldots,x_N)} \sum_{i=1}^{N} f_i(x_i) \quad \text{s.t.} \quad \sum_{i=1}^{N} g_i(x_i) = a, \quad h_i(x_i) \leq b_i, i = 1, \ldots, N \quad (1)$$

where $a, b_i \in \mathbb{R}$ and the cost function $\sum_i f_i$ is a sum of weighted norms of three factors: overload, energy cost and tardiness of the current state x. The first constraint is the only coupling object: g_i denotes the peak profile of each user and the global load of the district must attain a given curve $a = a(t)$ depending on time. All the functions f_i, g_i, h_i implicitly depend on time (they span a day), discretized in minutes or hours. The inequalities involving h_i are local time and energy (usually 3 kW) constraints of each user. The Lagrange function is $\mathcal{L}(\boldsymbol{x}, \mu, \lambda_i) = \sum_{i=1}^{N} [f_i(x_i) + \lambda_i(b_i - h_i(x_i))] + \mu(g_i(x_i) - a)$ where $\lambda_i \geq 0, \mu$ are called *Lagrange multipliers*. Since λ_i can be computed locally, the Lagrange multiplier of our interest is μ, associated to the only coupling constraint. From now on, we neglect the local constraints as they can be included directly in the cost functions f_i. As detailed in [4], the corresponding relaxed *dual problem* becomes unconstrained: $\max_\mu \min_{\boldsymbol{x}=(x_1,\dots,x_N)} \mathcal{L}(\boldsymbol{x}, \mu)$. The standard algorithm is as follows: given an initial estimate of μ, each user computes its best ECS x_i^* such that $\boldsymbol{x}^* = \arg\min_{\boldsymbol{x}} \mathcal{L}(\boldsymbol{x}, \mu)$. Then, $\boldsymbol{x}^*$ is sent to the central unit, and a sub-gradient of $\min_{\boldsymbol{x}} \mathcal{L}(\boldsymbol{x}, \mu)$ as function of μ is available. The central unit computes and sends to agents at iteration k: $\mu^{(k)} = \mu^{(k-1)} + \alpha^{(k-1)} \left(\sum_i g_i(x_i^*) - a \right)$, where $\alpha^{(k-1)}$ is the step length of the gradient descent algorithm. Since the Lagrange multiplier μ can be interpreted as the energy price, in order to decentralize the given dual problem., we split $\mu = \sum_{i=1}^{N} \mu_i$. A distributed algorithm that can be applied acts as the previous one with the only difference: agent i solves the optimization problem

$$\min_{x_i} f_i(x_i) + \mu_i \left(N g_i(x_i) - a \right), \tag{2}$$

where $N g_i(x_i) - a$ approximates the global overload $\sum_j g_j(x_j) - a$. The only computational effort of the central unit is the gradient descent step for μ. The latter optimization problem is solved by means of the population-based metaheuristic method QPSOL, see [3], that reduces a NP-hard combinatorial optimization problem to an adaptive algorithm requiring limited computational power.

The underlying idea is to split the optimization algorithm on 2 time scales: (1) the micro-scale concerns the improvement along the day of the day-ahead proposed ECS; (2) the macro-scale involves the reputation-reward mechanisms of the agents, described below, and their collective behavior.

3   Swarm Simulator Description

This simulation studies energy distribution to a city district managing its total daily power consumption without power peaks and achieving a given aggregate load curve. Users should follow utility suggestions and receive incentives according to their flexibility. Every day users compute local best ECS in a distributed way, according to their needs and utility constraints, as described in Sect. 2. In this Section we focus on the reputation mechanism defining the emerging learning process. Consider best ECS as daily input data. Agents actions define local effective ECS. Two indices evaluate end-users behaviors: (1) reputation depending on start times of effective ECS, (2) reward depending on the distance between best and effective (both local and global) load.

Reputation Definition. Each agent may accept or decline n_i suggestions, with n_i number of appliances. Denote by x_i^* the best (sub)-optimal ECS found for Eq. 2 at the end of each day, and denote by $\hat{x}_i$ the effective ECS decided by user i. Formally, the reputation of user i along the day is $r_i = 1 - \frac{|x_i^* - \hat{x}_i|}{n_i} \in [0, 1]$, where $|\cdot|$ denotes the distance between the best and effective i-th ECS in terms of start times of appliances, i.e., reputation decreases as violation rate gets high.

Reward Definition. The reward is defined in terms of credits: each agent may earn up to 24 credits each day, comparing hourly the best (b) and effective (e) two quantities: global load and local load. Formally the credits of user i at hour h is defined as $c_{ih} = 1 - \frac{|\text{glob\_load}_b - \text{glob\_load}_e|}{\text{glob\_load}_b + \text{glob\_load}_e} - \frac{|\text{loc\_load}_b - \text{loc\_load}_e|}{\text{loc\_load}_b + \text{loc\_load}_e}$. At the end of each day, credits $c_i \in [0,1]$ are re-normalized and create rank lists.

Behavior and Learning Process Modeling. Each agent acts based on his own behavior profile, shaped according to (1) favorite start times to schedule appliances; (2) relevance given to reward and reputation by means of the weight parameter $\alpha_i \in [0,1]$, to define reaction to feedback; (3) natural predisposition to follow advice, to set the violation probability, defined by standard deviation σ_i of a Gaussian distribution. Best ECS for utility are denoted by the start times vector x_i^* and actions are samples from Gaussian distributions $\hat{x}_i \sim \mathcal{N}(x_i^*, \sigma_i^2)$ with mean given by x_i^* and standard deviation σ_i representing flexibility. Profiles are modeled according to σ_i that is initially sampled uniformly in a given interval $[\sigma_1, \sigma_2]$. For large σ_i agents tend to selfish behaviors and do not accept suggested ECS. Another learning parameter is the weight $\alpha_i \in [0,1]$ each agent gives to reward and reputation as feedback, i.e., after each observation period user i evaluates the linear combination of its mean reputation $\bar{r}_i$ and its mean reward $\bar{c}_i : q_i = \alpha_i \bar{r}_i + (1 - \alpha_i)\bar{c}_i$. Given the *satisfaction threshold* ϵ (in numerical experiments $\epsilon = 0.6$), if $q_i > \epsilon$, agent i is satisfied and there is a certain probability that relaxes decreasing its standard deviation σ_i, otherwise it increases according to a fixed discrete random distribution. In conclusion, behavior of agent i is defined by the Gaussian probability density function $f = f(x_i^*, \sigma_i, \alpha_i)$. At each feedback iteration the behavior parameter σ_i is updated. Houses with best and worse reputations and rewards are listed as another daily feedback, and emerging collective beahvior is described in Sect. 4.2.

4 Numerical Results

4.1 Micro-Scale Simulation

In this numerical experiments, using MATLAB software we run the simulator for small residential neighborhoods, i.e., $N = 5, N = 10$ agents and through QPSOL and Lagrangian relaxation described in Sect. 2, few iterations are sufficient to get a significant reduction of the global overload, as shown in Fig. 1. The output of such distributed algorithm are the daily suggested ECS, and the macro-scale simulator deals with the learning process acting on human decisions for ECS.

4.2 Macro-Scale Simulation

Software used for the development of macro-scale simulation is GAMA-platform [7], an agent-based, spatially explicit, modeling and simulation platform. Models

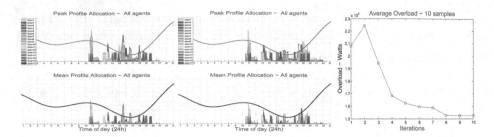

Fig. 1. In the left and center plot, the peak (upper plot) and mean (lower plot) power load (Watts) of a 5 agents neighborhood is displayed at the first and last iteration ($t = 10$) of the distributed algorithm proposed in Sect. 2. All agents are flexible during 10 am-9 pm. The right panel displays the average overload (over 10 samples), i.e., the distance between best and effective global load, as function of algorithm iterations.

are written in the GAML agent-oriented language, so that each house is considered to be an agent. We consider a district composed by $N = 100$ houses and a scheduled annual load for each resident about 1200–1400 kWh.

Appliances are distributed according to the following percentages: 99 % of houses have a WM, 70 % have a DW and 30 % have a TD. There are also some differences between user habits and families. These are modelled varying the maximum number of possible daily cycles for each appliance. In particular 40 % of residents will use every appliance no more than once a day, 50 % no more than twice and 10 % no more than three times a day. Some exceptions are considered.

The system evolution stabilizes in the presence of perturbative phenomena on the input parameters, i.e., differences between effective and best ECS. Using default value of parameters we can reach a mean percentage difference (over the best load) between the best total load and the effective total load converges to 20 % as in Fig. 2 (left).

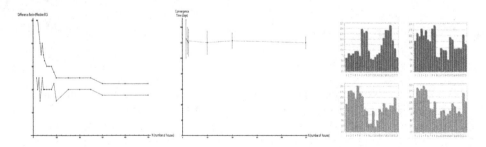

Fig. 2. The left plot shows the maximum (blue) and minimum (red) difference in percentage (converging to 20 %) between best and effective total load varying the number of houses. The central plot refers to necessary time to the district to reach a stable state (3–6 months) and a stable difference between the two loads, compared to the number of houses. Finally, the right chart is an example of total effective load (red) and total best load (green) when simulation starts (left) and at its stabilization (right) (Color figure online).

Varying the number of houses, the difference between effective and best load profile stabilizes starting from 100 houses in the district, as shown in Fig. 2 (center). Convergence time varies between 3 and 6 months. Reported values are the average over 10 simulations with the same number N of homes. Variance is greater if we consider few houses, while stabilization time increases with N.

5 Conclusions

In this paper we provide a mathematical model and a simulator of an energy distribution system applied to a residential district. Once end-users compute local optima in a distributed way, human decisions are modeled and a reputation-reward mechanism is performed on large numbers. Numerical results prove the efficiency of our algorithm: on the macroscale with few houses (150) the difference between best and effective ECS converges to 20 %, and with an average time of 3 months the district stabilizes. Future research may be devoted to apply Lagrangian Relaxation methods also to the macro time-scale, updating individual energy prices each day, as a function of the difference between best and effective ECS. Another advance is to develop asynchronous versions of the proposed algorithms adapting optimal ECS to asynchronous end-users decisions.

Acknowledgments. Authours would like to thank Ennio Grasso for the scientific hints on the mathematical modeling and numerical implementation.

References

1. Baharlouei, Z., Hashemi, M., Narimani, H., Mohsenian-Rad, H.: Achieving optimality and fairness in autonomous demand response: benchmarks and billing mechanisms. IEEE Trans. Smart Grid **4**(2), 968–975 (2013)
2. Borean, C., Ricci, A., Merlonghi, G.: Energyhome: a user-centric energy management system. Metering Int. **3**, 52 (2011)
3. Borean, C., Grasso, E.: QPSOL: quantum particle swarm optimization with levys flight. In: ICCGI 2014, Seville (2014)
4. Boyd, S., Vandenberghe, L.: Convex Optimization. Cambridge University Press, UK (2004)
5. Campos-Nanez, E., Garcia, A., Li, C.: A game-theoretic approach to efficient power management in sensor networks. Operat. Res. **56**(3), 552 (2008)
6. Caron, S., Kesidis, G.: Incentive-based energy consumption scheduling algorithms for the smart grid. In: Proceedings of the 1st IEEE International Conference on Smart Grid Communications (SmartGridComm), pp. 391–396 (2010)
7. GAMA-platform. https://code.google.com/p/gama-platform/
8. Hart, G.W.: Nonintrusive appliance load monitoring. Proc. IEEE **80**(12), 1870 (1992)
9. INTrEPID, FP7-ICT project. http://www.fp7-intrepid.eu/
10. Joo, J.-Y., Ilic, M.D.: Multi-layered optimization of demand resources using lagrange dual decomposition. IEEE Trans. Smart Grid. **4**(4), 2081–2088 (2013)

11. Krause, J., et al.: A survey of swarm algorithms applied to discrete optimization problems. In: Yang, X.-S., Cui, Z., Xiao, R., Gandomi, A.H., Karamanoglu, M. (eds.) Swarm Intelligence and Bio-Inspired Computation. Theory and Applications, pp. 169–191. Elsevier Science & Technology Books, UK (2013)
12. Liyan, J., Lang, T.: Day ahead dynamic pricing for demand response in dynamic environments. In: IEEE Conference on Decision and Control (CDC), pp. 5608–5613 (2013)
13. Pinyol, I., Sabater-Mir, J.: Computational trust and reputation models for open multi-agent systems: a review. Artif. Intell. Rev. **40**(1), 1–25 (2013)
14. Tuyls, K., Nowe, A.: Evolutionary game theory and multi-agent reinforcement learning. Knowl. Eng. Rev. **20**(01), 63–90 (2005)
15. Vinyals, M., et al.: Coalitional energy purchasing in the smart grid In: Proceedings of the IEEE International on Energy Conference and Exhibition, pp. 848–853 (2012)

Eliciting Affordances for Smart Objects in IoT Era

Assunta Matassa[1(✉)] and Rossana Simeoni[2]

[1] Department of Computer Science, University of Torino,
10149 Turin, Italy
matassa@di.unito.it
[2] Open Innovation Research, Telecom Italia,
10148 Turin, Italy
rossana.simeoni@telecomitalia.it

Abstract. In this paper we suggest a design research method for eliciting affordances and new meanings for Smart Objects in the Internet of Things Era. After an introduction to the topic and the description of some open issues, we propose to adopt a Critical Design approach, where the role of Ambiguity is twofold: on the one hand, it is the objective of the observation for defining a set of ambiguous objects or affordances; on the other hand, it is the result of a design conceptualization of smart objects aiming at provoking cognitive dissonance and finalized to understand people adaptation processes and behaviors.

Keywords: Human-Computer interaction · Critical design · Cognitive dissonance

1 Introduction: Object, Smart Object, IoT

Until recently, people have been used to considering physical objects as material to interact with for performing various tasks. The human capabilities for completing a task are enabled by the object's properties. We refer to these properties as 'natural elements' existing in objects and which help people to interact with the objects themselves. Moreover, these natural elements define a shared knowledge that people gain while interacting with the objects without activating of expensive learning processes.

In the last decades a new paradigm has been introduced in the conceptualization of physical objects [1]. The growth of embedded technology [2] in everyday objects [3], and their organization in a nexus of elements, is introducing a new meaning for objects and it is a suggesting new ways of interaction with them. Internet of Things (IoT) is the concept under which we collocate these new nexus of physical objects and interactions.

The IoT [4] allows going beyond what people foresee and it opens a new opportunities in exploiting objects' properties. In this perspective, the evolution is going in the direction of changing the shape and the appearance of objects augmenting their natural function with something new. Furthermore, the existing affordances in connected and technologically augmented objects are becoming unable to immediately communicate to people their actual values and meanings.

© Institute for Computer Sciences, Social Informatics and Telecommunications Engineering 2015
R. Giaffreda et al. (Eds.): IoT360 2014, Part I, LNICST 150, pp. 77–81, 2015.
DOI: 10.1007/978-3-319-19656-5_12

This new type of object is called Smart Object. The capabilities of a Smart Object go beyond what its aspect shows and what people can image, combining knowledge and insights derived from the original physical object.

The impossibility of establishing a clear connection between objects and functionalities could become a threat for humans, since they are missing their innate ability to understand what they can do only based on their knowledge and perception of the surrounding context. As an extreme consequence, with the spreading of the IoT and smart objects people could loose the ability to use everyday objects to accomplish their tasks. How can we solve this extreme situation?

2 Theoretical Background

The concept of physical affordance appears for the first time in Gibson's research [5], where he defines an affordance as a clear coupling between the meaning of an object and the actions that it allows. Norman [6] simplifies the term introducing the idea that affordance is a property that suggests what users can do with the object. Stimulating people's actions, the affordance suggests the correct way to interact with an object, inviting people to do something. Norman also introduces the existence of a combination between what an object suggests, what people perceive to be able to do and what really happens. In a successful case, there is a total combination between these aspects, in a negative case, instead, he describes the existence of gaps ("gulfs") between what people are thinking to do and what they are actually doing.

3 Cognitive Dissonance in Iot Era

The distance [7] between physical affordance - object properties suggesting interaction- and cognitive affordance - the way people perceive how they could interact with an object - can be formalized using the psychological definition of cognitive dissonance. The lack of a clear coupling of physical and cognitive affordances makes the situation confused and weak. The perceived inconsistency between knowledge, feelings and behavior establishes an inner state of discomfort - cognitive dissonance - that people try to reduce [8]. If this inconvenience is very common, it becomes more than common in IoT and Smart objects. People are continuously stressed by a new and unexpected use of components of surrounding environment that they are disabling to have a deeper comprehension of it.

The dissonance is perceived as psychologically uncomfortable, thereby people are stimulated to reduce or delete it, thus it are stimulated to reduce or delete it changing their behaviors and their beliefs about context and their components.

This theory is based on the recognition of the existence of knowledge [9] on which people build their behavior, and, more generally, build themselves. If something damages this balance, people immediately perceive a tension, a cognitive dissonance, and they try to react to it.

In a world of IoT and Ubiquitous computing, when "technologists" build smart objects, technologists tried to adopt the natural affordances present in objects to allow people to understand the way in with get in contact and use them [1, 2]. However, when we, as "designer", are thinking about an object provided with more powerful capabilities and functions, we are thinking about something that could go beyond the usual way of interaction. Anyway, Smart objects make hard the people understanding of the real values and meanings of objects through their affordances. What we are observing is the growth up of dissonance perceptions. The emergence of discordance between meanings and coupling [10] appears almost evident.

4   A Critical Design and Smart Objects

Starting with cognitive dissonance as an issue, we suggest to use it as a positive resource for designing smart objects with suitable affordances. With this aim, we propose to introduce cognitive dissonance as part of a methodological approach exploiting Critical Design. Dunne and Raby propose Critical design as a new form of research [11] aimed at provoking critical attention from users about how the design of objects, their shape and their representations influence values, ideologies and their behavior. Supporting Dunne and Raby's research idea about design [11], we adopt this innovative approach to provoke people's reaction and to stimulate their 'critical sensibility' in analyzing their relation with the surrounding environment. In fact, stimulating the development of critical attitudes in users, we are able to study the outcomes for defining critical and innovative insights about future concepts. Stressing cognitive dissonance we would like to introduce ambiguity in Smart Objects and then provoke reaction in users for studying them [8].

5   Eliciting Affordances for Smart Objects

We intend to exploit the lack of clear principles for eliciting affordances or new meanings in smart objects by suggesting a design research method, on top of the critical design approach, where the role of ambiguity is twofold: on the one hand it is the objective of the observation to define a set of "ambiguous" objects or "affordance"; on the other hand it is the result of a design conceptualization of smart objects aiming at provoking "cognitive dissonance" and finalized to understand "adaptation" processes and behavior [9].

Critical Design approach is receiving much attention in the Human Computer Interaction and Design research and its adoption is controversial and many ongoing discussions [12] focus on how to define a critical design theory suitable for HCI research and practice. Within this new trend we intend to propose a design research method capable of "informing", gathering information, useful in the conceptualization of Smart Objects.

For assessing our research method we are setting up a two steps experiment:

(a)   First, we define a set of everyday objects (i.e. a pencil) and then observe in which way people interact with them, how they adopt affordances and how they apply different interpretation while getting in touch with them. The observation is carried on as ethnography [13] a sociological method, for understanding the objects in the "context of use" and highlighting the existing interrelationships between users and objects, and users and users with objects.

(b) Second, we introduce "in the wild" a set of smart objects (i.e. a smart pencil), strictly related to the objects of the previous step, containing ambiguity in meaning and affordances and then observe the 'adaptive behavior' that people adopt as natural consequences of a state of cognitive dissonance [14].

This study will benefit from previous work concerning the embodiment of the interaction into smart objects [15–17] and critical design experiments [18].

References

1. Weiser, M.: The computer for the 21st century. Sci. Am. **265**(3), 94–104 (1991)
2. Weiser, M., Gold, R., Brown, J.S.: The origins of ubiquitous computing research at PARC in the late 1980s. IBM syst. J. **38**(4), 693–696 (1999)
3. Bleecker, J.: A manifesto for networked objects—cohabiting with pigeons, arphids and aibos in the Internet of things (2006)
4. McEwen, A., Cassimally, H.: Designing the Internet of Things. Wiley, Chichester (2013)
5. Gibson, J.J.: The Ecological Approach to Visual Perception. Psychology Press, New York (2013)
6. Norman, D.: The Design of Everyday Things. Doubleday, New York (1988)
7. Norman, D.: Affordances. Conv. Des. Interact. **6**(3), 38–42 (1999)
8. Gaver, W., Beaver, J., Benford, S.: Ambiguity as a resource for design. In: Proceedings of the SIGCHI Conference on Human Factors in Computing Systems, p. 233. ACM, New York, NY, USA (2003)
9. Oshikawa, S.: The theory of cognitive dissonance and experimental research. J. Mark. Res. **5**(4), 429–430 (1968)
10. Dourish, P.: Where the action is: the foundations of embodied interaction. MIT press, Cambridge (2004)
11. Dunne, A., Raby, F.: Critical Design FAQ (2007). Accessed on 1 September 2012
12. Bardzell, J., Bardzell, S., Stolterman, E.: Reading critical designs: supporting reasoned interpretations of critical design. In: Proceedings of the 32nd ACM Conference on Human Factors in Computing Systems, pp. 1951–1960, April 2014
13. Blomberg, J., Giacomi, J., Mosher, A., Swenton-Wall, P.: Ethnographic field methods and their relation to design. In: Dchuler, D., Namioka, A. (eds.) Participatory Design: Principles and Practices. Erlbaum, New Jersey (1993)
14. Draycott, S., Dabbs, A.: Cognitive dissonance 1: an overview of the literature and its integration into theory and practice in clinical psychology. Br. J. Clin. Psychol. **37**(3), 341–353 (1998)
15. Nowacka, D., Kirk, D.: Tangible autonomous interfaces (tais): exploring autonomous behaviors in this. In: Proceedings of the 8th International Conference on Tangible, Embedded and Embodied Interaction, pp. 1–8. ACM (2014)
16. Zimmermann, S., Rümelin, S., Butz, A.: I feel it in my fingers: haptic guidance on touch surfaces. In: Proceedings of the 8th International Conference on Tangible, Embedded and Embodied Interaction, pp. 9–12. ACM (2014)

17. Gross, S., Bardzell, J., Bardzell, S.: Skeu the evolution: skeuomorphs, style, and the material of tangible interactions. In: Proceedings of the 8th International Conference on Tangible, Embedded and Embodied Interaction, pp. 53–60. ACM (2014)
18. Bowen, S., Petrelli, D.: Remembering today tomorrow: exploring the human-centered design of digital mementos. Int. J. Hum. Comput. Stud. **69**(5), 324–337 (2011)

The Role of Affordance in Cyber-Physical Systems for Behavioral Change

Federica Cena[1(✉)], Amon Rapp[1], Alessandro Marcengo[2],
Adelina Brizio[3], Dize Hilviu[3], and Maurizio Tirassa[3]

[1] Department of Computer Science, University of Torino, Turin, Italy
{cena, rapp}@di.unito.it
[2] Telecom Italia - Research and Prototyping, Turin, Italy
alessandro.marcengo@telecomitalia.it
[3] Department of Psychology and Center for Cognitive Science,
University of Torino, Turin, Italy
adelina.brizio@yahoo.it,
dize.hilviu@gmail.com,
maurizio.tirassa@unito.it

Abstract. Cyber-Physical Systems are the next generation of embedded ICT systems, interconnected through the Internet of Things and endowed with data gathering functions and able to provide some output to users. Thanks to their features, if opportunely designed, they can affect user behavior on two levels: by means of the data gathered, promoting self-awareness to motivate change in the long term, and by means of direct physical cues, inviting users to perform some action in real time. The concept of affordance becomes crucial to the latter aspect: it is necessary to design novel, intuitive object affordances that foster a particular behavior.

Keywords: Cyber-Physical systems · Internet of things · Affordance · Behavioral change

1 Introduction

Cyber-Physical Systems (CPS) are the next generation of embedded ICT systems, interconnected through the Internet of Things and endowed with data gathering and communication functions. These systems are not technological devices as PC or smartphone, but everyday objects ad hoc enhanced with some reasoning capabilities. Due to their integration in the user environment and/or in the user body, they can track a variety of user data: physiological states (such as blood glucose level), psychological states (such as mood), behaviors (such as movements), and habits (such as food, sleep); but also environmental parameters (such as CO_2) and contextual information (such as places). All these data, related to different aspects of people daily lives, can provide the user with a "mirror" of herself, a complex representation of interests, habits, activities, etc. in her life [1]. This can support new forms of **self**-*awareness* and *self-knowledge*, which can foster behavior change, promoting more sustainable or healthier behaviors, discouraging bad habits, sustaining therapeutic compliance, managing chronic diseases

R. Giaffreda et al. (Eds.): IoT360 2014, Part I, LNICST 150, pp. 82–86, 2015.
DOI: 10.1007/978-3-319-19656-5_13

[2, 3]. Self-monitoring is an effective strategy to increase a person's awareness of a targeted behavior and its level of achievement [4]. Cadmus Bertram et al. [5] have proved the efficacy of electronic self-monitoring in adopting healthier life styles.

Thus, CPSs have the potentiality to promote some degree of change in users' behaviors, and several CPSs have been developed in order to try to modify a behavior by means of self-monitoring, such as [6, 7]. This may happen at two levels:

- an immediate behavioral activation by means of cues from the object, i.e., physical output such as light, vibrations, heat, etc., which may invite the user to reflect on her current situation, thus possibly triggering a corrective action. For example, a vibration can notify the user about a wrong sitting posture;
- a long-term behavioral change, by affecting the user self-awareness via the data gathered. For example, having data about my food practice might make me aware of my bad habits and thus motivate me to change them.

As regards the former level, *affordances* [8] can play a crucial role. According to Gibson, objects naturally offer a set of functionalities to the external world: the nature of the activities that they afford depends on how a specific individual or type of individuals (like all the members of a species, or those that belong 'to a certain sub-group, characterized e.g. by a certain culture) can conceive of the interaction with them. Affordances thus are at the interface between the individual(s) and the world. In the case of CPSs, how to design the affordances that they offer in such a way that users may be motivated change some of their behaviors, leveraging the potentialities of the CPSs, is still an open issue in the literature. In this paper we aim at (i) presenting a complex CPS capable of promoting behavior change at the two levels mentioned above, (ii) pointing out reflections for the design of affordances in CPSs.

2   A CPS for Impacting User Behavior

To design a CPS that may promote some kind of behavioral change we need three elements:

- a smart object integrated in the everyday life of people, able to gather user data in a transparent way, and to provide some intuitive feedback to users
- a complex data structure that integrates the gathered data
- a reasoning engine able to correlate different data and to provide meaningful data visualizations and complex recommendations.

In the following, we will present a use case for showing how a CPS with the above features may promote a particular behavior, in particular *decrease sedentary habits*. A sedentary lifestyle is one of the most devious features of life in affluent societies since it causes a relapse of disease of varying severity in the population with high costs for health care services. Despite the many attempts to overcome this problem, with or without the use of ICT ad hoc solutions, sedentary habits still are a major issue in contemporary society [9]. To tackle this problem, we want to design a novel CPS exploiting e-textile, i.e., materials that enable digital components and electronics to be embedded in fabrics (e.g., clothes, covers, ...), which represents the new frontier for integrating CPS in everyday life. E-textile allows to continuously and transparently gather a wealth of user behavioral data, not only about user's movements, but also about the physical environments by means of sensors embedded in the fabrics. The CPS should also have a knowledge structure to integrate these data, and advanced forms of reasoning about them so to correlate different aspects of the user's behavior from day to day (for example, to correlate mood with physical activities). To foster the behavior, CPS should provide two types of feedback: (i) on the physical level, simple feedback from the object as affordance to do a specific action: this might be a vibration or a change in the color of the object aimed at inviting the user to stand up; (ii) on the virtual level, more complex feedbacks for triggering long-term behavior change: such as recommendations and data visualization.

An open issue in this scenario is the role of affordance, as discussed in the next section.

3 Affordances in CPSs

Digital interactive systems rely on dematerialized affordances like icons, pointers, textual messages, etc., often based on metaphors from everyday activities like sitting at a desktop, watching through a window, etc. Affordances offered by CPSs, on the other hand, actually do belong to the physical world of everyday life. This opens a variety of new possibilities and issues in the design of interactive systems.

Alan Cooper in an affordance sees a stronger correlation between user and action [10]. In his view, affordances may be designed to provide users with information about the actions or activities that can or should be performed on, or with, the artifact. Everyday objects can now be endowed with computational capabilities enhancing not only their "reasoning" skills, but also their "communication" skills, their ability to invite users to perform certain actions in specific ways. The question then is how designers can integrate the physical affordances of everyday objects with some kind of new affordances that can communicate more information to the user. Can these additional information invite users to act towards specific directions, so to improve their lifestyles and wellbeing?

Part of the problem is that an individual's activities and the actions that she performs within them, and therefore her preparedness and will to perceive and act upon a specific (type of) affordance, are in turn circularly interwoven with her cultural background and her narrative situation, so that each term of these dynamics mutually defines and shapes the others [11–13]. That an artifacts like a CPS is designed from scratch is both its strength (because of the freedom that is thus granted to both the designer and the user) and its weakness (because there may exist only a thin layer of already established habits relevant to it).

One way to imagine how these novel kinds of affordances could be integrated in physical objects is provided by the notion of *phatic cue*. This may be envisaged as an affordance that communicates continuously a state and its change in time to the user. It leaves the communication channel open, establishing a continuous "phatic communication" [14] between the user and the object. Such affordance would not use "atomic messages", such as texts, to urge users to perform specific behaviors. Instead, they would use physical communication channels, such as lights, sounds, vibrations, heat, to constantly be in touch with the user. Leaving this communication channel always open can leverage the object physical features, e.g. varying its color, temperature, sound emission, to communicate a variation of its internal status or a change in the user's state.

In the use case presented, an *e-textile* can use modulations of colors or temperature of its surface to constantly keep in touch with the user. In this way, it can suggest a certain behaviors or change of behaviors to the user not through imperative linguistic messages, but via evocative, indirect and continuous affordances. For example, the e-textile in the form of a cover or a pillow, placed on the user's chair, might change its colors to communicate how much the user has been sedentary that day.

Designers and researchers should investigate how to leverage the physical characteristics of everyday objects to create these new kinds of affordances, to give life to new CPSs that, fully integrated in the user's everyday context, are constantly in touch with her.

References

1. Marcengo, A., Buriano, L., Geymonat, M.: Specch.io: a personal QS mirror for life patterns discovery and "Self" reshaping. In: Stephanidis, C., Antona, M. (eds.) UAHCI 2014, Part IV. LNCS, vol. 8516, pp. 215–226. Springer, Heidelberg (2014)
2. Bandura, A.: Social cognitive theory of self-regulation. Organ. Behav. Hum. Decis. Process. **50**, 248–287 (1991)
3. Nakajima, T., Lehdonvirta, V., Tokunaga, E., Kimura, H.: Reflecting human behavior to motivate desirable lifestyle. In: Conference of Designing Interactive Systems, pp. 405–414 (2008)
4. Burke, L.E., Wang, J., Sevick, M.A.: Self-monitoring in weight loss: a systematic review of the literature. J. Am. Diet. Assoc. **111**(1), 92–102 (2011)
5. Cadmus Bertram, L., Wang, J.B., Patterson, R.E., Newman, V.A., Parker, B.A., Pierce, J.P.: Web-based self monitoring for weight loss among overweight/obese women at increased risk for breast cancer: the HELP pilot study. PsychoOncology **22**(8), 1821–1828 (2013)
6. Froehlich, J., Dillahunt, T., Klasnja, P., Mankoff, J., Consolvo, S., Harrison, B., Landay, J.: UbiGreen: investigating a mobile tool for tracking and supporting green transportation habits. In: Proceedings of the SIGCHI Conference on Human Factors in Computing Systems, pp. 1043–1052. ACM, New York, USA (2009)
7. Kay, M., Choe, E.K., Shepherd, J., Greenstein, B., Watson, N., Consolvo, S., Kientz, J.A.: Lullaby: a capture & access system for understanding the sleep environment. In: 2012 ACM Conference on Ubiquitous Computing, pp. 226–234. ACM, New York, USA (2012)
8. Gibson, J.: The theory of affordances. In: Shaw, R.E., Bransford, J. (eds.) Perceiving, Acting, and Knowing: Toward an Ecological Psychology, pp. 67–82. Lawrence Erlbaum Associates Inc, Hillsdale (1977)
9. Cipriani, F., Baldasseroni, A., Franks, S.: Combating a sedentary lifestyle and physical activity promotion. Line – Help. SNLG (2011)
10. Cooper, A.: About Face: The Essentials of User Interface Design. Hungry Minds Inc, New York (1995)

11. Carassa, A., Morganti, F., Tirassa, M.: Movement, action, and situation: presence in virtual environments. In: Raya, M.A., Solaz, B.R. (eds.) Proceedings of the 7th Annual International Workshop on Presence (Presence 2004 – Valencia, Spain, 13–15 October 2004), pp. 7–12 (2004)
12. Carassa, A., Morganti, F., Tirassa, M.: A situated cognition perspective on presence. In: Bara, B.G., Barsalou, L., Bucciarelli, M. (eds.) Proceedings of the 27th Annual Conference of the Cognitive Science Society (Stresa, Italy, 21–23 July 2005), pp. 384–389 (2005)
13. Tirassa, M., Bosco, F.M.: On the nature and role of intersubjectivity in human communication. Emerg. Commun. Stud. New Technol. Pract. Commun. **10**, 81–95 (2008)
14. Jakobson, R.: Saggi di linguistica generale. Feltrinelli, Milano (1996)

Cognitive Load Detection on Commercial EEG Devices: An Optimized Signal Processing Chain

Arijit Sinharay, Debatri Chatterjee[(✉)], and Arpan Pal

TCS Innovation Lab, Kolkata, India
{arijit.sinharay,debatri.chatterjee,
arpan.pal}@tcs.com

Abstract. Use of Electroencephalography (EEG) to detect cognitive load is a well-practiced technique. Cognitive load reflects the mental load imparted on a person providing a crucial parameter for applications like personalized education and usability testing. There are several approaches to process the EEG signals and thus choosing an optimal signal processing chain is not a straight forward job. The scenario becomes even more interesting while using commercial low-cost, low resolution EEG devices connected to cloud through Internet of Things (IoT) platform. This paper proposes an optimized signal processing chain offering maximum classification accuracy and minimum computational complexity for measuring the cognitive load using low resolution EEG devices.

Keywords: Cognitive load · Mental workload · EEG signal processing · Emotiv

1 Introduction

Mental workload imposed on a person is an important component for human behavior modeling as it gives a direct representation of mental state of the person [1]. Cognitive load (CL) is the total amount of mental activity imposed on our working memory while doing any cognitive process. High CL can significantly influence the performance, leading to poor outcome, stress, or anxiety [1]. This CL information if made available on IoT platform in real-time [2, 3], can be utilized for different applications like personalized education [4], usability testing [5] etc. as depicted in Fig. 1.

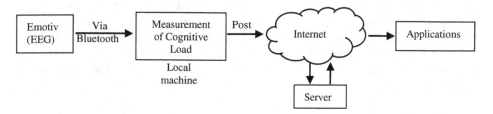

Fig. 1. Mental workload estimation and modeling through IoT

© Institute for Computer Sciences, Social Informatics and Telecommunications Engineering 2015
R. Giaffreda et al. (Eds.): IoT360 2014, Part I, LNICST 150, pp. 87–92, 2015.
DOI: 10.1007/978-3-319-19656-5_14

Thus measuring CL while doing any task has been of increasing interest. Subjective measures of CL, including self-reporting like NASA-TLX [6], measurement of error rates etc., are mostly self-biased compared to *object-indirect* (e.g. physiological, behavioral measurements) and *objective-direct* (e.g. brain activity measurement, dual task performance analysis) measurement methods. Physiological measures like brain signals, Galvanic Skin Response, functional Magnetic Resonance Imaging etc. can be used to access CL [7]. We have used electroencephalogram (EEG) technique as it is relatively in-expensive, non-invasive and have excellent temporal resolution. The frontal and central brain are mostly indicative of CL for tasks like problem solving, decision making, and language skills etc. [8, 9]. Different preprocessing steps, features and classifiers can be used for EEG signal analysis. Time-domain [10], frequency-domain [11], and statistical parameters have been used to access the CL. Here we tried detecting CL with commercially available low cost and low resolution Emotiv[1] EEG device. Hence, appropriate signal processing, machine learning steps are needed to get desired information.

The main contribution of this paper lies in proposing an optimal signal processing chain via comparative study among various existing algorithmic approaches using low-resolution devices like Emotiv. EEG signals are very susceptible to artifacts like eye-blinks, facial muscle movements etc., hence we used Hilbert-Huang Transform (HHT) [13] for required correction. The accuracy of classification can be increased by using a spatial filter [14]. We have used advanced Tikhonov-Regularized Common Spatial Pattern (TRCSP) [15]. Results show that it is possible to get good classification accuracy with Emotiv if processing steps are chosen properly.

The paper is organized as follows: Sect. 2 details the experiments and the data collection methods, followed by signal processing steps in Sect. 3. Section 4 presents the results with discussions. Finally, the paper is concluded in Sect. 5.

2 Experiments and Data Collection

For the present study we designed two types of reading tasks similar to [12] with slight modifications, pertaining low and high CL. For *low load* condition, subjects were asked to mentally count the number of two letter words (except 'of') while reading an English passage and report the number at the end. For *high load* condition, subjects were instructed to count two-letter words as well as three-letter words separately (except 'of' and 'the').

A group of 10 participants (aged between 25–30 years) were selected. All of them were right-handed male and had English as second language. These ensures minimum variance in the level of expertise and brain lateralization across all the subjects.

The stimulus were presented on a 9.7-in. iPad. Participant were given two sets of stimulus to work with (i.e. 2 high-load tasks and 2 low-load tasks). The EEG data corresponding to first set of stimulus were used as the training data and the second set were used as the test data and vice versa. An average of these two observations were used as the final result.

---

[1] www.emotiv.com.

3   EEG Signal Processing

Different algorithmic approaches tried are shown in Fig. 2 and the details are given in Table 1. The numbers provided in the construction of various *paths* in Table 1 are referred to signal processing blocks shown in Fig. 2. We used a feature vector comprising of variance, Hjorth parameters [10], alpha (δ), beta (β), theta (θ), delta (δ), gamma (γ) band powers and ratios of band powers $\beta/_\theta$ and $\alpha/_\delta$.

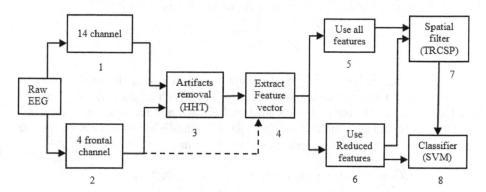

Fig. 2. Different approaches adopted for analyzing EEG signals

Table 1. Details of different Algorithm chains adopted

Motivation	Algorithm chain	Approach used
Choice of brain lobe to be probed :- to examine if a subset of all channels can be used with compromising on accuracy	*Path1:* 1→3→4→5→7→8	i) Probing all the brain lobes(using all 14 channels) ii) Using full feature vector set iii) Using TRCSP on feature vector set iv) SVM for final classification
	Path2: 2→3→4→5→7→8	i) Probing only left-frontal brain(AF3, F7, F3, FC5) [16] ii) Using full feature set on above channels iii) Using TRCSP on feature vector set iv) SVM for final classification
Choice of features to be used :- to examine if a reduced feature set can lead to same accuracy	*Path3:* 1→3→4→6→7→8	i) Probing all the brain lobes ii) Using only alpha and theta band power [16] iii) This reduced feature set fed to TRCSP iv) SVM for final classification
	Path4: 2→3→4→6→7→8	i) Probing only left-frontal brain ii) Using only alpha and theta band power [16] iii)This reduced feature set fed to TRCSP iv) SVM for final classification
Use of spatial filters:- to examine the need of CSP as Emotiv does not have neighboring electrode in true sense	*Path 5:* 1→3→4→6→8	i) Probing all the brain lobes ii) Using only alpha and theta band power iii) Reduced feature set to SVM [12]
	Path 6: 2→3→4→6→8	i) Probing only left-frontal brain ii) Using only alpha and theta band power iii) Reduced feature set to SVM
*Effect of HHT:-*Eye-blink lies in (0.4-4 Hz) & features in (4-12 Hz). So, tried to examine usefulness of artifacts removal	Preferred path with HHT	i) Selected preferred path from *Path1* through *Path6*
	Preferred path without HHT	ii) Selected same path but without using HHT

3.1 Comparison of Algorithms

Algorithms were compared based on: (i) the cognitive score (CS) obtained while classifying the EEG signals following a particular signal processing path, and (ii) the computational complexity (CC) of that particular algorithm.

CS is defined in (1). Features (reduced feature/output of TRCSP) extracted from training data were used to train SVM. Same features were calculated from test data also and fed to SVM. The analysis was done in a non-overlapping window (5 s) basis. Finally, the over-all cognitive score for a particular trial is given by

$$CS = \frac{\sum m_i \times w_i}{n} \tag{1}$$

where, m_i is the number of windows reported as class i, n is the total number of windows in a test trial and w_i is a weight-factor. For high load class $w_i = 100$ and for low load class $w_i = 0$. Hence for low load trial $CS \approx 0$ and for high trial $CS \approx 100$.

The computational complexity (CC) of an algorithm is the number of processing steps required for a particular input. In our work we have defined CC as

$$CC = n_c \times (L + C_{HHT}) + n_c \times (m_f \times F) + (n_c \times m_f) \times C_{CSP} \tag{2}$$

where, n_c is the number of channels selected, L is the computational complexity for a single channels, C_{HHT} is the computational complexity of HHT filter, m_f is the number of features selected, F is the complexity for extracting a particular feature, C_{CSP} is the computational complexity of using TRCSP filter. Thus (1) and (2) gives a measure of cognitive score and computational complexity for a particular algorithm.

4 Results and Discussions

Table 2 shows the cognitive score of low (L) and high (H) cognitive tasks following *Path1* through *Path6*. Maximum separation between H and L have been marked in 'blue'. The entries for $CS_{High} < CS_{Low}$, have been marked in red. We observed this reverse trend for 3 subjects while following *Path4* and for 1 subject while following *Path1*. Both *Path1* and *Path4* used TRCSP algorithm. Further investigation is needed to conclude whether TRCSP leads to this effect for low resolution EEG device. Figure 3a gives one-way ANOVA analysis of the results given in Table 2. Plot shows *Path6* gives highest difference between mean CS_{High} and CS_{Low} while having minimal intra-class variance. *Path1* gives maximum separation between CS_{High} and CS_{Low} for 6 subjects compared to *Path6* which gives maximum separation between for 1 subject. However, the ANOVA results indicate that the *Path6* is the preferred path as opposed to *Path1*, as the variance for CS_{High} is maximum for the same, which is undesirable.

Thus, we see *Path6* as the best possible approach in terms of classification accuracy while using Emotiv. *Path6* is also the path of least complexity as it: (i) uses only 4 channels instead of 14 channels, (ii) uses reduced feature set – using only these two features saves computational time for feature extraction and (iii) bypasses TRCSP.

Table 2. Comparison of different algorithms in terms of cognitive score

Sub	Path 1		Path 2		Path 3		Path 4		Path 5		Path 6	
	CS (H)	CS (L)	CS (H)	CS (L)	CS (H)	CS (L)	CS (H)	CS (L)	CS (H)	CS (L)	CS (H)	CS (L)
1	79.8	8.7	100	75	58.3	54.2	29	43	56	50	100	4
2	97.4	15.2	89.7	20.4	82.1	23.5	74.3	10.2	85.2	15.2	84.6	18.9
3	12	8.8	34.2	17.6	82.2	76.1	79	73	58	44	61	50
4	84	21	96.3	71.4	81.1	80.2	64.2	50	89	83	89	71
5	100	44	98	51.7	74.5	51.4	65	78	86	55	74	51
6	71.4	29	89.8	70.3	81.6	66.6	83	62	97	48	89	40
7	33.3	52	77.7	23.5	50	29.4	80.5	76.4	86	58	75	58
8	100	23.3	98.4	25.3	80.4	13.6	84	25.2	86	26.5	96	30.2
9	28.5	20.1	54.2	50.1	57.5	42.3	17.5	41.1	35.2	32.1	40.2	26.8
10	67.3	24.6	82.3	45s	71.9	48.5	64.1	50.9	75.4	45.7	78.5	38.8

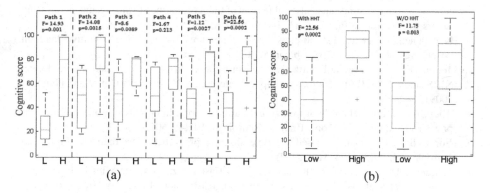

Fig. 3. (a) Boxplot of different algorithms: *Path6* is the chosen path as it offers maximum F-value and minimum p-value, (b) Effect of artifacts removal: maximum F-value is obtained while using HHT filters .

Next we investigated usefulness of HHT filters. Figure 3b shows the CS for both tasks with or without HHT. The separation between average CS for H and L is greater and variance for H and L is lowest for artifact removed signals using HHT.

5   Conclusion

In this paper, we proposed the optimal signal processing chain specifically suitable for low-resolution EEG devices like Emotiv. We have introduced a performance score for evaluating different algorithms to choose the optimal signal processing chain for similar low cost devices. The results show that, using Emotiv or similar low-cost low reso-lution devices, it is possible to measure the CL by probing left frontal brain lobe for a combined text reading and counting memory task. It also shows that the alpha and theta band powers, directly fed to SVM, are sufficient to capture the imparted CL. The proposed optimum signal processing chain also requires least computational resources thereby making it suitable for cognitive load related IoT applications.

References

1. Chen, F., Ruiz, N., Choi, E., Epps, J., Khawaja, M.A., Taib, R., Wang, Y.: Multimodal behavior and interaction as indicators of cognitive load. ACM Trans. Interact. Intell. Syst. (TiiS) **2**(4), 22 (2012)
2. Gubbi, J., et al.: Internet of Things (IoT): a vision, architectural elements, and future directions. Future Gener. Comput. Syst. **29**(7), 1645–1660 (2013)
3. Misra, P., et al.: A computing platform for development and deployment of sensor data based applications and services, Patent No. WO2013072925 A2
4. Fok, A.W., Ip, H.H.-S.: Personalized education: an exploratory study of learning pedagogies in relation to personalization technologies. In: Liu, W., Shi, Y., Li, Q. (eds.) ICWL 2004. LNCS, vol. 3143, pp. 407–415. Springer, Heidelberg (2004)
5. Pal, A., Chatterjee, D., kar, D.: Evaluation and Improvements of on-screen keyboard for Television and Set-top Box, ISCE, Singapore, 14–17 June 2011
6. Hitt, J.M., Kring, J.P., Daskarolise, E., Morris, C., Mouloua, M.: Assessing mental workload with subjective measures: an analytical review of the nasa-tlx index since its inception. Hum. Factors Ergon. Soc. Ann. Meet. **43**, 1404 (1999)
7. Haapalainen, E., et al.: Psycho-physiological measures for assessing cognitive load. In: Proceedings of the 12th ACM Ubicomp (2010)
8. Molteni, E., et al.: Frontal brain activation during a working memory task: a time-domain fNIRS study. SPIE BiOS: Biomedical Optics. International Society for Optics and Photonics (2009)
9. Brody, B.A., et al.: The role of frontal and parietal cortex in cognitive processing: tests of spatial and sequence functions. Brain J. Neurology **101**(4), 607–633 (1978)
10. Hjorth, B.: EEG analysis based on time domain properties. Electroencephalogr. Clin. Neurophysiol. **29**(3), 306–310 (1970)
11. Chatterjee, D., Sinharay, A., Konar, A.: EEG-Based fuzzy cognitive load classification during logical analysis of program segments. In: IEEE International Conference on Fuzzy Systems (FUZZ-IEEE), 7–10 July 2013
12. Zarjam, P., Epps, J., Chen, F.: Evaluation of working memory load using EEG signals In: Proceedings of APSIPA Annual Summit and Conference, pp. 715–719 (2010)
13. Wang, Y.L., Liu, J.H., Liu, Y.C.: Automatic removal of ocular artifacts from electroencephalogram using Hilbert-Huang transform. In: The 2nd International Conference on Bioinformatics and Biomedical Engineering, 2008. ICBBE 2008, pp. 2138–2141 (2008)
14. Wojcikiewicz, W., Vidaurre, C., Kawanabe, M.: Stationary common spatial patterns: towards robust classification of non-stationary eeg signals, In: 2011 IEEE International Conference on Acoustics, Speech and Signal Processing (ICASSP), pp. 577–580.(2011)
15. Lotte, F., Guan, C.: Regularizing common spatial patterns to improve BCI designs: unified theory and new algorithms. IEEE Trans. Biomed. Eng. **58**(2), 355–362 (2011)
16. Sauseng, P., Klimesch, W., Schabus, M., Doppelmayr, M.: Fronto-parietal EEG coherence in theta and upper alpha reflect central executive functions of working memory. Int. J. Psychophysiol. **57**(2), 97–103 (2005)

From Language to Action: Extraction and Disambiguation of Affordances in ModelAct

Irene Russo[1]([✉]) and Livio Robaldo[2]

[1] ILC CNR Pisa, Pisa, Italy
irene.russo@ilc.cnr.it
[2] Dipartimento di Informatica, Universita' di Torino, Torino, Italy
robaldo@di.unito.it

Abstract. In this paper we focus on how information about concrete actions performed on food should be provided to IoT devices in terms of affordances extracted from corpora. Natural language processing has a role in defining which kind of knowledge devices interacting with machines and appliances should handle when humans send requests through natural language interfaces.

We propose a model for the extraction of affordances of food from corpora and their role in sequences of procedural (sub)actions. The food processor of the future can find helpful this knowledge to interact with users suggesting alternatives in food processing in recipes steps and basic reasoning about preconditions and consequences in making meals.

Keywords: Affordances · Natural language processing · Verbs' disambiguation

1 One Verb, More Action Types

The way human beings talk about basic and concrete actions can conceal the evidence that a verb like *to open* refers to different procedural sequences of sub-actions, dependent on the features of the objects: *open the window* is akin to *open the door*, but very different with respect to *open the nut*. In fact no one to one correspondence can be established between verbs and action concepts, causing huge problems for natural language understanding. Language processing required in tasks such as automatic translation and human machine interaction is difficult to achieve when reference to concrete actions is concerned, since the language labels used to indicate action concepts may pick up many different action types and each language shows a different variation potential.

This is one of the crucial reasons for which natural language instructions are not clear for a machine in an open domain communication scenario. The explicit understanding of the language conditions enabling the interpretation of simple sentences requires both a solid knowledge of the range of variation of verbs referring to action and a clear definition of the conceptual structures embodied by each language. Without these premises the overall language processing problem constituted by the linguistic categorization of action cannot be grounded. These issues

© Institute for Computer Sciences, Social Informatics and Telecommunications Engineering 2015
R. Giaffreda et al. (Eds.): IoT360 2014, Part I, LNICST 150, pp. 93–96, 2015.
DOI: 10.1007/978-3-319-19656-5_15

are relevant for the IoT paradigm, since this kind of knowledge should be provided to devices interacting with machines and appliances and with humans through natural language interfaces. How this knowledge should be represented? How can it be extracted from language? These are some of the questions that ModelAct (modelact.lablita.it), a FIRB project funded by MIUR, wants to address. ModelAct aims at providing a cognitive-based model for human categorization of actions. Since the same verb like *to open* can denote different sequences of (sub)actions - different sequences of body movements performed by an agent - it is essential for devices to disambiguate between these denotations and to reason on them, processing linguistic instructions with the awareness of movements implied. In particular, the definition of a natural language disambiguation module able to guess which sequences of (sub)actions is required to open a box instead of a nut is important. ModelAct exploits the ImagAct ontology (www.imagact.it), which identifies the action categories by means of prototypical scenes. Scenes are short 3D videos, they are language independent and their semantic value can be naturally understood, allowing the appropriate encoding in different languages (English, Italian, Spanish and Mandarin Chinese).

In this context, the notion of affordance can bridge the gap between ecological psychology studies and AI approaches to knowledge management. Affordances have been theorized by [3] as the possibilities for action that every environmental object offers. They are different and unique for every living being, in that they are not strictly related to objective properties; rather, they lie on possible ways in which living beings can interact with objects themselves. Affordance is defined as the quality of an object that enables an action: it concerns the relation between a perceptual property of the object and what an agent can do with it. In embodied robotics affordances are often conceptualized as a quality of an object, or of an environment, which allow an artificial agent to perform an action. Environment for artificial agents can be seen as a source of information that help the robot in performing actions, thus reducing the complexity of representation and reasoning [4], exactly in the same way an object showing such properties that afford sitting (e.g. a chair) will help us understand how we can use it (sitting).

Conceptual information concerning objects affordances can be acquired through language. Our focus is on verb-direct object pairs as the linguistic realizations of the relations between actions performed by an agent on objects. We distinguish between general affordances that can be potentially displayed by every objects - more generic verbs like *to take*, *to bring* etc. - and specific affordances as canonical/peculiar activities a specific object is involved in, like *open* for *bottle*. Affordance verbs as verbs that select a distinctive action for a specific object can be discovered through statistical measures in corpora [6].

2   A Possible Application: Food's Affordances for Food Processors

ModelAct analyses data from ImagAct, a previous project that, through manual annotation, clustered sets of sentences distinguishing senses of a verb in terms of (sub)sequences of movements. 800 verbs, both for Italian and English, have been studied and more than 3000 objects' mentions are included in the dataset. In this paper we want to focus on the affordances of a specific class of objects, e.g. the one that are involved in making food. In the near future a food processor can be a complex appliance connected to our smartphones, able to make the best use of the available ingredients, assembling them following steps in a recipe that we choose [1]. Information from sensors monitoring the temperature, the weight and the moisture level of the food can interact with information in recipe's steps. It will be possible to monitor the processor from a smartphone and food's affordances can suggest alternatives at a certain stage (e.g. "Now they are boiled. Do you prefer your zucchini as soup or in puree?"). For this reason, a knowledge base covering a wide range of possibilities and a basic set of reasoning rules on them should be provided to devices; acquiring it through language means helping in the settings of naturale language interfaces interacting with devices.

From ImagAct we can extract basic affordances for food nouns (see Fig. 1):

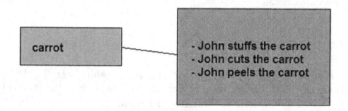

Fig. 1. ImagAct affordances for carrot

However, this knowledge base should be improved including more possibilities. From a corpus of more than 5000 recipes crawled from instructables.com and parsed with Stanford CoreNLP tools [5] we can add valuable knowledge to our model, discovering affordances and extracting sequences of actions, expressing the kind of action(s) that precede or follow the affordance we are focusing on.

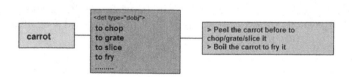

Fig. 2. Corpus extracted affordances for carrot

With respect to the knowledge we have in ImagAct, we can add that a carrot can be the patient of other actions, both generic and specific affordances (see Fig. 2). Intersecting the list of nouns in ImagAct that have food as hypernyms in WordNet 3.0 [2] and selecting the ones with frequency more than 100 in our recipes corpus, we obtained a list of 78 nouns. For each of them basic affordances, local affordances sequences and global affordances sequences can be extracted. With basic affordances we mean the full list of action verbs the noun can be direct object of (e.g. for carrot *to cut, to chop, to grate, to slice*; for milk *to add, to pour, to stir, to whisk*; for sugar *to add, to burn, to dissolve, to mix, to sprinkle*). With local affordances sequences we mean a pair of action verbs that in the same sentence are coordinated and have the noun as direct object (e.g. *Take the carrot and dip it* or *Add a pinch of sugar and stir it*). With global affordances sequences we mean a temporal ordered list of action verbs that have the noun as direct object in the context of the same recipe (e.g. *Take the carrot, clean the carrot, shave the carrot on the salad*). From recipes it's possible to locate each action in a sequence, enabling reasoning on actions sequences in the future in terms of preconditions and consequences (e.g. a carrot should boiled before to make a pure). This knowledge is not static but deeply influence by saliency and probability; with a different corpus (e.g. a corpus composed by just Asian recipes) it could change radically, implying that the information can be adapted for special needs.

References

1. Beetz, M., Klank, U., Kresse, I., Maldonado, A., Msenlechner, L., Pangercic, D., Rhr, T., Tenorth, M.: Robotic roommates making pancakes. In: 2011 11th IEEE-RAS International Conference on Humanoid Robots (2011)
2. Fellbaum, C. (ed.): WordNet: An Electronic Lexical Database. MIT Press, Cambridge (1998)
3. Gibson, J.J.: The Ecological Approach to Visual Perception. Houghton Mifflin, Boston (1979)
4. Horton, T.E., Chakraborty, A., St. Amant R.: Affordances for robots: a brief survey. Avant **3**(2), 70–84 (2012)
5. Manning, C.D., Surdeanu, M., Bauer, J., Finkel, J., Bethard, S.J., McClosky, D.: The Stanford CoreNLP natural language processing toolkit. In: Proceedings of the 52nd Annual Meeting of the Association for Computational Linguistics: System Demonstrations, pp. 55–60 (2014)
6. Russo, I., De Felice, I., Frontini, F., Khan, F., Monachini, M.: (Fore)seeing actions in objects. Acquiring distinctive affordances from language. In: Proceedings of the 10th International Workshop on Natural Language Processing and Cognitive Science - NLPCS 2013, pp. 151–161 (2013)

PERGAMES 2014

Understanding Stroke Patients' Motivation for Motivation-Driven Rehabilitative Game Design

Aung Pyae[2(✉)], Mika Luimula[1], and Jouni Smed[2]

[1] Turku University of Applied Sciences, Turku, Finland
mika.luimula@turkuamk.fi
[2] University of Turku, Turku, Finland
{aung.pyae,jouni.smed}@utu.fi

Abstract. Stroke is one of the major problems in medical and healthcare that can cause severe disability and death of patients especially for older population. Rehabilitation plays an important role in stroke therapy. However, most of the rehabilitative exercises are monotonous and tiring for the patients. For a particular time, they can easily get bored in doing these exercises. The role of patient's motivation in rehabilitation is vital. Motivation and rehabilitative outcomes are strongly related. Digital games are promising to help stroke patients to feel motivated and more engaged in rehabilitative training through motivational gameplay. Most of the commercial games available in the market are not well-designed for stroke patients and their motivational needs in rehabilitation. This study aims at understanding the motivational requirements of stroke patients in doing rehabilitative exercises and living in a post-stroke life. Based on the findings from the literature review, we report that there are many factors that can influence the stroke patients' level of motivation such as social functioning, patient-therapist relationship, goal-setting, and music. These findings are insightful and useful for ideating and designing interactive motivation-driven games for stroke patients. The motivational factors of stroke patients in rehabilitation may help the game designers to design motivation-driven game contexts, contents, and gameplay. Moreover, these findings may help not only game designers but also healthcare professionals who concern stroke patient's motivation in rehabilitative context.

Keywords: rehabilitation · motivation · digital games · human-computer interaction · user requirements

1 Introduction

Stroke is one of the major medical and healthcare problems that can cause severe disability, partial paralysis, memory loss, and even death of sufferers. According to Burke et al. [1], 85 % of patients live with impaired upper and lower limbs after suffering from stroke. The World Health Organization (WHO) states that every year there are 15 million people who suffer from stroke in the world. Among them, 5 million patients die and another 5 million are living with permanent disability that negatively

© Institute for Computer Sciences, Social Informatics and Telecommunications Engineering 2015
R. Giaffreda et al. (Eds.): IoT360 2014, Part I, LNICST 150, pp. 99–111, 2015.
DOI: 10.1007/978-3-319-19656-5_16

impacts their quality of life. Stroke survivors may experience limitations in range of motions, fine motor skills, gross motor skills, reaching, and manipulation. These deficits can dramatically change the patient's daily life that has to be dependent on others (e.g. family members or caregivers) in doing personal management such as showering, feeding, changing clothes, house chores, and ADL (Activities of Daily Living) tasks. Because of these physical limitations after stroke can reduce patient's participation in social and leisure activities, community programs, and work activities [2]. As a result, it may lead to depression, social isolation, and loneliness in life. Rehabilitation training, in which repetitive exercises are involved, can help the stroke patients with motor impairments of lower and upper limbs to overcome the physical limitations following stroke [2]. Rehabilitation is the essential part of the stroke recovery for stroke survivors because repetitive and rehabilitative exercises can support the brain to get sufficient stimuli to remodel and to regain better motor control. Moreover, rehabilitation can help the patients retrain their functional abilities in walking, transferring, balancing, and doing ADLs.

However, stroke therapy involves daily rehabilitative exercises, which include repetitive movements of the affected limbs. Patients typically complain that these exercises are monotonous, tiring, and boring. Chang et al. [2] pointed out that only 31% of patients who have post-stroke motor deficiencies perform the therapeutic exercises as prescribed by the physiotherapists. Early termination of stroke rehabilitation may lead to permanent disability in life. Motivation and therapeutic outcomes are strongly linked [3]. Healthcare professionals generally believe that patient's motivation plays an important role and it can largely determine therapeutic outcomes. There are other factors that can negatively impact on the patient's motivation in rehabilitative process such as lack of social support from family members and friends, expensive fees of stroke therapy, difficulty in travelling to rehabilitative center, and lack of caregiver who can look after them.

2 Background

Recent studies show that healthcare professionals are more and more interested in using computer games for stroke rehabilitation [1]. In general, video games are known to be an engaging platform for the players and gamers because of entertaining, motivating, and fun activities. Virtual rehabilitation has received a great interest from many researchers and healthcare professionals because it can provide a real world environment (e.g. tennis court in sport game or ski resort in leisure game) where players can forget about their surroundings and situation and pay attention to a task in a simulated virtual environment [5]. By playing digital game-based rehabilitative exercises, stroke patients may have improvements in the upper and lower limb mobility as well as higher level of motivation and fun. Among the commercial games available in the market, Nintendo Wii seems to be the most promising technology to be used as a therapeutic tool in stroke rehabilitation. Because of its low-cost hardware and physical game activities, many researchers have tried to use Wii games in stroke therapy. Basically, Wii encourages game players to use physical movements and natural actions in gameplay (e.g., playing tennis in Wii Sports). It has gained positive feedback and support from the therapists because of its ease of use, entertaining game contents, and a wide variety of games available which can help patients to perform therapeutic training and physical exercises [6]. Although Nintendo Wii is useful and usable in rehabilitation, there are some usability issues that can be critical to the patients who play the games for rehabilitative purpose. For instance, the players cannot customize the level of difficulties in the game itself to meet the needs of different levels of disability. Besides, it does not convey therapeutic feedback to the patients and it does not monitor the patient's progress in every session. The other game consoles available in the market such as Microsoft Xbox, Sony PlayStation, and Eye Toy are also not designed for rehabilitation and therapeutic training because these games are only targeted for young and healthy users. Furthermore, these games are mainly for fun, entertainment, and recreation. The game content in these game systems is not targeted for stroke patients. Thus, physical movements in the gameplay are difficult and not suitable for stroke patients. As these games are solely aimed for healthy players, the motivational content of the games is also not suitable for the motivational needs of the stroke patients. Therefore, all these gaps between rehabilitative and motivational needs of stroke patients and existing gaming technologies should be bridged. In this study, we aim at understanding and having empathy on the needs of the stroke patients' motivation in rehabilitation for designing rehabilitative games for them.

3   Motivational Factors

To design and develop interactive motivation-driven games for stroke rehabilitation, it is important to understand and to have empathy for the problems, needs, motivation, pain points, and goals of stroke patients. In this study, we conducted a literature review to explore and to understand the motivational factors that can influence stroke patients in rehabilitation. According to the literature, there are many factors that can have an impact on the stroke patients' motivation in doing rehabilitative exercises and living post-stroke life positively. Social and emotional support from family members, patient-therapist relationship, role changes in family, understanding in rehabilitative process, long and short term goals, and music are some of the important motivational elements that can affect the patient's level of motivation in performing and continuing their rehabilitation that can lead to faster recovery from the stroke. Motivation has been variously described in terms of innate and internal drives or needs, inner stimuli and responses, and goals or the directions of the motivation. The motivation concerns the intrinsic and extrinsic conditions responsible for variations in the intensity, quality, and direction of on-going behaviour [7]. To understand a patient's motivation, one must also consider the environmental pressures that can impact on the patient and include the demands of his or her condition after stroke. In fact, there are environmental factors associated with most of the patients' needs or drives. Research on the stroke patients' motivation is necessary to focus either on the inner needs of the patients, or on the environmental pressures and demands.

3.1 Social Functioning

Social functioning such as social support, social contact, and social integration, plays in an important role for the post-stroke patients. Social contact and social support may not only improve the physical recovery of the patients but also enhance the level of motivation in rehabilitation. Moreover, it may encourage the stroke patients to actively engage in the rehabilitative training. Patients who receive social support from family members are likely to get higher motivation in rehabilitation. In contrast, socially isolated patients are likely to have less motivation in rehabilitation and they are pessimistic about the post-stroke life. Dombovy et al. [8] state that stroke rehabilitation is the combination and coordination of social, medical, educational, and vocational measures for training a patient to regain the highest level of functional recovery and ability. They continue to say that encouraging the socialization of a stroke patient is one of the factors of well-established principles of rehabilitation for stroke. Santus et al. [9] point out that the family is a natural source of social support for a stroke patient and it may influence his or her functional recovery by providing companionship and an opportunity for a normal life. They highlight that the rehabilitation program should emphasize not only the training for physical improvement but also education of family members and society how to support the patient socially and physically. Deteriorating relationships after the stroke are common phenomena for the stroke patients and social communication remains the most stressful issue. Changes in social activities, vocational interests, and role assignments also affect the family system of a stroke patient. Barry [16] points out that stroke patient's expectations on one hand and his or her significant others' expectations on the other hand can strongly influence on his or her level of motivation. The people who play a key role in the stroke patient's rehabilitation are not only the therapists but also his or her family members, friends, associates in whatever situation or setting he or she may live and work.

Evans et al. [11] advocate that social support and functional rehabilitative outcome after stroke are positively linked, suggesting that the support and involvement of family members in rehabilitation are important to speed up the recovery from the stroke. Although family encouragement was one of the factors that can positively affect the stroke patient's motivation, pushing too hard to make improvements in rehabilitation can lead to lower level of patient's motivation in therapeutic training [3]. In addition to this, overprotection can reduce the patient's level of motivation. Social connection with family members and friends is an important factor for patients after stroke but it is very challenging for them to communicate with other people such as understanding what people say, expressing their emotions, talking to other people, walking, eating out, and shopping. It can make the stroke patients feel depressed, discouraged, disconnected, and isolated at a time when they need more social support from family members, friends, and relatives [10]. It is true to say that everyone needs social support and stroke patients cannot be excluded from their social needs. There are many ways that family members and friends can socially support the stroke patients such as companionship from family members, peer's support in rehabilitation, sharing information about stroke rehabilitation and recovery, trying new things for them, listening to their concerns and frustration, sharing their stories, keeping connection with old friends, helping in social outing, participating in social events and activities, and making new friends. Shimoda and Robinson [12] state that a lack of social support can prevent the stroke patients from regularly attending rehabilitative training or lead to a lack of motivation in doing rehabilitative exercises. Most stroke patients can get their motivation through interaction with their beloved ones such as playing with their grandchildren (e.g. intergenerational games), eating out with partners, going cinema with their friends, and socializing with neighbours [13]. Krause et al. [17] states that in general, social support covers the terms such as affective support, information support, and tangible support [17].

3.2   Patient-Therapist Relationship

One of the most important motivating factors is the use of the therapist's relationship with the patient as a form of bringing about the patient's recovery, readjustment, and rehabilitation after stroke [16]. The relationship between the stroke patient and the therapist forms one of the motivational elements in rehabilitation. Maclean et al. [3] mention that if a therapist has low expectations of how a patient will perform in rehabilitative tasks, it may cause a negative effect on the patient's motivation. Positive feedback, support, and encouragement from the therapist are important for the stroke patients to gain confidence and positive emotions in rehabilitation. The therapists can encourage stroke patients to feel more confident and motivated to continue to do rehabilitative exercises in the process of stroke recovery whereas giving confusing messages to the patients about the role of therapists in rehabilitation could lead to unnecessary misunderstanding in therapy and it may negatively impact on the patient's motivation in continuing rehabilitation process. The therapist can increase the motivation of stroke patients by striking up a rapport with patients and discussing about their lives before and after stroke [3]. Generally, the therapists not only help the patients improve in physical rehabilitation but they can also consult the patient's social and family issues. Therefore, the relationship between therapists and stroke patients are crucial in stroke rehabilitation.

3.3   Setting Relevant Rehabilitative Goal

Post-stroke rehabilitation is described as a long-term process where the patient and the healthcare team try to get an agreement on the activities to be focused and the goals to be achieved through interaction, negotiation, and collaboration between the stroke patient and the healthcare professionals such as doctors, therapists, and caregivers. Setting a relevant rehabilitative goal can positively affect on the stroke patient's motivation. However, the goals should be meaningful, realistic, achievable, and measurable. The smaller goals for stroke patients should be related to real-life goals which are meaningful, achievable, and realistic. Moreover, the personalized rehabilitation goals may enhance the level of motivation of stroke patients in rehabilitation. These personalized goals may vary from patient to patient. For example, a particular stroke patient may want to re-enter into the working life or to drive a car when he or she recovers from the stroke whereas another stroke patient may want to be more independent in doing ADLs.

Therefore, a goal that can link to individual needs and wants may positively impact on the stroke patient's motivation and engagement in rehabilitation. Therapists and caregivers need to help the stroke patients to achieve the smaller goals of therapy such as better movements of limbs followed by the bigger goals such as re-integrating into community and going back to work [13].

3.4 Rehabilitative Setting and Environment

Rehabilitative environment is regarded as one of the important factors for patients' motivation in rehabilitation. Generally, it involves well-designed and patient-friendly rehabilitation room, communal meals, and group training sessions where the stroke patients can share their experiences about rehabilitation and learn each other's progress in training, are the positive factors of motivation that fasten recovery from stroke. Almost every stroke patient has to go through a rehabilitation process after they have gone through an acute hospital. They have to spend most of their time at a rehabilitation centre before they regain the functional abilities of the impaired limbs. Therefore, the role of the rehabilitative environment such as a rehabilitation training room, a setting of the gymnasium, and people in this environment, is important for the stroke patients to feel comfortable, convenient, and secure. In addition to personal factors such as health history and condition, gender, role changes in family, sex, social background, and educational background, individual patient's motivation may be impacted also by environmental influences that involve physical condition, social and emotional condition, and individual attitudes for rehabilitation [18].

3.5 Information from Healthcare Professionals

Highly motivated patients feel that education and information provided by the healthcare professionals can change their thinking about therapy. They may see it as not only a helpful solution but also the necessity of an important role in stroke rehabilitation [14]. Before a particular patient starts his or her rehabilitation program, it is important for the therapists to explain the information about rehabilitation and therapeutic exercises. In this way, the patients can understand the process of rehabilitation and the benefits of the exercises. Moreover, understanding the process of rehabilitation and its benefits can enhance the patients' level of motivation and engagement in rehabilitation. The information of rehabilitation process from the therapists and their explanation are important for the stroke patients to understand their condition, process, and progress very well, and which may lead to a higher motivation in rehabilitation and faster recovery from stroke.

3.6 Meaningful Rehabilitative Task

Occupational therapy (OT) includes relearning skills for doing activities of daily living for the patients to get independence in their daily lives. For example, personal grooming, showering, toileting, meal preparation, and money management are some of the ADL tasks in occupational therapy. These OT exercises are meaningful and they reflect the social lifestyles of the stroke patients. By doing activity based exercises (e.g., ADL-based rehabilitative exercises), the patients may feel motivated and more engaged in the exercises. Flores et al. [15] advocate that meaningful tasks should be integrated into the rehabilitation. By doing meaningful rehabilitative tasks, patients can get a direct relationship between the use of impaired limbs in the therapeutic training and the use in their activities of daily living.

3.7 Individual Needs and Customization

As motoric impairment can be different from one patient to another, successful rehabilitative program requires personalization or customization for the individual patients to address their problems, to meet their needs, and to adapt individual's motoric level. Adaptability is one of the important factors for individual patients so that the difficulty level can be increased when the patient's motoric abilities improve in a particular period [15]. Understanding individual stroke patient's needs, focusing on personalized or customized motivation, looking beyond simple fun elements to provide engaging and correct upper or lower limb movements and activities are the difficult challenges in stroke rehabilitation.

3.8 Positive Feedback from Therapist

The encouragement from medical professionals such as doctors, therapists, and nurses, plays a vital role in stroke rehabilitation. Often, the therapists have to not only explain the information about rehabilitation but support them with positive feedback so that the patients can feel more confident, motivated, and engaged in what they are doing. The feedback from the therapist to the patients should be positive to encourage them to actively engage in the rehabilitation. It may help them feel more motivated in performing the rehabilitative tasks and encourage them to be more engaged, active, and confident. Feedback plays an important role in rehabilitative training to maintain and sustain the motivation of individual patient during the rehabilitation process. Extrinsic feedback or external response can encourage the persistence to perform better in a situation of physical education [19].

3.9 Music for Rehabilitation

Everyday many people expose music for different reasons such as relaxation, interest, and motivation. Generally, people use music to achieve different types of goals in everyday life such as to motivate in doing exercises, to get relaxation, to pass time when driving for long hours or taking bus for long distance. Music is an interesting area for the healthcare professionals and researchers to study on how it may affect the stroke patient's motivation in therapeutic way. Music therapy may be effective in reducing negative emotions such as anger, depression, and anxiety, whereas promoting positive affections such as happiness, joy, and pleasant. Music Therapy can be used as listening therapy for the stroke patients to listen to a list of songs that caregiver or music therapist has selected for them to match a mood or to bring back memories [13]. Music can trigger the positive emotions of the stroke patients that may lead to more engagement in doing rehabilitative exercises. Music can be used as a healing tool in the social and personal context that can have a positive impact on the emotion of individual patient who is recovering from a stroke. Moreover, it can enable social interaction between the therapist and the patient or among a group of people in a rehabilitative training session [20]. Music may affect the physical, mental, and social components of the post-stroke rehabilitation process in many ways such as therapeutic listening and rhythmic movements.

3.10   Recreational Activities for Stroke Patients

Recreational activities such as playing digital games or board games, singing songs, participating in social outings, and going out for shopping, are recognized as motivational elements for the stroke patients that enable better social connection and re-integration with peers, friends, therapists, and communities. By participating in recreational activities, the stroke patients may regain a sense of social reintegration and better social ties with other people. Moreover, it may overcome the issues of social isolation and depression and it may help the stroke patients to feel more motivated in rehabilitation training and improve their quality of life. There are many benefits of leisure activities that can positively affect individual well-being and quality of life. Recreational activities also help the stroke patients to enhance their physical and mental health condition, together with personal growth and social communication. Leisure activities are suitable for everyone who can experience positive moments from doing these activities regardless of what state of health he or she is in. While the types of the recreational activities a person has done before the stroke might be different from the leisure activities that he or she is currently doing in post-stroke life, the feeling of wellbeing that one gets from these recreational activities will not be different [21].

4   Discussion

Understanding the stroke patient's motivation in doing rehabilitative exercises is an important step in designing digital games for stroke patients and rehabilitation. Thus, the findings from understanding motivational elements of stroke patients in rehabilitation can be applied as design inputs and considerations in the game design process. According to the literature review, social functioning such as social ties with friends, peers, and family members and social communication, is one of the most important motivational factors for the stroke patients to get motivated in doing the rehabilitative exercises which is why it is one of the most important design inputs for designing a game for stroke rehabilitation. In designing a digital game for rehabilitative purpose, we can design multiplayer game where two or more players can play the game together so that they can socially connect with each other through the gameplay. By playing multiplayer games, the stroke patients can build up the social ties with peers and have a mutual understanding between patients in a similar situation. Moreover, not only the patients but also the therapists or other healthcare professionals can monitor or even participate in the multiplayer game. To achieve the idea of improving socialization of the stroke patients, we can also design intergenerational games for them to maintain the social connection between the patients and their family members. According to Llyod [24], intergenerational communication between older adults and younger generation can decrease the prevalence of ageing and it can considerably support to improve the mental health and physical well-being amongst the elderly group. With regard to the digital game-based socialization, Theng et al. [25] insist that generally computer-mediated games can provide inter-generational gameplay (e.g. Multiplayer Sport Games). Moreover, it can support entertaining and socializing features that are used as tools to promote positive mental health, social health, and physical well-being of the older adults. To design digital games for stroke patient's rehabilitation, the concept of "Patient-Therapist relationship" can be used as a basis for the relationship between virtual therapist and the player. Virtual therapist can be a narrator or a virtual coach in the rehabilitative training in the game itself. In addition to this, the customization of the avatar's identity selected by the player can be integrated in the game so that the player may have stronger connection to the virtual therapist in the game. According to Kenny et al. [26], Virtual Human Agent technology has been used by the researchers to develop 2D or 3D characters that are used in virtual reality games and applications. For example, these virtual characters can be designed as virtual therapists, virtual nurses, and caregivers in the context of stroke rehabilitation.

With regard to the setting a relevant and achievable goal in the rehabilitation, we can account this as a goal-based game for the stroke patients. It is important that the goals are realistic and achievable and meet the individual's needs. In designing a goal-based game, we can allow the player to set a particular goal to achieve at particular levels or to get certain ranks or to earn certain points or scores in the game. In this way, the player can feel more motivated and engaged in the gameplay. Well-maintained and clean rooms, friendly social interaction, and stroke patient friendly facilities are amongst the important settings in the rehabilitative context that can have an impact on the level of motivation. For the game design, game environment or context should be more realistic and familiar to the players and should reflect their social lifestyle. By designing a game environment reflecting the stroke patients' social lifestyle, it can help them to feel more engaged in the game itself, which can improve the level of their motivation. For example, we can design a virtual shopping game environment in which the players can do shopping activities that they used to do before the stroke. Pyae et al. [27] advocate that in designing game for stroke patients, game environment should be meaningful and it should reflect the player's social background.

Information provided by the healthcare professionals such as doctors, therapists, and nurses, is important for the stroke patient in stroke rehabilitation. In the game design, we can use this concept as a help system; for example, virtual training by a virtual therapist, and information provided by a virtual nurse or caregiver on how to conduct the game. In addition, a virtual character (e.g. virtual therapist) can provide the progress of the gameplay, game scores, and game incentives in real-time during the gameplay. Physical therapy focuses on regaining strength and mobility of the upper or lower limbs by doing therapeutic exercises whereas occupational therapy focuses on relearning real activities (e.g. ADL, community reintegration, personal management and cognitive skills) that a patient has lost after suffering from the stroke. These ADL-based tasks are basically meaningful and realistic to the patients. In a game environment, we can also include real world tasks in the game activities. For example, we can design a cooking game for the stroke patients where they can prepare and cook the meal and at the same time, they perform therapeutic movements followed by cognitive skills such as choosing the right ingredients for the food and manage the cooking time. Furthermore, we can design a game that based on real-world activities such as simulation for driving a car, virtual shopping tasks, use of mobile phone or ATM or public phone, purchase of a public transport ticket, and other social activities. According to Pyae et al. [27], by playing meaningful game tasks, the stroke patients may feel more engaged, motivated, and active in the rehabilitative training.

In stroke rehabilitation, the individual needs may vary from patient to patient. Thus, the therapists and nurses have to customize the rehabilitation based on the individual requirements and goals. As a game design consideration, it is important to implement the player's personalization and customization in the game itself such as user profile, game levels, game scores, and ranks. When designing games for stroke patients, we can customize the game-based therapeutic activities or tasks to reflect the individual needs and resistances such as strength, mobility, and endurance of upper limbs. User profile, avatar customization, and game level setup (e.g. easy, hard, and master) can be included in the game design which allows the therapists or the patients to customize the games to meet their individual needs. By achieving certain levels the players may feel more engaged and motivated in the gameplay. Real-time game feedback is considered as one of the most important elements in general game design. In stroke rehabilitation, positive feedback from therapists in rehabilitative training should encourage the stroke patients. In the game design, it should emphasize giving positive and encouraging feedback such as progression level, positive feedback in audio or visual display by the game itself, and certain scores as incentives for the players in whatever situation they are. By getting encouraging feedback or incentives from the game, the players may actively involve in the gameplay and it is bound to increase their level of motivation. Music therapy is helpful for stroke survivors not only for entertaining but also for therapeutic purpose. Since music can be used as an emotionally stimulating tool, music therapy can also help to enhance or maintain one's mental health and physical well-being, communication, social well-being, and quality of life [23]. The role of music is vital in designing digital games. The background music and audio feedback form important game elements to judge if a particular game is interactive, engaging, and enjoyable. When designing and developing interactive games for stroke patients, it is important to choose the right genre of music and audio feedback so that the patients feel more engaged and active in the gameplay. Finally, recreational activities (e.g. chess games, singing games, shopping games, card games, and puzzle) can be integrated into the game design to improve the stroke patient's motivation in the gameplay.

After considering all the motivational factors that can have an impact on the stroke patient's level of motivation and rehabilitative outcome, we can suggest game design guidelines and ideas for designing and developing interactive games for stroke patients and rehabilitation. Table 1 lists the motivational factors of stroke patients and game design inputs and considerations for the game designers.

Table 1. Indication to the game design principles.

Motivational Factors	Game Design Consideration
Social Functioning	• Multiplayer game • Intergenerational game • Virtual friend • Video chat in game • Social-networking game
Patient-Therapist Relationship	• Virtual therapist • Virtual nurse • Virtual Coach
Goal Setting	• Level design • Perceivable and achievable goals
Rehabilitative Setting and Environment	• Game theme and scenery • Difficulty of the game • Complexity of the game
Information from Healthcare Professionals	• Game tutorials • Game introduction • Help system • Computer-controlled assistant

5 Conclusion

We listed motivational factors of stroke patients' rehabilitation based on the literature. The factors are useful and insightful when designing digital games for stroke patients and their rehabilitation. We outlined game design considerations based on the motivational factors. At the moment, we are implementing motivation-driven functional games, which will be followed user testing and evaluation with stroke patients and therapists. This practical work will help us to evaluate and improve the approach we have outlined in this paper.

Acknowledgments. We would like to thank our collaborators and partners in the project called Gamified Solutions in Healthcare (GSH). This on-going project was supported and funded by Finnish Funding Agency for Technology and Innovation (Tekes), City of Turku, and several technological companies.

References

1. Burke, J.W., McNeill, M.D.J., Charles, D.K., Morrow, P.J., Crosbie, J.H., McDonough, S.M.: Designing Engaging, Playable Games for Rehabilitation. In: International Conference Series On Disability, Virtual Reality And Associated Technologies (ICDVRAT) (2010)
2. Chang, Y.J, Cheang, S.F, Huang, J.D.: A Kinect-Based System for Physical Rehabilitation. A Pilot Study for Young Adults with Motor Disabilities. Research in Development Disabilities, 32, 2566-2570 (2011)

3. Maclean, N., Pound, P., Wolfe, C., Rudd, A.: The Concept of Patient Motivation: A Qualitative Analysis of Stroke Professionals' Attitudes. Stroke **33**, 444–448 (2002)
4. Shen, Y., Ong, S.K., Nee, A.Y.C.: An Augmented Reality System for Hand Movement Rehabilitation. In: Proc. iCREATe '08, pp. 189-192 (2008)
5. Halton, J.: Virtual Rehabilitation with Video Games. A New Frontier for Occupational Therapy. Occupational Therapy Now, vol. 9(6), pp. 12-14 (2008)
6. Anderson, F., Annett, M., Bischof, W.F.: Lean on Wii: Physical Rehabilitation With Virtual Reality and Wii Peripherals. Annual Review of CyberTherapy and Telemedicine **8**, 181–184 (2010)
7. Maclean, N., Pound, P., Wolfe, C., Rudd, A.: Qualitative Analysis of Stroke Patients' Motivation for Rehabilitation. Bmj 2000, 321 (7268):1051-1054 (2000)
8. Domboyy, M.L., Sandok, B.A., Basford, J.R.: Rehabilitation for Stroke: A Review. Stroke **17**, 363–369 (1986)
9. Sanntus, G.A., Ranzenigo, A., Caregnato, R., Maria, R.I.: Social and Family Integration of Hemiplegic Elderly Patients 1 Year after Stroke. Stroke **21**, 1019–1022 (1990)
10. Recovery after Stroke: Social Support, www.stroke.org
11. Evans, R.L., Matlock, A.-L., Bishop, D.S., Stranahan, S., Pederson, C.: Family Intervention After Stroke: Does Counseling or Education Help? Stroke **19**, 1243–1249 (1988)
12. Shimoda, K., Robinson, R.G.: The Relationship between Social Impairment and Recovery from Stroke. Psychiatry **61**, 101–111 (1998)
13. Finding Motivation after Stroke or Brain Damage, http://sueb.hubpages.com/hub/Finding-Motivation-after-Stroke-or-Brain-Damage
14. White, G.N., Cordato, D.J., O'Rourke, F., Mendis, R.L., Ghia, D., Chang, D.K.: Validation of the Stroke Rehabilitation Motivation Scale: A Pilot Study. Asian J Gerontol Geriatr **7**, 80–87 (2012)
15. Flores, E., Tobon, G., Cavallaro, E., Cavallaro, F.I., Perry, J.C., Keller, T.: Improving Patient Motivation in Game Development for Motor Deficit Rehabilitation. In: Intl. Conf. on Adva.in Comp. Entert, Tech., ACM, 381-384 (2008)
16. Barry, J.: Patient Motivation for Rehabilitation. Cleft Palate J. **2**, 62–68 (1965)
17. Krause, N., Frank, J.W., Dasinger, L.K., Sullivan, J.J., Sinclair, S.J.: Determinants of Duration of Disability and Return-to-work After Work-related Injury and Illness: Challenges for Future Research. AMJ Industrial Med **40**(4), 464–484 (2001)
18. Holmqvish, L.W., Koch, L.: Environmental Factors in Stroke Rehabilitation, Being in Hospital itself Demotivates Patients. British Medical Journal **322**, 1501–1502 (2001)
19. Van-Vliet, P.M., Wulf, G.: Extrinsic Feedback for Motor Learning after Stroke: What is the Evidence? Disabil Rehabil **28**, 831–840 (2006)
20. Knight, A.J., Wiese, N.: Therapeutic Music and Nursing in Poststroke Rehabilitation. Rehabilitation Nursing **36**(5), 200–215 (2011)
21. Leisure and Participation Information for Patients and Families, www.strokeengine.org
22. Roth, E.A., Wisser, S.: Music Therapy: The Rhythm of Recovery. The Case Manager **15**(3), 52–56 (2004)
23. Music Therapy, www.strokengine.ca
24. Lloyd, J.: The State of Intergenerational Relations Today. ILC-UK (2008)
25. Theng, Y.L., Chua, P.H., Pham, T.P.: Wii as Entertainment and Socialization Aids for Mental and Social Health of Elderly. In: Proc. CHI'12 Extended Abstracts, (New York: ACM), 691-702
26. Kenny, P., Parsons, T., Gratch, J., Rizzo, A.: Virtual Humans for Assisted Healthcare. In: 1st Int. Conf. on Pervasive Technology Related to Assistive Environments 1-4, ACM Press, New York (2008)

27. Pyae, A., Tan, B.Y., Gossage, M.: Understanding Stroke Patients' Needs for Designing User-Centered Rehabilitative Games. Proceedings of the 7th Annual International Conference on Computer Games Multimedia and Allied Technologies, pp.151-156 (2013)
28. Mao, J.Y., Vredenbur, K., Smith, P.W.: User-centered Design Methods In Practice: A Survey of the State of the Art. Proc. Center for Advanced Studies on Collaborative Research, pp. 12 (2001)
29. Boulet, G.: Rapid Prototyping: An Efficient Way to Collaboratively Design and Develop E-Learning Content, http://www.guyboulet.net/site/docs/Rapid_prototyping.pdf
30. Malmivirta, H.: Art as Bridge for Personal and Professional Growth. Acta Universitatis Tamperensis 1629. Tampere: Juvenes Print
31. Malmivirta, H.: Yellow cottage and patch of potatoes. In: Malmivirta, H., Kivelä, S. (eds.) Art and Culture – Keys for better Brain health. Turku University of Applied Sciences. Education materials 89. Turku University of Applied Sciences, 91– 26 (2014)

A Game-Based Solution for In-Home Rehabilitation

Silvia Gabrielli[1(✉)], Rosa Maimone[1], Cristina Costa[1],
Antonio Ascolese[2], Johanna Jonsdottir[3], Wolfhard Klein[4],
and Gabriel Bendersky[5]

[1] CREATE-NET, Via Alla Cascata 56/D, Trento, Italy
{silvia.gabrielli,rosa.maimone,
cristina.costa}@create-net.org
[2] Imaginary Srl, Milan, Italy
giancarlo.bo@i-maginary.it
[3] Fondazione Don Carlo Gnocchi Onlus, Milan, Italy
jjonsdottir@dongnocchi.it
[4] Neurological Therapeutic Centre Gmundnerberg, Altmünster, Austria
wolfhard.klein@ntgb.at
[5] Edna Pasher Ph.D and Associates, Management Consultants, Tel Aviv, Israel
hadas@pasher.co.il

Abstract. This paper presents initial concepts from the REHAB@HOME project investigating the patient-centered design of game environments aimed to raising patients' motivation and compliance with motor-cognitive rehabilitation programs. During the initial phase of the project a patient's client was developed to deploy five rehabilitation games through main gaming platforms and interaction devices (Kinect, LeapMotion, Sifteo Cubes). Also, a professional client was designed to enable clinicians the remote monitoring of patients' progress in home settings. We discuss main features developed for both clients that can inform the future realization of game-based solutions for upper body rehabilitation programs.

Keywords: Serious games · Motor-cognitive rehabilitation · Patient-centred design · Professional clients

1 Introduction

Stroke is the second most common cause of death in Europe (EU Cardiovascular Disease statistics, 2012) and it affects about 15 million people worldwide each year. Stroke survivors experience a broad range of problems that can impact their cognitive and motor systems, leading to chronic disability (e.g., hemiparesis) more often affecting the upper body (i.e., arms, Dobkin, 2005). The goal of rehabilitation is to help survivors become as independent as possible and to attain the best possible quality of life. For over half of stroke patients, rehabilitation will be a long-term process requiring work supervised by therapists, supported by specialized equipment, lasting several months. However, increasing cost pressure on the healthcare system is leading to shorter periods of intensive rehabilitation at specialized facilities. Therefore the

© Institute for Computer Sciences, Social Informatics and Telecommunications Engineering 2015
R. Giaffreda et al. (Eds.): IoT360 2014, Part I, LNICST 150, pp. 112–117, 2015.
DOI: 10.1007/978-3-319-19656-5_17

adoption of suitable technologies for in home rehabilitation, together with a proper training about the execution of a personalized program of exercises, can help reduce the patient's stay at the hospital, as well as the need and cost of reaching the rehabilitation facilities and helping in relapse prevention or improving the patient's state to his potential. In this work, we present early concepts for a patient client and a professional client, realized in the REHAB@HOME European project in collaboration with therapists and patients in Italy and Austria, aimed at supporting in-home rehabilitation of the upper body.

2   Related Work

In the area of rehabilitation research and practice, there have been previous attempts to leverage on low cost gaming platforms, such as Wii (Deutsch et al., 2008) and Playstation 2 EyeToy (Flynn et al., 2007), to support post-stroke therapy. However, these solutions are difficult to deploy with patients in earlier stages of recovery when they have only limited range of motion. For this type of patients other more specific game-based solutions have been recently proposed. Huber et al. (2008) and Jack et al. (2001) developed haptic glove based games in which users scare away butterflies, play the piano, and squeeze virtual pistons to improve the player's finger flexion and extension. Burke et al. (2009) built two webcam color tracked games similar to whack-a mole. In addition, they created a physics-based orange catching game and a whack-a-mouse game, both controlled with magnetic sensors and a vibraphone game, using a Wii remote as a pointing device. Game concepts and solutions more related to everyday tasks and activities of daily living have been explored to increase patients' motivation to play, by providing more meaningful settings (Sanchez et al. 2006; Burke et al. 2009). Flores et al. (2008) identified game design criteria that stem from stroke rehabilitation and elderly entertainment. Vandermaesen et al. (2013) developed the Lifta-cube prototype for training of the upper extremities and tested it with four patients (affected by cerebrovascular accident or paraplegia) finding encouraging results and benefits regarding patients' motivation.

In our work, instead of focusing on developing games for specific ranges of disability we aim to realize solutions that can be adapted for use by patients at different levels of recovery (a similar approach was proposed in Alankus, 2011). By informing our design with requirements from therapists and patients, we aim to realize a rehabilitation platform enabling therapists to select and tailor games for individual patients' programs.

3   Game Design for Motor Rehabilitation

During the first year of the REHAB@HOME project we conducted a patient centered design process to realize a set of rehabilitation games targeting post-stroke and multiple sclerosis patients in need of upper body motor rehabilitation. The design process also involved requirements collected by interviewing a number of therapists at Fondazione Don Gnocchi (Italy) and Neurological Therapeutic Centre Gmundnerberg (Austria).

We ended up developing a patient client providing access to four games, three of which could be played with the Kinect gaming platform, one with the SifteoCubes platform. We also decided to include in the experimentation an available game for the novel LeapMotion device (a sensor controller that supports hand and finger motions as input, analogous to a mouse, but requiring no hand contact or touching). The criteria for inclusion and development of these 5 games, was to assess their benefits for deployment in the context of arm/hand motor rehabilitation sessions. The specific movements required by the games were the following: shoulder abduction, adduction, flexion, extension, wrist flexion, extension, supination, opening/closing of hand, reaching movements and finger movements of precision. In the following we briefly describe the games realized and deployed in the first two years of the project (Fig. 1 shows the menu screen on the patient client for selecting the Kinect games developed):

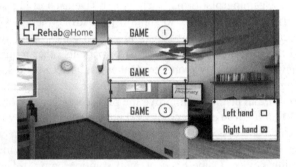

Fig. 1. Screenshot of the menu to select the Kinect games.

(1) Bombs & Flowers minigame [Kinect]: the patient interacts in a living room environment where s/he has to touch flowers items and avoid bombs. S/he is required to use both hands moving them from the center of the body to the sides and is provided instructions, visual feedback, and total score achieved during the session.

(2) Can minigame [Kinect]: the patient needs to move cans from a central table to the correct shelf, by matching corresponding colors which change position during the game; s/he can use just one hand per session (s/he can change hands between sessions) and get instructions, visual feedback and overall score achieved.

(3) Blackboard minigame [Kinect]: the patient needs to move different shapes from the left side to colored spots on the right side, by following a random path using only one hand. Random pairings are proposed (e.g. star-blue, square-red) on the top of the screen, red dots appear along the path, which should be collected; instructions, visual feedback and overall score are also provided.

(4) Caterpillar game [LeapMotion]: the patient needs to guide a caterpillar around the screen with one finger to collect numbers in a sequential order, achieve levels and eventually become a butterfly; instructions, visual and auditory feedback are provided.

(5) Simon game [Sifteo Cubes, Fig. 2]: 3 (1.7 in) cubes are provided in fixed positions on a table which display colours randomly assigned by the system; the patient is

asked to tilt a fourth cube to select a colour on its display and put the cube in contact with the corresponding cube (same colour) in the fixed positions; visual, auditory feedback, number of sessions played and score are provided through the cubes displays; typically the patient plays by using one hand for 3 consecutive sessions.

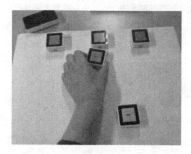

Fig. 2. Simon game played with Sifteo Cubes

3.1 The Professional Client

In order to remote monitoring the rehabilitation process and manage the patients, a web application has been envisioned. The Web based graphical interface has two main views:

The professional station view, which has two main functions. As therapy management tool, it allows the continuous monitoring, management and communication with patients during their rehabilitation activities. It can be used by clinical staff to personalize and schedule the program of exercises for each patient, and tuning on the fly the rehabilitation program when needed. Besides this, it supports long-term and statistical analysis of collected data and information, taking into account the data collected by the patient station during his interaction with the games, such as motion data, games data and usage information. The analysis of the collected data supports therapists and clinicians in understanding the level of progress during the rehabilitation process and in choosing possible adjustments, both in the short and long term, thus providing, at the same time, a solid ground for a more effective planning of the rehabilitation process.

The design of the Professional client was conducted by following the results of the user requirements collection and analysis in the first year of the project. In particular, we complied with the Rehabilitation Plan of Care indications provided by therapists at the two clinics involved in the project. The Professional client interface is divided into four distinct areas (Fig. 3), each associated to a different colour, as follows:

- My Patients: including all functionalities for managing patients, like the assignment and configuration of exercises through the games, and the visualization of relevant data about progress with the rehabilitation process (Fig. 4).
- My Profile: providing all functionalities related to the staff profile, and tools to communicate with other staff involved in managing a patient.

- Games: an inventory of the available games, with their full description.
- Equipment: an inventory of the available equipments/devices, with their full description.

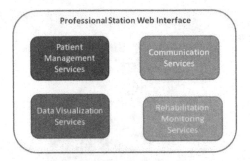

Fig. 3. Services integrated into the Professional Client Interface

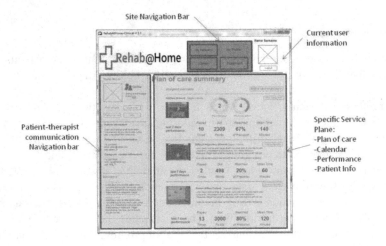

Fig. 4. Screenshot of main features provided by the Professional Client Interface

4 Conclusion

This work has presented initial design concepts for a patient client and a professional client to be used for in-home upper body rehabilitation and its remote monitoring by clinics. We are currently in the process of conducting pilot studies to assess the level of usability and satisfaction of patients and therapists with the games and interfaces realized. The architecture of the overall REHAB@HOME solution will also include a family client to support the involvement of family members and caregivers in the in-home rehabilitation process (e.g., providing possibility of playing co-located games to sustain motivation of the patient, and to get an overview of patient's progress with therapy), which will be designed according to information collected from users. In addition the overall solution will include Web2.0 social and communication tools, which will support the communication between the patient and his medical professionals and promote communication with other patients using the system. A longitudinal evaluation of the integrated REHAB@HOME solution will be conducted in 2015 involving a large group of patients and therapists in Italy and Austria.

Acknowledgments. This work has been supported by the FP7 STREP Project REHAB@-HOME N. 306113.

References

Alankus, G.: Motion-based video games for stroke rehabilitation with reduced compensatory motions. Doctoral Dissertation, Department of Computer Science and Engineering, Washington University in St. Louis (2011)

Burke, J.W., et al.: Serious games for upper limb rehabilitation following stroke, pp. 103–110 (2009)

Deutsch, J.E., et al.: Use of a low-cost, commercially available gaming console (Wii) for rehabilitation of an adolescent with cerebral palsy. Phys. Ther. **88**(10), 1196–1207 (2008)

Dobkin, B.H.: Rehabilitation after Stroke. N. Engl. J. Med. **352**, 1677–1684 (2005). doi:10.1056/NEJMcp043511

European Cardiovascular Disease Statistics (2012). http://www.escardio.org/about/documents/eu-cardiovascular-disease-statistics-2012.pdf

Flores, E., Tobon, G., Cavallaro, E., Cavallaro, F.I., Perry, J., Keller, T.: Improving patient motivation in game development for motor deficit rehabilitation. In: Proceedings of the 2008 International Conference on Advances in Computer Entertainment Technology, Yokohama, Japan, pp. 381–384 (2008)

Flynn, S., et al.: Feasibility of using the Sony PlayStation 2 gaming platform for an individual poststroke: a case report. J. Neurol. Phys. Ther. JNPT **31**(4), 180–189 (2007)

Huber, M., et al.: PlayStation 3-based tele-rehabilitation for children with hemiplegia, pp. 105–112 (2008)

Jack, D., et al.: Virtual reality-enhanced stroke rehabilitation. IEEE Trans. Neural Sys. Rehabil. Eng. **9**(3), 308–318 (2001)

Sanchez, R.J., et al.: Automating arm movement training following severe stroke: functional exercises with quantitative feedback in a gravity-reduced environment. IEEE Trans. Neural Sys. Rehabil. Eng. **14**(3), 378–389 (2006)

Vandermaesen, M., et al.: Liftacube: a pervasive prototype for rehabilitation in a residential setting. In: Proceedings of the 6th International Conference on Pervasive Technologies Related to Assistive Environments (PETRA 2013), May 2013

Evaluation of Pervasive Games: Recruitment of Qualified Participants Through Preparatory Game Phases

Vlasios Kasapakis(✉), Damianos Gavalas, and Thomas Chatzidimitris

Department of Cultural Technology and Communication,
University of the Aegean, Mytilene, Greece
{v.kasapakis, d.gavalas, tchatz}@aegean.com

Abstract. In this paper we present the evaluation process for *Barbarossa*, a pervasive role playing game. *Barbarossa* involves an invitational (preparatory) and a main execution phase. The former is freely available though Google Play store and may be played anytime/anywhere. The latter defines three inter-dependent player roles acted by players who need to collaborate in a treasure hunting game. The eligibility of players for participating in the main game phase is restricted among those ranked relatively high in the invitational phase. Herein, we investigate the impact of the invitational game mode on the players overall game experience. The main hypothesis tested is that game awareness (gained from participating in a preliminary game phase) may serve as a means for recruiting the most suitable subjects for user trials on pervasive game research prototypes.

Keywords: Pervasive games · Evaluation · User trials

1 Introduction

As pervasive game prototypes proliferate and gamers' awareness on this emerging gaming genre consolidates, research focus is increasingly diverted towards under-standing the human factors which are mostly influential to the overall players' experience. Along this line, several challenges surface with respect to pervasive games evaluation and several evaluation methods have been proposed and tested in order to support designers' comprehension on the aspects that impact the overall quality of experience in pervasive games [1, 2]. Game evaluation trials serve as a valuable instrument for measuring the enjoyment and immersion perceived by players; however, they typically involve a lengthy and expensive multi-phase process (preparatory activities, subjects' recruitment, trials orchestration and monitoring, execution and compilation of surveys, etc.). The evaluation process is even more demanding when considering pervasive game trials, wherein trials are executed in the physical space, far from a supervised laboratory environment. As a result, user trials should be well prepared and carefully orchestrated to ensure their flawless execution.

The focal objective of evaluations trials is to receive unbiased feedback from neutral, 'external' subjects about the usability, playability and experience perceived

© Institute for Computer Sciences, Social Informatics and Telecommunications Engineering 2015
R. Giaffreda et al. (Eds.): IoT360 2014, Part I, LNICST 150, pp. 118–124, 2015.
DOI: 10.1007/978-3-319-19656-5_18

throughout the game sessions. The recording of neutral views expressed by the evaluators may indicate technical flaws or even suggest essential script, usability or technical improvements. Hence, the recruitment of qualified participants is regarded as one of the most critical and challenging aspects of user evaluation trials [2]. Another crucial, yet commonly overlooked, aspect of pervasive games evaluation relates with players invitations. Montola argues that the participation awareness level of a player during game sessions commonly shifts from the 'unaware' to the 'aware' state. The level of awareness may be influenced by the invitation method employed to recruit players. Furthermore, addressing invitations to prospective players (i.e. those that belong to the game's potential target group) may allow them to gain game experiences while increasing participation awareness [3].

The pervasive game prototypes evaluated in the past have utilized a variety of invitation methods for recruiting participants like e-mails [4, 5], personal contacts [6], announcements/advertisements [4, 7], recruitment of colleagues/organization employees [8], Jones and Marsden tabulated a list of advantages and disadvantages inherent in the above subject recruitment methods [9].

Notably, none of the above referenced evaluated pervasive games utilized invitation methods that enhance players' game awareness. That is, experiences are missing in assessing evaluation methods which actually introduce the players into the game; even more so, no methods have been proposed to allow game designers monitoring and 'screening' the players and provide them the means to select the most eligible players to participate into the evaluation process.

The main hypothesis investigated in this article is that a preparatory game phase (acting as a 'qualification round') would designate the players mostly interested in participating in the main game phase; hence, these players would be the most appropriate evaluators as they could be regarded as representative sample of the game's potential target group. The above hypothesis has been validated in the evaluation of *Barbarossa*. Along this line we opted to implement a freely available invitational game mode in the Android application market - Google Play, enabling players worldwide to participate into the game, thereby ensuring openness and neutrality in the recruitment process. Also by strongly linking the invitational phase game to the overall game scenario, the players have been seamlessly introduced into the game and gained a better understanding of its concept and goals.

2 Game Scenario and Implementation

Barbarossa [10] is a two-phase trans-reality role playing game. The first game phase is available from the Google Play app store under the title "The Conqueror".[1] In the first phase scenario the Barbarossa pirate brothers Aruj, Khzir and Ilyas (known for their pirate raids throughout the Aegean sea during 1600−1650 A.D.), following a battle against the Knights of St. John outside the castle of Mytilene and assisted by some traitors within the castle walls, conquered the city. In this phase the players act as

---

[1] https://play.google.com/store/apps/details?id=zarc.crash.conqueror&hl=en.

Knights of the St. John who try to free the conquered city. Acting so, the players use a custom Android application which utilizes Google Maps and a turn-based role-playing game which allows them to complete and create quests located into the surrounding area of Mytilene. Upon completing quests the players gain experience points that indicate their commitment and attribution to the game.

The players ranked higher (in experience points) in the first phase are invited to participate in the second game phase called "The Interplay"; in the latter, Mytilene is freed and the Knights rush in the castle to catch Aruj, Ilyas and Khzir. At the crypts of the castle the three Pirates knowing that the Knights are looking for them, hide all their treasures to a treasure chest. Aruj and Ilyas lock the chest with one combination lock each, while Khzir takes it and ridding his horse leaves the crypts to hide it. In a while, the Knights arrive at the crypts and manage to catch Aruj as a prisoner. Ilyas, though, manages to flee and a Knight chases after him.

In order to complete the second game phase, three players should cooperate to unlock the treasure chest hid by Khzir somewhere in the city. It is noted that the "The Conqueror" application detects the distance of the players from the Mytilene center (located on Lesvos island, Greece) while playing, grouping players into two separate experience rankings categories, the Insiders who play in Mytilene (≤ 3.5 km from the city center) and the Outlanders who play away from the city. One of the Outlanders and another of the Insiders as well as a guest (selected by the Insider player) are invited into the second phase based on their total experience points, collected in the first phase. The three players utilize custom Android applications integrating a variety of technologies, including QR-Code scanning, environment sound level recording, augmented reality, location-based gaming, the Google Directions service, sensor devices (SunSPOTs), etc. The players aim at completing their assigned missions (based on separate, yet, supplementary scenarios) to locate the locked chest and the two lock combinations and unlock the chest. Full implementation details of *Barbarossa* may be found in the official website of the game at www.BarbarossaRPG.com.

3   Evaluation Method and Results

So far, questionnaires, interviews and log data (i.e. data capturing the mobility and interaction activity of players throughout the game sessions) have been the methods most commonly employed in pervasive games evaluation. The same practice has been followed in *Barbarossa*. We have conducted user evaluation trials using all the three abovementioned evaluation methods; log data have been a critical element in the evaluation process in order to cross-check them (when available) against player answers (as compiled by questionnaires and interviews) and extract more safe and reliable conclusions. Below we describe the evaluation process in full detail. For the questionnaires we used linkert scale and yes/no questions.

The evaluation process of the game commenced in October 29th, 2013 by releasing the invitational game mode though Google Play as well as a website wherein the players could check their rankings. We provided players sufficient time (21 days) to play the first game phase; thereafter we started contacting the highest ranked players among the Outlanders and the Insiders in order to form the 3-player teams required to proceed to the second game phase. We have invited one team at a time, a practice that enhanced competition among Phase I players who wished to participate in the second game phase.

Prior to proceeding to the second game phase we have asked all members of the 3-player teams that qualified from Phase I (i.e. those acting as Treasure Hunters and Knights) to complete a questionnaire about their experiences in the first phase. Then, we introduced the players into the second game phase and allowed them a week to play the game session and collaboratively locate and unlock the treasure chest. Having completed the second phase, we have invited all players to complete an additional questionnaire tailored to the scenario they pursued in the second game phase. Finally, each player has been interviewed about her overall game experience. In parallel, we have collected log data (e.g. total completed and created quests, game session duration, distance travelled and speed) about the players game actions throughout the game sessions.

Currently (July 2014) *Barbarossa* features more than 1500 downloads and a average rating of 4.04/5 in Google Play. Furthermore, 874 players registered in *Barbarossa*; according to our log data, 262 among them performed at least one in game action, such as undertaking a quest.

Before investigating the impact of the invitational phase on the overall game experience, the usability aspects of the invitational game mode had to be evaluated to ensure that no serious flaws prevented players state transition towards game awareness. Table 1 presents the responses of evaluators with respect to their gaming background. Almost all players stated that they are regular video game players, while only two first phase participants have had previous experience with games similar to *Barbarossa*.

Table 1. Demographic questions.

Do you play video games regularly?		
Yes (Y)	15	75.00 %
No (N)	5	25.00 %
Have you played a game similar to Barbarossa in the past?		
Yes (Y)	2	10.00 %
No (N)	18	90.00 %

We have also addressed several questions to participants to understand their perception of game usability aspects of the first phase game mode (see Table 2).

Our evaluation results revealed that the invitational game mode performed well without any serious flaws that could affect players' experience. The above finding is backed by the only 6 error reports submitted by players to the Google Play Developer Console. Besides, the results indicate easy access to the invitational game mode. Finally, all players responded positively with respect to the games learnability (i.e. their ability to recall how to perform basic game actions).

After the completion of the second game phase we invited the players to complete questionnaires about the scenario they pursued in that phase followed by an interview. In order to assess the impact of the invitational mode to the players' comprehension of the game goals we asked the players to express their perception about the clarity of the

Table 2. Usability questions.

Overall, the game system performed well with no serious errors or flaws		
Strongly agree	9	45.00 %
Agree	10	50.00 %
Neutral	1	5.00 %
Disagree	0	0.00 %
Strongly disagree	0	0.00 %
It was easy to find, download, install and start the game		
Strongly agree	17	85.00 %
Agree	3	15.00 %
Neutral	0	0.00 %
Disagree	0	0.00 %
Strongly disagree	0	0.00 %
It was easy to learn and recall how to perform basic actions in the game		
Strongly agree	15	75.00 %
Agree	5	25.00 %
Neutral	0	0.00 %
Disagree	0	0.00 %
Strongly disagree	0	0.00 %

game goals. As illustrated in Table 3, the players (even the Knights who did not met their co-players in person and played far from the game stage location) were aware of the game goals and also felt responsible to complete their mission to support the success of their team.

Table 3. Overall game play experience & social/multiplayer aspects questions.

The game goal was comprehensible and unambiguous				
	Knight		Treasure Hunter	
Strongly agree	9	90.00 %	10	100.00 %
Agree	1	10.00 %	0	0.00 %
Neutral	0	0.00 %	0	0.00 %
Disagree	0	0.00 %	0	0.00 %
Strongly disagree	0	0.00 %	0	0.00 %
I felt responsible to complete my mission for my team to succeed				
	Knight		Treasure Hunter	
Strongly agree	7	70.00 %	9	90.00 %
Agree	2	20.00 %	1	10.00 %
Neutral	1	10.00 %	0	0.00 %
Disagree	0	0.00 %	0	0.00 %
Strongly disagree	0	0.00 %	0	0.00 %

Table 4. Interview questions about the invitation phase.

Question	Was the first phase of the game useful in order to understand the whole game concept?	Did the first phase of the game eased the second phase of the game completion?	Having played the first phase of the game, have you developed interest on how the game would progress?
Treasure Hunters	Yes (100 %)	Yes (100 %)	Yes (100 %)
Knights	Yes (100 %)	Yes (100 %)	Yes (100 %)

The most interesting questions investigating the impact of the first game phase have been asked during the interview, as we opted to allow participants to freely and fully express their views. In Table 4 we present the interview results concerning players' opinion on the utility of the invitational phase. Compiled participant answers are presented as a percentage of positive and negative answers. Answers are grouped by the player assigned roles into the second phase. The Pirate players have not been inquired about the first game phase as they have not participated to it (they have been invited into the second phase by their Treasure Hunters friends).

The results clearly indicate that all players admitted the invitational game mode impact in raising their awareness on the overall game concept as well as assisting the completion of the second phase scenario. Finally the invitational game mode triggered players' interest on the game's progression, thereby increasing their keenness to participate in Phase II.

4   Conclusion

Pervasive game prototype developers traditionally relied on emails, personal contacts and announcements/advertising to invite participants and perform user trials. In *Barbarossa*, we utilized an invitational game mode to recruit qualified participants for the user evaluation trials. The recruited participants provided valuable feedback and represented both players located worldwide (as the first phase of *Barbarossa* has been freely available online) and also located in the area where the game has been actually staged (Mytilene).

The evaluation results confirmed that the execution of a preparatory game mode, when applicable, can help developers to recruit highly qualified participants, truly enthusiastic to playing the game. Further, invitational game modes may serve as a useful instrument for developers to train evaluation participants on any technological equipment used in the game and also enhance their awareness on the overall game goal, scenario and gameplay.

References

1. Jegers, K.: Pervasive GameFlow: Identifying and Exploring the Mechanisms of Player Enjoyment in Pervasive Games. Department of informatics, Umeå university, Umea(2009)
2. Saarenpää, H.: Data Gathering Methods for Evaluating Playability of Pervasive Mobile Games (2008)
3. Montola, M., Stenros, J., Wærn, A.: Pervasive Games: Theory and Design. Morgan Kaufmann Publishers, Burlington (2009)
4. Fischer, J., Lindt, I., Stenros, J.: Final crossmedia report (Part II) – Epidemic Menace II evaluation report (2006)
5. Guo, B., Fujimura, R., Zhang, D., Imai, M.: Design-in-play: improving the variability of indoor pervasive games. Multimedia Tools Appl. **59**, 259–277 (2012)
6. Kirman, B., Linehan, C., Lawson, S.: Blowtooth: a provocative pervasive game for smuggling virtual drugs through real airport security. Pers. Ubiquit. Comput. **16**, 755–767 (2012)
7. Benford, S., Flintham, M., Drozd, A., Anastasi, R., Rowland, D., Tandavanitj, N., Adams, M., Row-Farr, J., Oldroyd, A., Sutton, J.: Uncle Roy all around you: implicating the city in a location-based performance. In: Proceedings of Advanced Computer Entertainment, ACM (2004)
8. Hannamari, S., Kuittinen, J., Montola, M.: Insectopia evaluation report (2007)
9. Jones, M., Marsden, G.: Mobile Interaction Design. Wiley, Chichester (2006)
10. Kasapakis, V., Gavalas, D., Bubaris, N.: Addressing openness and portability in outdoor pervasive role-playing games. In: Third International Conference on Communications and Information Technology (ICCIT), pp. 93–97 (2013)

Internet of Things Based Multiplayer Pervasive Games: An Architectural Analysis

André MacDowell$^{(\boxtimes)}$ and Markus Endler

Department of Informatics, Pontifícia Universidade Católica do Rio de Janeiro
(PUC-Rio) Rio de Janeiro, Rio de Janeiro, Brazil
{adowell, endler}@inf.puc-rio.br

Abstract. Recent advances, increasing affordability and popularity of Internet of Things (IoT) technologies are opening exciting new ways of interaction and sensing for mobile device users. Furthermore, the great acceptance of smart mobile devices in our daily lives makes possible various ludic experiences, which could be greatly improved with IoT technologies. This new setting opens many opportunities for design and development of Pervasive Games for the IoT. In this work, we propose a palette of canonic interaction models and gamification tactics that can be combined for the design of new Pervasive IoT Game experiences. Subsequently, we present the methodology and results of a validation interview regarding our model with experienced game designers. Finally, we present a case study for a Pervasive IoT Game, also giving an overview of our middleware for mobile communication as well as its extension for IoT, discussing the possibilities of implementing new Pervasive IoT Games using it.

Keywords: Pervasive games · Internet of things · Gamification · Middleware · Mobile · Collaborative · Multiplayer · Sensor tracking · Location based services · Sensing

1 Introduction

The recent emergence and increased deployment of Internet of Things (IoT) technologies are opening new avenues of research and development opportunities in Pervasive Games design. According to Gartner Group [1], IoT is "the network of physical objects that contains embedded technology to communicate and sense or interact with the objects' internal state or the external environment." One example of such IoT-enabling technology is Bluetooth® Smart (Bluetooth 4.0), which is rapidly expanding in the smartphone segment.[1] Nowadays, smartphones running the latest Android version, iPhones, Windows phones and Blackberry phones already support Bluetooth® Smart. In parallel, many companies are designing and producing several sorts of peripheral devices such as toys, watches, tennis shoes, heart-rate monitors and SensorTags[2] that are able to connect to Bluetooth® Smart Ready mobile phones.

---

[1] List of devices as of August-2014 at: http://www.bluetooth.com/Pages/Bluetooth-Smart-Devices.aspx.

[2] Texas Instruments, CC2541 Sensor Tags, April 2013. More information at: http://www.ti.com/lit/ml/swru324b/swru324b.pdf.

© Institute for Computer Sciences, Social Informatics and Telecommunications Engineering 2015
R. Giaffreda et al. (Eds.): IoT360 2014, Part I, LNICST 150, pp. 125–138, 2015.
DOI: 10.1007/978-3-319-19656-5_19

Therefore, very soon, many applications will revolve around the interaction with smart things, and games will be no exception. In fact, we envision that in the near future a huge variety of everyday objects, including toys, appliances, tools and other portable gadgets, will become *smart* and *connected* and will be silently incorporated on our daily lives and on our entertainment.

The referred smart objects usually feature some short-range wireless communication capability, as well as some limited processing and/or storage capability. Several of these objects will also have some embedded sensors (e.g., proximity, temperature, sound, light, acceleration, etc.) which will enable the objects to "sense and figure out what is happening in their environment".

Most importantly, these objects will be primarily low-energy, small, light-weight, and hence long-lived and portable. These last characteristics will lead, in our opinion, to an increasing incorporation of these smart objects as central elements in next-generation *Pervasive Games*, that is, games in which the traditional boundaries bestowed by traditional computer games are expanded in the social, temporal and spatial dimensions [2].

The era in which Pervasive and Mixed Reality Games will be part of our daily lives is already starting [3], and with these new technologies, the gameplay possibilities can be extended even further. Also, the increasing usage of *smartphones*[3] is a positive setting for a future in which *smart personal devices* can interact with *smart things*. In fact, we think that smart things and smartphones will be used *together* in future Pervasive IoT Games, where the latter will function as the player's window to the cyber-physical gameplay.

2 Towards Designing Pervasive IoT Games

We open the discussion with the question: *Should Pervasive IoT game design be significantly different from current mobile game design?* This is relevant because we are handling new and not widely tested (marketwise) technology. To answer that, it is interesting to separate two important concepts of game design: the *Base Interaction Model*, which is directly related to the gameplay mechanics, and the *Gamification Tactics*, which are tools and strategies to hold the attention of the player and immerse him onto the experience, thus transforming the player interaction into a proper game.

For the rest of this section, we propose a *model* for designing Pervasive IoT games through separation of the core elements of the game experience. We have to acknowledge the contribution, as base inspiration for this model, the works of [4–8]. The model was validated through a qualitative interview described in Sect. 3 of this work.

2.1 Interaction Models

As it would be in a mobile game played nowadays, or in any other console or computer game by all means, there are base interaction models that are combined to give a certain

---

[3] According to eMarketer: http://www.emarketer.com/Article/Smartphone-Users-Worldwide-Will-Total-175-Billion-2014/1010536.

gameplay experience to the player. The player could control a character in a tri-dimensional scenario using keyboard and mouse, or a controller, for instance. The player could also interact directly to a screen with his hands and control a certain object, or draw a certain pattern. These are all base interaction strategies that are applied, and combined many times, to give the player a more complex way to interact with the game and have a certain experience envisioned by the designer.

These interactions can differ deeply from each other depending on the category of the game being analyzed. During this work, we use several definitions regarding these game categories that are defined in our *Game Design and Interaction Analysis*, accessible at http://www.lac-rio.com/projects/pervasive-iot-games.

Below, we present a few of the interaction models we identified as possible for future IoT Pervasive Games using smart tokens as sensors/things, those of which are capable only of announcing their presence/proximity:

1. Find the Thing (e.g. Mobile Geocaching Game)
Tokens: Fixed or movable
Main Idea: Users search for smart tokens. When a certain token is found, this action is
   registered on the user's smart device and/or a cloud service (if the game is multiplayer). A user can also pick up a token and bring it somewhere else or do a
   certain action with it. If the token is being moved, its coordinates could be updated
   to the cloud service by the user's smart device's own GPS. The user's interaction
   with the token directly influences the type of gameplay a game with this base
   interaction might have.

2. Guess where Things will be (e.g. Radar Tag Game)
Tokens: Movable
Main Idea: Tokens are always on the move. Tokens could be owned by certain users or
   be entirely independent. Players might need to guess a pattern of movement or
   discern the tokens next position/destination. Players could interact with the tokens
   when around them in a way to facilitate this movement prediction.

3. Bring lonely Things together (e.g. Smart Tag Game)
Tokens: Movable
Main Idea: Tokens are owned by certain users. In certain moments of the game, some
   users might be required to match their tokens with another token, which might be
   in possession of another player. This other player might be required to match his
   token with this same user, or the contrary, he could have to avoid this user for a
   certain period of time. These play mechanics will of course vary depending of the
   real proposition of the game.

4. Things that color other Things (e.g. Zombie Infection or Area Control Game)
Tokens: Fixed or Movable
Main Idea: Tokens are emitters of a certain type of frequency/data. When a player with
   a smart device and/or a movable token enters the actuation diameter of said emitter,
   the player is then "colored" or "infected" and is now visible to the game as a player
   of a certain type/color. The player could now act as a movable emitter to other
   players or fixed tokens. This type of interaction could lead to interesting tag/area

control games, dealing with other gameplay mechanics such as map/area strategy on an urban area and teamwork.

5. Change the Thing

Tokens: Fixed or Movable

Main Idea: When the player interacts with the token, it writes certain data on it. From then on, the token may behave differently than before, or start broadcasting a different type of data.

2.2 Gamification Tactics for Pervasive Games

For this work, we define *Gamification Tactics* as features that are capable of transforming an otherwise common action, task or interaction with a game element into an enjoyable ludic activity. This definition is used normally for non-gaming contexts [9], but we will maintain it for this work since the main idea still is *to "gamify" an otherwise non-ludic interactive experience.*

The employed tactics normally are what differentiates a successful game from a failure. Some of them are meta-game features, which means that they add to the game experience although they act directly from other features of the same game (e.g. game achievements). Some of them are:

- *Improve Certain User Perks when the Player is Doing Well.* Each time a user guesses right, the user gets gameplay points to increase his/her radar cell diameter, or else, use more radar cells to better surround the token [e.g. *"Guess were Things will be"*].
- *Achievements:* Each time the user accomplishes a hard task or passes a specific milestone in the game, he is notified that he "achieved" this goal. The user can accompany his list of goals in another screen on the game or in another place.
- *Customization:* The player can customize certain aspects of the game (normally related to graphical assets) at his will or from a certain pre-defined list of assets.
- *Storytelling/Environment Setting/Graphics/Music:* The game has artistic components that complement the overall game experience by themselves. These are usually very important on computer and console gaming, but a little less on mobile.
- *In-game Fictional Currency:* The player gets a fictional currency on the game after doing certain objectives or achieving certain milestones, which he can use to unlock or improve other aspects of the game (like the ones related to these other tactics).
- *In-game Purchases:* Successful on both mobile and console games (Digital Games), the player has the possibility to buy for real money something related to one of these others tactics (including fictional currency), which simplifies the acquisition of new content if the player is not willing to pass through the previously defined method by the designer.
- *Point-Based Ranking or Leaderboard:* Also present on Analog Games (e.g. Sports) and Digital Games generally, the fact that your progress and feedback is scored by points and those scores can be compared to those of other players induces competitiveness and further interest to the game.

2.3   Pervasive Storytelling

Storytelling as commonly known in today's games could be used in new innovative ways when applied in IoT Pervasive Games. A game with immersive and dynamic storytelling could make use of the *"Find the Thing"* base interaction, for example, and unfold its own story to the player following the data retrieved by him during inter-actions with placed tokens on an environment. It could also send a specific signal to the token, so that the story will be different when the next user arrives at said token (e.g. *"Change the Thing"*).

These are experiences that could be, in the near future we envision, very common in our daily lives and could be very well used for advertising, public events, social interactions, massive urban games, and more.

2.4   Game Mechanics and the Overall Player Experience

The design of a game in terms of its playability derives from various types of smaller simpler interactions. When these interactions are mixed with gamification tactics (notably environmental setting and storytelling), the game gives the player a sense of immersion and a complex experience that is usually greater than the sum of its smaller parts.

This principle is a key factor in general game design, but it is especially important in games that are dealing with new types of technologies, those of which usually lead to new base interactions such as the ones described previously as IoT/Pervasive mobile nodes and sensors interaction. When these factors are well worked, it means that the overall experience given by the game is a concise experience that will most likely be well absorbed by the player and, thus, lead to a successful game.

3   Validating Our Model – Qualitative Interviews

The goal of this evaluation is to inquire if the proposed method to abstract the inter-action and gamification tactics for the design of Pervasive IoT Games into independent architectural elements is valid for those who will most likely use it, *game developers*. To validate this architectural proposition, we would like to assess if the proposed set of game elements is sufficient to abstract an independent game experience.

3.1   Methodology

Since our goal is to serve as guideline for game developers interested in pervasive mobile games and IoT, we aim with this interview to validate that, in a game developer view's, the model is sufficiently concise and robust to abstract the game elements of different categories of game experiences. On other level, we also search if the model is sufficient not only to abstract the game experience, but to fully describe it. Our goal is to have some confirmation from the developers that the model is at least sufficient for the abstraction of the experience, not directly aiming for the second "fully description" goal.

There are very few popular pervasive games on the market for us to define them as a specific game category for the interview. Because of that, we will use two other categories of games: *Analog Games* and *Digital Games* (both mobile and console).[4] These categories represent well the mixture of physical games in the real world and digital games on a virtual world in a way that fits what is accepted to be a Pervasive Game, since it breaks the known temporal and spatial boundaries of most games [2, 4, 6].

The interview was conducted with eight game developers, and it was proposed for the interviewee to analyze three different games. The games were *"Tag Game"* (Analog), *"Grand Theft Auto IV"* (Digital/Console Game) and *"Angry Birds"* (Digital/ Mobile Game). The subject was asked to abstract the interaction and gamification tactics from the games according to the proposed elements of both categories in an annex of the interview.[5] After the analysis of each game, the interviewee was asked some questions about his acquiescence with the abstraction he/she just did, and also asked to comment further about it, making suggestions and critics for the model.

The interview was sent by email and Facebook for the interviewees, together with a small explanation about it, which comprehended: *That it was to prove or disprove a model to abstract game experiences; That criticism was highly acceptable; That in it they would analyze three games - and then proceeded listing them; That they had to check in Page 2 and 3 of the interview about the elements they would want to use to abstract the game experiences; That if they felt like it wasn't enough, they should explain why, and if necessary, propose other elements; and That when in doubt, just do what you think it's right.*

3.2 Result Analysis[6]

The eight interviewees were all Brazilians, male, average of 25 years old, 4.5 years of game developing experience and 20 years of experience as gamers. They all succeeded in choosing interactions and gamification tactics from the balloons in the annex to abstract each game, differing in their arguments on why they choose one or another balloon and on the abstraction itself.

Also, as it was expected, the acceptance of the model as "adequate" to abstract the player experience (Question 2–58 %) was higher than the acceptance of the model as being capable of "fully characterizing the player experience" (Question 3–30 %). By analyzing the structure of the negative feedback, we identified two main problems: a *structural problem* and a *content problem*. The structural problem is related to the structure of the model, which is either too abstract or too specialized on the types of interactions and gamification tactics. This is reflected on comments like this:

"The balloons were a bit confusing from a game development point, and some of them felt very specific to describe the games in question. This would prove to be a problem if the objective is to create descriptions that can apply to any game.!"

---

[4] More information can be found in the *Game Design and Interaction Analysis* at http://www.lac-rio.com/projects/pervasive-iot-games.

[5] The model of the interview, proposed interactive and gamification elements, full results and interview transcripts can be also accessed at http://www.lac-rio.com/projects/pervasive-iot-games.

[6] As was commented previously, the full and uncommented results of the interviews can be found at the LAC website, at the footnotes on the last page.

The other type of problem is a content problem, which happened when the interviewee could not find a specific interaction or tactic within the balloons:

"'Identify roles', or 'Identify others logical state'. Something related to each participant in a way to identify all the others as runners or chasers."

Which was most of the time because either the interviewee was confused and couldn't find a balloon that expressed what he wanted, or that balloon actually wasn't there, thus, expressing a "lack of content" problem. The content problem doesn't goes against the model, since it can be easily solved by simply increasing the variety of interactions and/or gamification tactics, which is not a structural problem with the model. By considering as negative acceptance only the structural problems, we see an increase in both acceptance rates for our "adequate" (67 %) and "fully characterizes" (63 %) game experiences.

It's also interesting that, from all three types of games, the one with the highest acceptance rate for the model is "Angry Birds", a mobile game with many strong gamification elements. The lowest was the "Tag Game", mainly because of the difficulty in visualizing gamification tactics for an Analog Game.

Although we discussed acceptance rates, our focus wasn't really on the statistics from the interviews, but for the actual feedback as how well the model can be used to abstract these experiences. In general, it was met with positive feedback, since all of the content problems are positive for the model validation. Like this answer for Question 2:

"No. They give great insight about the ambience of the game and player motivation, but lack one important aspect of gameplay that molds the whole player experience which are the puzzles that must be solved on each level. The scenarios present multiple obstacles that challenge the player both mentally (as he must discover the solution) and skillfully (as he must aim correctly to implement his strategy). Suggested balloons are: 'Puzzle' and 'Obstacle' (relation status with other elements)"

By suggesting the inclusion of balloons like "Puzzle" and "Obstacle", they are actually affirming that they understood the main concept, which is to mold the player experience with these interaction and gamification elements, which is even doable with the current suggested balloons, since the both experiences can be derived by smaller and simpler elements.

It is apparent for us that, after the interviews, the model is *sufficient* to abstract game experiences, dividing them into interaction elements and gamification elements, but not entirely adequate to fully describe all game's nuances and every possible iteration of player experience, since it is, as it was observed looking at the results, a *very different experience for each person*.

4 Case Study – Area Control Game with Mobile IoT

As part of a case study for our architectural analysis of Pervasive IoT games, we designed a game with enough features as to represent the proposed model. The game is still under development and its first version is due to the end of 2014.

The game is similar to the analog playground game known as *capture the flag*. It is a local multiplayer session game, meaning it is played by a certain number of people in a specific area and time, and it has finite duration. The players will carry *smart devices* supporting Bluetooth® Smart technology, and the flags will be *mobile objects with sensors* (such as the previously mentioned Texas Instruments Sensor Tag) capable of capturing contextual information from their environment and transmitting these sensed data through their Bluetooth® Smart interfaces.

4.1 Playability

Players are divided in two or three teams, each of which owns one or more flags. Flags are initially placed within a pre-determined area belonging to each team (Fig. 1).

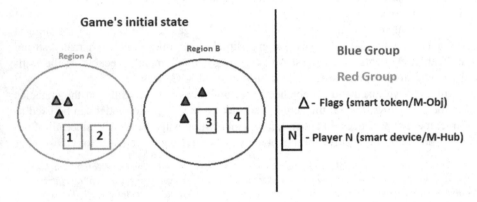

Fig. 1. A simple mockup of the game's initial state

The goal of each team is to take all the other team's flags and move them to their own region, but an opponent player can take flags only if they are unguarded. Players can guard their own flags by staying in the same region as theirs or by carrying them around the game area.

When players from different groups meet or a flag-taking attempt happens, the involved players engage in a battle. The battle winners can take a flag if the losers are carrying/guarding one, and the losers can't fight or steal flags for a period of time. The game ends when all the flags are owned by a single team.

Since the game's theme surrounds the idea of controlling an enemy's area and slowly advancing your position (it can be modified so that each group has several control areas, or maybe with control areas previously un-owned by both groups), its tentative codename is *Area Control Game with Mobile IoT*.

4.2 Tentative System Architecture

Players are viewed by the system as mobile devices and flags as mobile smart objects. The smart objects are not capable of direct connection with the server, so their location/state is only updated upon interaction with the players.

The server infers flag ownership considering the flag's last known location, last owner and last battle in which it was involved. The players are always sharing location information with the server and listening to broadcasts from the smart sensors (through Bluetooth). The server will notify a player if another player from a different group is nearby and their direction. If they are close enough, they can engage in battle, and only then the players will know if one of them is carrying a flag, being notified on their smart devices.

Player battles will occur through their smart devices following a *weighted rock-paper-scissors* method. Players will have experience points that will be counted as a weight on their attack choice, so a high level player can win a battle even choosing a weapon weak against the other players'. Players get more experience points by winning individual battles, capturing flags and winning games.

The system architecture on a lower level will follow the ContextNet Architecture for IoMT Collaborative Applications [14, 15]. This architecture will be further described in the Sect. 5 of this work.

4.3   IoT Pervasive Game Model Analysis

Being an IoT Pervasive game, the Area Control IoT Game should be abstractable through our Interaction/Gamification model:

Interaction Models. The game has direct interaction between players and things in a way that: Players have to *"Find Things"* and *"Change Things"*. Also, things interact with players in a way to broadcast their proximity, while player information is constantly updated to the server, which updates other players with the information, which interacts with other things. This means that, in a way, the interaction possibilities between things can mimic one of the *"Things color other things"* interaction.

Gamification Tactics. Since the players have experience points that influence on the game mechanics, we have the *"Improve certain user perks when the player is doing well"* aspect. Also, *"Achievements"*, *"Customization"*, *"Storytelling"*, *"Environment Setting"* and *"Graphics"* are all aspects that could act positively in the final gaming experience.

Re-construction of the Game Experience Experiment. The idea is that if we change an interaction and/or a gamification tactic to some other, the game experience will still be concise, but the final game will be entirely different.

For example, if we remove the *"Change the Thing"* interaction and add *"Guess where things will be"*, we can come up with a game in which some sensors are fixed and visible to the player (broadcasting proximity) and others are movable but untraceable. The players have to find (*"Find the Thing"*) the fixed sensor to receive a clue about the whereabouts of the movable thing. After that, the player will follow the clue so than it can reach the movable thing close enough, and by doing that he receives a point.

A ranking (*"Point-based leaderboard"*) of the players with most findings can be updated daily do that the players can compete with each other (removing the *"Improve user perks"* in this case).

With this exercise, we can assess that by changing a few elements of the base interactions between game elements and the gamification tactics employed in the game, we can drastically change the final game experience for the player.

5 The ContextNet Architecture

Project ContextNet is primarily focused on developing middleware services and APIs aimed at facilitating the development of large-scale context-aware pervasive and mobile applications [10]. It is in constant evolution, but it has already been used for the development of some quite complex distributed mobile applications.[7] The code is freely available for download,[8] but not open source. This middleware and its recent extension for IoT will be used as the basis for developing multiplayer Pervasive IoT Games.

5.1 The Communication Middleware

ContextNet defines a high-performance mobile communication middleware, called *Scalable Data Distribution Layer (SDDL)* [11]. This middleware connects Stationary Nodes of a core network (*a.k.a.*, the *SDDL Core*) with all Mobile Nodes. While the former are desktops or servers executing in a cluster, or cloud, over the OMG DDS [12] middleware, the latter are mobile end user devices (i.e. smartphones and tablets).

The SDDL communication protocol for inbound-outbound communication between the SDDL Core and the mobile nodes is the Mobile Reliable UDP (MR-UDP) [13]. In a nutshell, MR-UDP is Reliable-UDP with mechanisms for tolerating intermittent connectivity, dynamic IP address changes of the Mobile nodes and reaching these nodes behind firewalls/NATs. It is used by the mobile nodes to connect with a special type of SDDL Core node called *Gateway*, of which any number can be deployed in the SDDL Core. Each Gateway maintains one independent MR-UDP connection with each mobile node, and is responsible for translating application-messages from MR-UDP to the intra-SDDL core protocol, and, in the opposite direction, converting core messages to MR-UDP messages and delivering them reliably to the corresponding mobile nodes.

The SDDL Core has several other specialized nodes (see Fig. 2): the *PoA-Manager*, which holds the addresses list of all currently active Gateways and eventually requests mobile nodes to switch Gateways; *GroupDefiners* evaluate the group-memberships of all mobile nodes (based on some attribute of their inbound application messages) and

---

[7] More information at http://www.lac-rio.com/projects.

[8] Accessible at http://www.lac-rio.com/software.

manage the reliable delivery of group-cast messages to the mobiles, and the *Controller*, which provides a Map-based user interface to visualize and interact with any mobile node of the system.

Finally, there is the *ClientLib (CNCLib)*, a Java library which establishes and manages a MR-UDP connection of a mobile node client (in Java, Android or Lua), and the Gateways. It hides most MR-UDP details end error handling from the application layer, and supports application-transparent handover of the mobile node between SDDL Gateways.

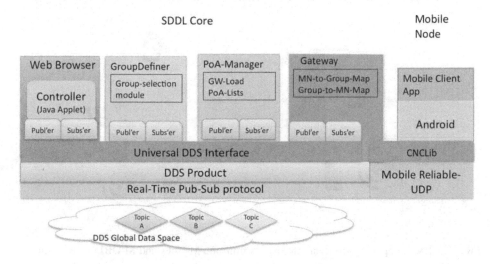

Fig. 2. Nodes and protocols used in SDDL, as seen in [11].

The SDDL has been extensively tested in lab experiments, mainly because we wanted to test the system with thousands of mobile nodes, and doing such large-scale tests in with real devices the field is not feasible. In our performance tests, we observed that the Gateways support up to 5000 simultaneous MR-UDP connections each and a total throughput of 5000 messages/s inbound. However, we have also tested the SDDL middleware over 2G/3G wireless Internet connections (while the testers roamed through the city), and obtained good results with respect to latency and message loss. More details of our performance tests can be found in Sect. 4 of [11].

5.2   SDDL as a Middleware for IoT Games

In the last couple of months, the ContextNet project embraced support for applications in the *Internet of Mobile Things* (IoMT). Therefore, the SDDL middleware was extended with the concept of a *Mobile Hub (M-Hub)* [14, 15]. In IoMT, a "smart thing or object" can/will be mobile, and is therefore called *Mobile Object (M-OBJ)*. M-OBJs have short-range wireless communication allowing them to interact with nearby Mobile Hubs. These M-Hubs are portable devices, such as smartphones, which: (a) have

MR-UDP connectivity with a Gateway of the SDDL Core in the a cloud; (b) have means of obtaining their current geographic position and (c) have a short-range wireless communication interface, allowing them to discover, connect and interact with close M-OBJs.

We plan to use this SDDL middleware extension for IoMT as the basis for our Pervasive IoT Game, the *Area Control Game*. Essentially, it will consists of mobile clients and one or more *Game Processing Nodes (GPN)*, to be deployed in the SDDL Core. The *GPN* will be responsible for the long-range communication as it processes the information passed by the gateways, primarily received from the M-Hubs (Fig. 3).

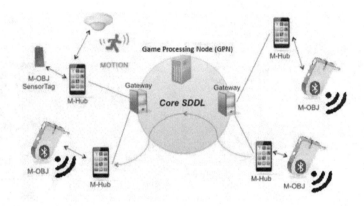

Fig. 3. GPNs computes contextual information from the M-Hubs and M-OBJs, like location.

Besides our Area Control Game case study, we idealized a few examples of perfectly implementable IoT Pervasive games using the ContextNet Middleware technology for mobile nodes communication. Below is the idealized architecture for these examples summarized:

- **Sensor and Token Structures (Mobile Object or M-ObJ)**
  - They have a UUID[9] and some set of attributes.
  - They can broadcast and unicast small packets of information to M-Hubs and to each other (but only through M-Hubs).
  - They will most likely use the Bluetooth® LE Technology, but can also use other types of communication technology, since the GPN is capable of abstracting the data it receives and pass it forth.
  - Most of them will also have some on-board sensors that reveal information of the object's current state and environment (e.g. temperature)
  - They can have memory, so they can store the information sent by the M-Hubs.

---

[9] A universally unique identifier is an identifier standard used in software construction, standardized by the Open Software Foundation as part of the Distributed Computing Environment: http://en.wikipedia.org/wiki/Universally_unique_identifier.

- **Mobile Hubs (M-Hub)**
  - The smart devices carried by the users. They must be able to "synch" with more than one M-Obj at the same time.
  - They must be capable of mixing information obtained from the Internet with information obtained from nearby M-Objs.
  - They should preferable have access to GPS, as most of the interesting applications are Location Based, but thats not mandatory.
  - They will communicate with other M-Hubs and possibly with a cloud service through the SDDL Middleware.
  - Have much greater storage, processing and battery capacity than M-Objs.
  - Acts as the long-haul communication intermediary for M-OBJs in its proximity, as well as a point of reference.

Also, we just finished a first prototype of M-Hub for Android. This prototype runs on our Moto E smart phone, which has Bluetooth® Smart and already detects and connects to nearby Bluetooth devices playing the role of a M-OBJ. The M-Hub already attaches its current GPS coordinate to the M-OBJ's sensor data, and sends a JSON message, via MR-UDP whenever it connects or disconnects from the M-OBJ.

We also observed that the discovery and connection times of a M-OBJ to a M-Hub takes at most 9 s when the Bluetooth Smart connects for the first time, but only 300 ms on all the following connections.

6 Conclusion

We believe that all technology needed to implement these ideas are already at hand. This work's main goal is to organize design patterns, strategies and important features that should exist in future IoT Pervasive games, so that future developers can properly use these ideas.

Another objective we have is to show through our case studies how IoT Gaming can have great social and cultural impact as they can be used to encourage participatory sensing for urban development, collective action, to report problems (like crackling sidewalks on urban areas), and urban environment. These can be achieved mainly through a clever use of both base interactions and gamification tactics.

Thus, by showing a few examples of case studies of such games using our ContextNet Architecture for IoMT applications, and by analyzing our feedback from the model validation interview, we are able to confirm that these strategies are capable of achieving their main goal: to build new engaging pervasive game experiences.

Acknowledgements. We acknowledge the partial financial support through fostering scholarship from CNPQ, process no. 153910/2013-5.

References

1. Perkins, E.: Gartner Group Getting Past the Word Games to Secure the Internet of Things. http://blogs.gartner.com/earl-perkins/2014/03/05/getting-past-the-word-games-to-secure-the-internet-of-things/ (2014). Accessed 4 July 2014

2. Montola, M.: Exploring the edge of the magic circle: defining pervasive games. In: Proceedings of DAC, p. 103, December 2005
3. Hodson, H.: Google's ingress game is a gold mine for augmented reality. New Sci. (1971) **216**(2893), 19 (2012). doi:10.1016/S0262-4079(12)63058-9
4. Magerkurth, C., Cheok, A.D., Mandryk, R.L., Nilsen, T.: Pervasive games: bringing computer entertainment back to the real world. Comput. Entertainment (CIE) **3**(3), 4 (2005)
5. Stenros, J., Montola, M., Mäyrä, F.: Pervasive games in ludic society. In: Proceedings of the 2007 Conference on Future Play, pp. 30–37. ACM, November 2007
6. Wetzel, R.: A case for design patterns supporting the development of mobile mixed reality games. In: Second Workshop on Design Patterns in Games (2013)
7. Antoniou, V., Schlieder, C.: Participation patterns, VGI and gamification. In: AGILE 2014 – Castellón, 3–6 June 2014
8. Ballagas, R., Kuntze, A., Walz, S.P.: Gaming tourism: lessons from evaluating REXplorer, a pervasive game for tourists. In: Indulska, J., Patterson, D.J., Rodden, T., Ott, M. (eds.) PERVASIVE 2008. LNCS, vol. 5013, pp. 244–261. Springer, Heidelberg (2008)
9. Deterding S., Sicart M., Nacke L., O'Hara, K., Dixon, D.: Gamification: using game-design elements in non-gaming contexts. In: CHI 2011 Extended Abstracts on Human Factors in Computing Systems (CHI EA 2011), pp. 2425–2428. ACM, New York, NY, USA, (2011). doi:10.1145/1979742.1979575
10. Endler M., Baptista G., David L., Vasconcelos R., Malcher M., Pantoja V., Pinheiro V., Viterbo J.: ContextNet: context reasoning and sharing middleware for large-scale pervasive collaboration and social networking. In: Proceedings of the Workshop on Posters and Demos Track (PDT 2011), Article 2, p. 2. ACM, New York, NY, USA (2011). doi:10.1145/2088960.2088962
11. David, L., Vasconcelos, R., Alves, L., André, R., Endler, M.: A DDS-based middleware for scalable tracking, communication and collaboration of mobile nodes. J. Internet Serv. Appl. **4**(1), 1–15 (2013). doi:10.1186/1869-0238-4-16
12. OMG: Data Distribution Service Portal. http://portals.omg.org/dds/. Accessed June 2014
13. Silva, L.D., Roriz, M., Endler, M.: MR-UDP: Yet another reliable user datagram protocol, now for mobile nodes, Monografias em Ciência da Computação, nr. MCC 06/13, Departamento de Informática, PUC-Rio (2013). ISSN 0103-9741
14. Endler, M. et al.: ContextNet reaches out to the Internet of Things. http://www.lac-rio.com/news/contextnet-reaches%C2%A0out-the%C2%A0internet-of%C2%A0things (2014). Accessed 4 Aug 2014
15. Talavera, L.E., Endler, M., Vasconcelos, I., Vasconcelos, R.,Cunha, M., Silva, F.S.: The Mobile Hub Concept: Enabling applications for the Internet of Mobile Things, Monografias em Ciência da Computação, nr. MCC 04/14, Departamento de Informática, PUC-Rio (2014). ISSN 0103-9741
16. Duan, J., Gao, D., Yang, D., Foh, C.H., Chen, H.H.: An energy-aware trust derivation scheme with game theoretic approach in wireless sensor networks for IoT applications. IEEE Internet Things J. **1**(1), 58–69 (2014). doi:10.1109/JIOT.2014.2314132

PacMap: Transferring PacMan
to the Physical Realm

Thomas Chatzidimitris[✉], Damianos Gavalas, and Vlasios Kasapakis

Department of Cultural Technology and Communication,
University of the Aegean, Mytilene, Greece
{tchatz, dgavalas, v.kasapakis}@aegean.gr

Abstract. This paper discusses the implementation of the pervasive game *PacMap*. Openness and portability have been the main design objectives for PacMap. We elaborate on programming techniques which may be applicable to a broad range of location-based games that involve the movement of virtual characters over map interfaces. In particular, we present techniques to execute shortest path algorithms on spatial environments bypassing the restrictions imposed by commercial mapping services. Last, we present ways to improve the movement and enhance the intelligence of virtual characters taking into consideration the actions and position of players in location-based games.

Keywords: Pacmap · Pacman · Pervasive games · Location-based games · Shortest path · Dijkstra

1 Introduction

Pervasive gaming is an emerging gaming genre that transfers gameplay from the virtual world to the real environment, leading to the spatial, temporal and social expansion of the magic circle [1]. The key element in these games is the awareness and incorporation of user context: depending on the location, environmental or social context the game's scenario and the gameplay are adjusted accordingly.

When this genre of games appeared, the use of wearable devices (like sensors and GPS) was deemed necessary to capture user and environmental context, although the use of such equipment has been reported to affect the user's immersion during the gameplay. The advent of smartphones with their advanced processing, networking and sensory capabilities overturned the abovementioned restrictions of wearable equipment and provided pervasive games developers the means for implementing computationally intensive, context-aware applications commonly incorporating augmented reality.

This paper introduces PacMap, a pervasive variant of the classical game PacMan. PacMap has been largely inspired by Human PacMan [2], a milestone pervasive game project released in 2004. From the technology perspective, PacMap makes use of infrastructure and resources still unavailable at the time that Human PacMan was protoyped: it uses widely available equipment (like smartphones), 3G or WiFi networks, GPS and sensors. Furthermore, our prototype incorporates programming techniques and principles applicable to a wide range of location-based hunting/chase games. In particular, the implementation of PacMap aims at creating appealing and

© Institute for Computer Sciences, Social Informatics and Telecommunications Engineering 2015
R. Giaffreda et al. (Eds.): IoT360 2014, Part I, LNICST 150, pp. 139–144, 2015.
DOI: 10.1007/978-3-319-19656-5_20

engaging game spaces, allowing anytime/anywhere gameplay, without any need for orchestration. The game stage is set around the actual location of the user and considers the actual surrounding road segments as game action 'corridors'. Moreover, we propose an implementation that utilizes the high level information granularity inherent in open map platforms and breaks the dependency on commercial map providers who set daily/monthly limits on the number of web service invocations. Finally, this paper suggests techniques for the smooth movement of virtual characters on map-based interfaces, which should adapt real-time on the actual player movement within the game space.

2   Related Work

Location-based games claim a major share in pervasive games market. Many research prototypes [2–6] as well as some commercial games, like Ingress[1] and Zombies Run,[2] use location-aware services to support their scenario, having the user's location as point of reference.

Human Pacman has been a milestone pervasive game (notably, one of the first to transfer the experience of an arcade game out to the physical world), which largely inspired the design of PacMap. Using a slightly modified game plot of the traditional Pacman, players are enrolled as pacmen, helpers and ghosts. The interaction, as well as the movement of players within the game space, requires the use of devices, like sensors and wireless LAN Cards, which are stored in a backpack. The players also carry head-mounted displays, whereon information about the plot of the game and augmented reality content are projected. The use of equipment, the need for orchestration (helpers) and the difficulty to set the game space at any location, seriously limits the portability and openness of the game.

The evolution of mobile computing (most notably, the emergence of mobile devices like smartphones, tablets, smart watches, etc.), has radically changed the design and development of pervasive games. The incorporation of technologies, like GPS, sensors (accelerometer, gyroscope, proximity, compass, barometer, gesture, heart rate, etc.) and built-in cameras provided game designers and developers the looked-for machinery to build location-based games with complex and appealing scenarios, and limited the requirement for specialized supplementary equipment. Notably, latest research prototypes commonly consume mapping services [5], like Google Maps, as well as relevant web services (e.g. directions for walking and transit transfers, points of interest, elevation, traffic and geocoding), which are provided by the service providers via specialized Application Programming Interfaces (APIs).

The use of several among the above mentioned services (e.g. the directions service) is subject to commercial usage. In practice, this limits the number of monthly invocations under a certain development license. This restriction raises a major challenge in the design of location-based games which involve heavy use of mapping services

---

[1] https://play.google.com/store/apps/details?id=com.nianticproject.ingress.

[2] https://play.goggle.com/store/apps/details?id=com.sixtostart.zombiesrun.

(e.g. chase/hunt games), especially those enrolling intelligent virtual characters and require execution of path finding algorithms for virtual hunters.

3 Game Scenario

The game scenario of PacMap adheres as much as possible to that of the classic arcade game Pacman. It is a location-based game, which requires Internet connection and enabled GPS receiver in the device. The game space is determined at startup, considering the actual road segments around the user's position as possible walking corridors for the pacman player. The user is supposed to collect all the cookies positioned across the streets. Unlike the pacman which us acted by a human player, the enemies (i.e. the ghosts) are virtual characters handled by the game engine. Similarly to the original arcade game, the ghosts are supposed to catch pacman, each following a different mobility pattern moving on the map, around the user's area. The purple, orange and blue ghosts execute random movements in the game space. The red ghost follows the user as the latter moves within the gamespace. Figure 1 illustrates a snapshot of the PacMap's gameplay.

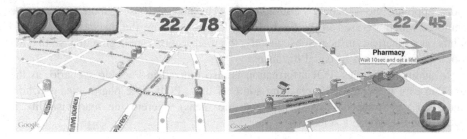

Fig. 1. PacMap gameplay screenshots.

4 Game Engine Architecture

PacMap's system's architecture adopts a typical client-server model. The server side part undertakes the fabrication of the game space, whereas the client side visualizes the game space and enables the interaction among the player and the game engine.

As illustrated in Fig. 2, the client sends out his location information to the game server in order to create the appropriate game space. The latter is confined by a circle around the user's location, with a radius of 200 m. The game server uses the geolocation information to contact a map server and retrieve the nodes and POIs lying within this imaginary circle (the communication is handled by the OpenStreetMap API[3]).

---

[3] OpenStreetMap is an open-source mapping service, providing developers with useful crowdsourced topographical information. Data contributors may register geospatial elements such as nodes and POIs along the street network. Among others, the OpenStreetMap web services allow exporting the vertices of rectilinear parts, comprising a road network.

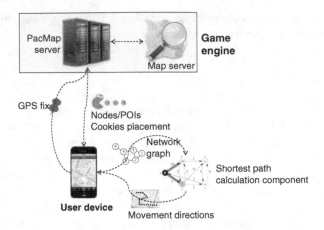

Fig. 2. PacMap system architecture.

The arrangement of game components within the game space (e.g. the placement of cookies) is carried out through utilizing the area nodes information. To ensure even distribution of cookies, the game engine firstly measures the distance between two nodes applying the Vincenty's formulae [7]. The latter is based upon two iterative methods, which are used in the field of Geodesy to measure the distance among two points on a spherical surface. Subsequently, the road sections are segmented, so that the cookies can be placed in equal distances.

In addition to nodes, POI information is also utilized in PacMap scenario, as the user can earn life credits, by reaching some of these POIs (like pharmacies and hospitals), or get "trapped" (e.g. in bar/nightlife areas) wherein the map visibility is reduced on the device's screen.

5   PacMap Implementation

The arcade game Pacman involves ghosts which chase the pacman, with their movement promptly adapting to that of pacman. In order to transfer such functionality to a map-based interface each ghost needs to receive a series of road segments to be traversed. Provided a start and an end location (e.g. the current location of the ghost and the player, respectively) a reasonable action for the ghost following the user is to invoke a 'direction' web service typically offered by commercial map data providers (e.g. the Directions service of the Google Maps API) and then faithfully follow the shortest path walking directions recommended by the service. However, if the user location changes too often, direction service invocations (passing the updated ghost/player location parameters) will increase accordingly and soon exceed the invocations limit set by commercial providers.

Enemies (i.e. ghosts) movement patterns fall into two types. Orange, blue and purple ghosts repeatedly execute a random movement around the map. To implement these movements, we derive two random pairs of coordinates over the arc of the imaginary circle centered at the user's current position. These two pairs of coordinates (representing the start/end nodes of each successive ghost movement) are submitted to the Directions API service of the map server, thus generating the actual path to be followed by each ghost. From the games research viewpoint, the movement of the red ghost is more challenging as it presumably applicable to many alike map/location-based chase games, since (according to the PacMap scenario) it is supposed to follow the user as s/he moves within the game space.

Ghosts movement respects the game space topography, namely the nodes exported from the game server during the game space generation phase (see Fig. 3a). Considering a graph transformation of the game space (connecting adjacent nodes which are connected through a road segment on the actual setting and calculating the distances among them), it is then straightforward to execute a shortest path algorithm to compute the path to be followed by the user (see Fig. 3b). PacMap's directions service implements the Dijkstra's algorithm,[4] wherein edge costs equal the physical distance among their connected end nodes. For example, the red ghost considers the node nearest to the ghost's current location as start node and the node the user currently heads to as end node (e.g. node B in Fig. 3a).

Shortest paths are derived whenever the user reaches a new edge or turns to another direction. To ensure prompt adaptation of ghost's movement to the player's movement, the device determines the nodes among which the user is currently located whenever his location (i.e. GPS fix) is updated.

(a)   **(b)**

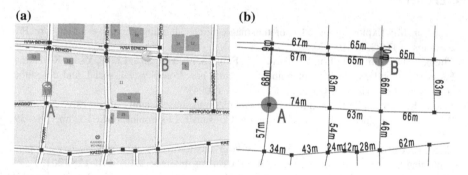

Fig. 3. (a) An example game space illustrating the extracted topology nodes; (b) shortest path derived by a directions service executing Dijkstra's algorithm upon a graph transformation of the game space (Color figure online).

The sole goal of the ghost is to "catch" pacman, i.e. to reach its currently assigned end node, having gone through the edge currently traversed by the user. In case that the ghost arrives at its end node without passing via the player's edge, the algorithm is re-executed, with the other end point of that edge set as the new end point for the requested directions.

---

[4] Dijkstra's algorithm is a graph search algorithm that solves the single-source shortest path problem for a graph with non-negative edge path costs, producing a shortest path tree.

It is noted that the shortest path algorithm is executed on the client side to eliminate the effect of network latency inherent in client-server interactions. On an average game space considering 420 nodes, the algorithm takes 95 ms to yield the shortest path when executed on a Samsung Galaxy S4 device (processor: ARMv7 – 1.8 GHz × 4 cores/ ram:1.8 GB).

6 Conclusion

We introduced the prototype pervasive game PacMap, one of the few attempts to migrate a classical arcade game onto the physical realm. We have proposed programming techniques largely applicable to nearly any map-based chase game scenario, the main objective being to ensure openness and portability. We have also discussed implementation techniques for path-finding on real urban settings which bypass the restrictions imposed by commercial Direction APIs. The use of those techniques enables programmers and designers to develop location/map-based games, with flexible scenarios that involve intelligent virtual characters dynamically adapting on players movement behavior during the game.

References

1. Montola, M.: Exploring the edge of the magic circle: defining pervasive games. In: Proceedings of DAC, p. 103 (2005)
2. Cheok, A.D., Goh, K.H., Liu, W., Farbiz, F., Fong, S.W., Teo, S.L., Li, Y., Yang, X.: Human Pacman: a mobile, wide-area entertainment system based on physical, social, and ubiquitous computing. Pers. Ubiquit. Comput. 8(2), 71–81 (2004)
3. Jantke, K.P., Arnold, O., Spundflasch, S.: Aliens on the bus: a family of pervasive games. In: Proceedings of 2nd Global Conference on Consumer Electronics (GCCE), pp. 387–391 (2013)
4. Chen, L., Chen, G., Benford, S.: Your way your missions: a location-aware pervasive game exploiting the routes of players. Int. J. Hum. Comput. Interact. 29(2), 110–128 (2013)
5. Kasapakis, V., Gavalas, D., Bubaris, N.: Addressing openness and portability in outdoor pervasive role-playing games. In: Proceedings of the 3rd International Conference on Communications and Information Technology (ICCIT 2013), pp. 93–97 (2013)
6. de Souza e silva, A.: Alien revolt (2005–2007): a case study of the first location-based mobile game in Brazil. IEEE Technol. Soc. Mag. 27(1), 18–28 (2008)
7. Vincenty, T.: Direct and inverse solutions of geodesics on the ellipsoid with application of nested equations. Surv. Rev. 23(176), 88–93 (1975)

Exergames for Elderly in Ambient Assisted Living Environments

Determinants for Performance Technology Acceptance

Philipp Brauner[(⊠)] and Martina Ziefle

Human-Computer Interaction Center, RWTH Aachen University,
Campus Boulevard 57, 52074 Aachen, Germany
{brauner,ziefle}@comm.rwth-aachen.de

Abstract. Ambient Assisted Living (AAL) environments offer a solution to the challenges of the demographic change by supporting elderly and chronically ill people inside their own home environments. Serious and pervasive games can change people's attitudes and can promote healthy behavior. However, both concepts are rarely combined and the integration of both concepts is insufficiently explored. We present a user study (n = 64) of an Exergame for AAL environments with the research foci performance and acceptance. Age is the predominant factor for performance, while the intention to use is determined by gaming frequency. Neither technical self-efficacy nor age had considerable influence on these measures. However, the interaction with the game had a considerable positive effect on the participant's perceived health and pain. The study shows that Exergames in AAL environments are a viable solution to support the autonomy and independence of people in an aging society.

Keywords: Serious games · Exergames · Ambient Assisted Living (AAL) · Self-Efficacy · Acceptance · User experience · Gaming frequency

1 Introduction and Related Work

Increased life expectancy in many western countries leads to a demographic change that will have a tremendous impact on the healthcare system. According to current predictions, a shrinking working population will have to support a growing number of retirees: In Europe, the share of people aged 65 years and over is projected to increase by more than 50 % from 17.1 % in 2008 to 30 % in 2060 [1]. Likewise, the share of people older than 80 years is projected to triple in the same timeframe. This will stress the healthcare systems significantly as the likelihood of chronic illnesses increases with age [2]. In contrast, the per capita expenses for healthcare is declining in many western societies [3]. Accordingly, in the near future less people will contribute to a healthcare system that more people depend on.

Two solutions alleviate the rising costs of the healthcare systems: First, Ambient Assisted Living (AAL) technologies that are integrated into the home environments of

© Institute for Computer Sciences, Social Informatics and Telecommunications Engineering 2015
R. Giaffreda et al. (Eds.): IoT360 2014, Part I, LNICST 150, pp. 145–150, 2015.
DOI: 10.1007/978-3-319-19656-5_21

elderly, chronically ill, or disabled people. These technologies can assist in several every day tasks and facilitate a comfortable and independent life in one's own home [4, 5]. Second, serious games can change people's attitudes towards health, can promote healthy behavior, and can increase physical agility [6–9].

Additionally, it is possible to combine these two solutions as serious games can be offered in AAL environments. Serious games and particularly Exergames harness the power of the psychological Premack principle [10]: They interlink physical activities (which are often perceived as unpleasant) with games (which are usually perceived as pleasant and entertaining). Specifically, exercise games require physical activities and body movements to progress within a game. Still, to unfold the potential positive effects users must utilize them frequently and on a regular basis. However, the individual factors influencing perceived usability, intention to use, and performance within serious Exergames in Ambient Assisted Living environments have been insufficiently explored so far. To fill this void, we present a serious game for AAL environments and a summative user study that detangles the influence of user factors on performance, acceptance, and perceived health status.

2 Game Concept and Development

The exercise game is designed to fit into our Ambient Assisted Living room that is designed as a research space to understand if and under which conditions users would adopt ambient assisted technology [11]. The room is a simulacrum of a comfortable 25 m^2 living room, with a large window, two couches, and two bookshelves, that is transparently augmented by several input and output devices such as a sensory floor for detecting falls, a Kinect-based movement and gesture detection system, and an infrared camera to check the inhabitant's health status. Also, the room is furnished with a wall-sized multi-touch display (4.8 × 2.4 m^2, see [12]).

The game itself is situated in a virtual garden environment that is presented on the large wall (see Fig. 1). The user's task is to pass through a series of consecutive levels with increasing complexity in which he or she collects different fruits and vegetables by performing different gestures with his or her body. A Microsoft Kinect™ sensor tracks the user's movements and the game evaluates whether the gestures are performed correctly. For example, in the first level the user's task is to pick apples from a tree by raising one arm. In the following level, another type of fruit and movement are added, in this case pears that require a grab and hold gesture. All required gestures within the game were developed in cooperation with medical professionals (orthopedists and ergo therapists) to ensure that essential and often neglected body movements are exercised during the game [6, 13].

A previous study evaluated an initial prototype of the game with 71 participants (between 20 and 86 years of age) in a doctor's office [6]. Although the performance within the game was much higher for younger users, users from all ages liked the game and expressed the wish to use it frequently. While interacting with the game increased the perceived physical exertion, the perceived pain levels decreased.

The second prototype was refined to reflect the user's feedback from the initial user study and was then integrated into the Ambient Assisted Living room (see Fig. 1).

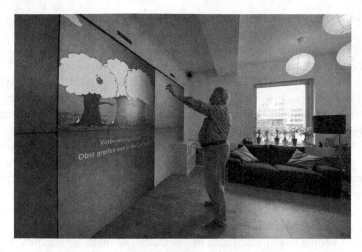

Fig. 1. Prototype of the Exergame in an AAL environment.

The following section describes the user study that was carried out to evaluate the second iteration of the game prototype.

3   Method

The exploratory study investigates how older adults interact with the exercise game integrated in the ambient assisted home environment and addresses three main research questions: First, what user factors contribute to performance within the Exergame? Second, which factors explain the intention to use the game? Third, has the game an impact on the perceived health of the users?

Procedure: The participants played the first three levels of the game in RWTH Aachen University's ambient assisted living lab (eHealth lab). Each of the three levels lasted 120 s. Before the interaction with the game a survey assessed the explanatory variables. After the game the subjective preferences regarding the game were measured. Log files captured the participants' performance within the game.

Explanatory variables (control variables) for modeling user factors were *self-efficacy in interacting with technology (SET), need for achievement (NArch), gaming frequency (GF), gender,* and *age. Self-efficacy in interaction with technology* [14] explains large portions of effectivity, efficiency, and user-satisfaction in interaction with information and communication technology and plays a mayor role for elderly interacting with technology [15]. *Gaming frequency* is measured as the average playing frequency of games (card, board, and movement games with and without computers). *Need for achievement* measures the desire to reach difficult and distant goals in domains such as sports or in the job [16]. The inclination towards games might transfer towards the movement games and people with high need for achievement might feel incited by the game.

<u>Depended variables</u> were *performance* within the game (measured as average number of *fruits/vegetables* collected in the first three levels), *perceived pain* and *perceived exertion* (difference before and after using the game), as well as *behavioral intention (BI)* from the Unified Theory of Acceptance and Use of Technology (UTAUT2) model [17] as the intention to use such a game in the future. The UTAUT2 model explains the adoption of technology depending on a set of promoting and hindering factors. *Perceived exertion* is measured before and after the game on a reduced Borg scale [18]. The scale is subjective, yet it correlates strongly with the heart rate ($r > .8$).

Except for in-game *performance*, all variables are surveyed on 6-point Likert scales. The data is analyzed using χ^2-tests, univariate analyses of variance with repeated-measures (repeated-measures ANOVA), and stepwise multiple linear regressions. Type I error rate (level of significance) is set to $\alpha = .05$. Type II error rate (power) is set to $(1 - \beta) = .8$. For linear regressions only valid models with no or moderate VIF are reported. The explained variance is reported as corrected r^2-values.

In total, 64 people have participated in the study (32 male, 32 female). The *age* of the participants ranged from 17 to 85 years ($M = 43.2$, $\sigma = 19.6$). 26 % reported chronic illnesses, mainly asthma, diabetes, cardiovascular diseases, but also depressions. To analyze age-related effects with factorial methods, the sample was divided into the groups *young* ($M = 25.7$, $\sigma = 4.5$) and *old* ($M = 60.6$, $\sigma = 11.4$). *Gender* was equally distributed among both age groups ($\chi^2(1, N = 64) = .250$, $p = .617 > .05$, n.s.).

4   Results

The results are presented as follows: First, the determinants for *performance* are reported. Second, the factors explaining the *behavioral intention* are presented. Finally, the effect of the game on *perceived pain* and *exertion* are shown.

4.1   Determinants for Performance

To identify factors explaining *performance*, a multiple regression analysis with the dependent variable *performance* and the independent variables a*ge, gaming frequency, need for achievement, perceived pain,* and *self-efficacy in interacting with technology* was carried out. The regression yielded three significant models: The first model, with the factor a*ge*, explains $r^2 = .508$ (50 %) of the variance in *performance* ($F(1, 57) = 58.960$, $p < .01$). The second model (*Age + NArch*) explains an additional 5 % ($r^2 = .559$) of the *performance* ($F(2, 56) = 37.819$, $p < .01$). The third and last model (*Age + NArch + Gender*) contributes an extra 4 % ($r^2 = .605$, $F(3, 55) = 30.671$, $p < .01$).

4.2   Determinants for Usage Intention (Behavioral Intention)

In addition to the previous set of independent variables, the users' average performance is considered in the regression model for *behavioral intention (BI)* from the UTAUT2 model. This regression yielded two significant models: The first, with the single factor *gaming frequency*, explains $r^2 = .206$ (20 %) of the *BI* (F(1, 57) = 16.059, p < .01). The second model, with *gaming frequency* and *performance*, explains an additional 6 % ($r^2 = .257$, F(2, 56) = 11.041, p < .01) of the *BI*.

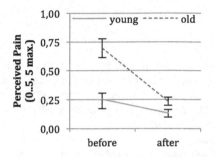 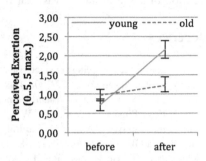

Fig. 2. Change of perceived pain (left) and perceived exertion (right).

4.3   Effect on Perceived Exertion and Perceived Pain

While the levels of *perceived exertion* increased significantly during the experiment (F(1, 62) = 14.571, p < .001, $\eta^2 = .190$), the levels of *perceived pain* decreased (F(1, 62) = 118.543, p < .001, $\eta^2 = .230$). For both measures a significant interaction with *age* is observed. (*Exertion*: F(1, 62) = 7.215, p = .009, $\eta^2 = .104$, *Pain*: F(1, 62) = 6.322, p = .025, $\eta^2 = .093$). Specifically, younger users reported higher levels of *perceived exertion* while older users reported stronger reductions in their *perceived pain* levels (see Fig. 2, left and right).

5   Discussion

The results of the user study fit well into the current research landscape. The study affirmed that age is the strongest predictor for performance within the game and that psychomotoric performance decreases with age. The remarkable revelation, however, is that no other personality factor has a considerable influence on performance. Game performance is only weakly affected by need for achievement and gender. Additionally, neither gaming frequency nor self-efficacy in interacting with technology has an influence on performance. The intention to use the serious game (Behavioral Intention) is influenced only by the current gaming frequency of the participants. This finding has both negative and positive aspects that need to be addressed in future research: On the negative side, the game seems to be only attractive to people who are already inclined to gaming and who play games on a regular basis. Therefore, people unattached to games might not use Exergames in ambient assisted living environments. They cannot profit from the benefits of these and have to find other ways to sustain their physical fitness. On the positive side, the intention to use Exergames in ambient assisted living environments is neither affected by age, need for achievement, nor by self-efficacy in interacting with technology. Consequently, Exergames seem to be a ubiquitous solution to increase the physical fitness of people living in AAL environments, at least if they like to play games.

Most importantly, even the short interaction with the Exergame motivated our test users to vigorously engage in physical activity. The short-term effect was a reduced perceived pain (especially for elderly) while a possible long-term effect might be the prevention of a rise of cardio-vascular diseases in elderly.

References

1. Giannakouris, K.: Ageing characterises the demographic perspectives of the European societies, Statistics in Focus, 72/2008, Luxembourg, Publications Office of the European Union (2008) http://ec.europa.eu/eurostat/documents/3433488/5583040/KS-SF-08-072-EN.PDF
2. Ho, K.K.L., Pinsky, J.L., Kannel, W.B., Levy, D.: The epidemiology of heart failure: the framingham study. J. Am. Coll. Cardiol. **22**, A6–A13 (1993)
3. Health at a Glance: Europe 2012. OECD Publishing (2012)
4. Kleinberger, T., Becker, M., Ras, E.: Ambient intelligence in assisted living: enable elderly people to handle future interfaces. In: Univers Access HCI, pp. 103–112 (2007)
5. Röcker, C.: Designing ambient assisted living applications : an overview over state-of-the-art implementation concepts. In: International Conference on Information and Digital Engineering (ICIDE 2011), pp. 167–172 (2011)
6. Brauner, P., Calero Valdez, A., Schroeder, U., Ziefle, M.: Increase physical fitness and create health awareness through exergames and gamification. In: Holzinger, A., Ziefle, M., Hitz, M., Debevc, M. (eds.) SouthCHI 2013. LNCS, vol. 7946, pp. 349–362. Springer, Heidelberg (2013)
7. Grimes, A., Kantroo, V., Grinter, R.E.: Let's play!: mobile health games for adults (2010)
8. Weisman, S.: Computer games for the frail elderly. Gerontologist **23**, 361–363 (1983)
9. Gerling, K., Schild, J., Masuch, M.: Exergame design for elderly users: the case study of SilverBalance. In: ACE 2010, pp. 66–69 (2010)
10. Premack, D.: Toward empirical behavior laws: I Positive reinforcement. Psychol. Rev. Psychol. Rev. **66**, 219 (1959)
11. Ziefle, M., Röcker, C., Wilkowska, W., Kasugai, K., Klack, L., Möllering, C., Beul, S.: A multi-disciplinary approach to ambient assisted living. In: Röcker, C., Ziefle, M. (eds.) E-Health, Assistive Technologies and Applications for Assisted Living: Challenges and Solutions, pp. 76–93. IGI Global, Hershey (2011)
12. Kasugai, K., Ziefle, M., Röcker, C., Russel, P.: Creating spatio-temporal contiguities between real and virtual rooms in an assistive living environment. In: Bonner, J., Smyth, S., O' Neill, S., Mival, O. (eds.) Proceedings of Create 10 Innovative Interactions, Loughborough, Elms Court, pp. 62–67 (2010)
13. Brauner, P., Rausch, C., Beul, S., Ziefle, M.: Alt schlägt Jung Bewegungsförderung für Ältere durch Serious Games. In: Jeschke, S., Kobbelt, L., Dröge, A. (eds.) Exploring Virtuality - Virtualität im interdisziplinären Diskurs, pp. 215–239. Springer, Wiesbaden (2014)
14. Beier, G.: Kontrollüberzeugungen im Umgang mit Technik [Locus of control when interacting with technology]. Rep. Psychol. **24**, 684–693 (1999)
15. Ziefle, M., Bay, S.: How older adults meet complexity: aging effects on the usability of different mobile phones. Behav. Inf. Technol. **24**, 375–389 (2005)
16. Schuler, H., Prochaska, M.: LMI: Leistungsmotivationsinventar [Dimensionen berufsbezogener Leistungsorientierung]. Hogrefe (2001)
17. Venkatesh, V., Morris, M.G., Davis, G.B., Davis, F.D.: User acceptance of information technology: toward a unified view. MIS Q. **27**, 425–478 (2003)
18. Borg, G.A.V.: Psychophysical bases of perceived exertion. Med. Sci. Sports Exerc. **14**, 377–381 (1982)

SafeMove – Safe Mobility of Elderly in the Vicinity of Their Home and on Journeys

Irit Luft Madar[1(✉)], Matt Smith[2], and Peter Knackfuss[3]

[1] Methodica, 12 Hachoma St. R. Letzion, POB 11853, 61116 Tel-Aviv, Israel
iritl@methodic.co.il
[2] e-Learning Studios, Innovation Village Cheetah Road,
Coventry CV1 2TL, UK
matt@e-learningstudios.com
[3] 3InfoConsult Gesellschaft für Informationstechnik mbH,
Stolzenauer Str. 3, 28207 Bremen, Germany
peter.knackfuss@infoconsult.net

Abstract. The demographic change that is foreseeable in the future will permeate all throughout society, and require new approaches to ageing and its concomitant challenges. Serious games are one of the answers towards this challenge. Herein, we describe ways how the SafeMove project plans to employ serious games in the context of helping elderly people with light dementia to operate on their own. Due to the multi-facetted approach of the SafeMove project, serious games are embedded in a holistic system for the elderly, which will ultimately help them stay active and ambulatory as long as possible, while feeling safe and well cared for. This will enable them to stay in the comfort of their own homes for as long as possible, while helping them stay active and socially connected. The serious games will provide the impetus to exercise more, as well as connect with others playing the same games.

Keywords: Light dementia · aMCI · Elderly · Mobility · Safe mobility · Social groups

1 Overview

By 2020, 25 % of the EU's population will be older than 65 years, which will lead to a shrinking of the European working-age population. This demographic and financial shift will increase the cost of the healthcare systems, as more people will need some sort of physical, social or mental care allowing them to remain an integrated and active part of society. One of the key factors, which enables a person to remain an active member of society and enjoy a high quality of living is the ability to freely, safely and easily travel from point to point. This ability becomes less available to people as they grow old and the capability to remain active and to maintain a high level of well-being becomes compromised.

There are many reasons, both physical and cognitive, why elderly people become reluctant or unable to travel or even take a walk. This lack of movement and motivation leads to social isolation and to an excessive need for personal care.

© Institute for Computer Sciences, Social Informatics and Telecommunications Engineering 2015
R. Giaffreda et al. (Eds.): IoT360 2014, Part I, LNICST 150, pp. 151–156, 2015.
DOI: 10.1007/978-3-319-19656-5_22

The SafeMove project vision is to enable elderly people with amnestic Mild Cognitive Impairment – (aMCI, i.e. light dementia) to stay active and in the comfort of their own homes for a longer period of time, while simultaneously being able to go out and to join social activities. The project aims to achieve this vision by assisting them to become well trained users of modern IT devices and by creating both a physical and a virtual community.

SafeMove aims to reach its goals by creating an integrative and personalised system comprised of three key synergetic elements:

1. **SafeMove@Home:** Home-based physical and cognitive training, also through serious games. IT training games and devices (based on the Kinect sensor) are being developed to enhance both the mental and physical fitness of the elderly in an interactive, effective and enjoyable way: The system allows the users to practice their outdoor routes at home, play serious games (that are being developed based on professional knowledge from various clinical researches on dementia). The system also addresses the development of social relationships by encouraging contact between users.
2. **SafeMove on Tour:** Location-based mobile assistance for outdoor life activities. An application for mobile devices is being developed in order to support elderly persons with aMCI to find their way outside their homes, navigate through public traffic or at social events etc. By using the real-time assistance provided by their mobile devices, they remember daily life routines such as dressing themselves according to the weather conditions, taking the keys with them when leaving the house or even making sure they're still on the route they planned in advance.
3. **SafeMove Assist:** Caregivers and family members have the opportunity to assess the health of their clients remotely and to support them in keeping them healthy and mobile. With the help of the SafeMove assist platform, caregivers receive valuable information concerning the users and are able to assist several users simultaneously.

The SafeMove project is funded by the Ambient Assisted Living (AAL) Joint Programme and is carried out by a collaborative interdisciplinary group of experts working including physicians, scientists, consultants, designers, health-care providers etc.

2   SafeMove Games

The games for the SafeMove project are being developed to inspire confidence in the user's physical and mental abilities.

Using the gesture based Microsoft Kinect, the elderly can play fun and challenging mini-games to keep their faculties sharp, interact with peers and enjoy gentle guided exercise all while in the safety of their own home.

It is our hope that these features will not replace their trips outdoors but that it would encourage them to be strong and confident when going out, preventing their lifestyle from declining and giving them the courage to keep going in the event of a fall or other troubling event.

The games will all be set in one environment, a park, where the user will be able to explore and launch mini-games which are each designed around Physical, Cognitive and Social elements.

Physical, Cognitive and Social elements are not mutually exclusive and we expect a significant amount of cross over in the mini games.

The combined activities are designed to provide a holistic approach to improving social interaction skills, providing an awareness of social skills and improve confidence and promote a feeling of wellbeing.

The mini-games which have so far been developed for the SafeMove project include:

Walking in a Virtual Park

This is a simple physical game which uses a walking gesture. This game is designed to give the users gentle and guided exercise.

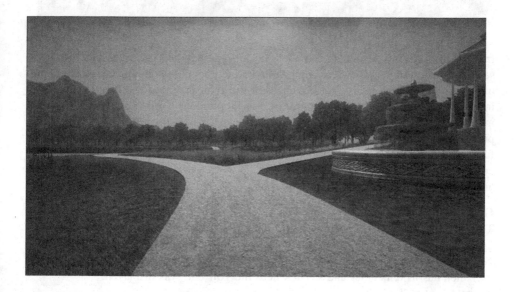

Hoopla

The user is faced with 3 colour posts in the ground at the same distance away. The colours are Red, Blue and Yellow. The user will be given hoops to throw to these posts.

There will be a tombola sign which spins around and will have one of the 3 colours written on it but it may be displayed in a different colour. For example, the word says **RED** but it is written in blue. The user must then throw the hoop to the blue post. So the user must throw the hoop at the correct post according to the colour of the word and not the word itself.

This game is a variant of the classic Stroop Test. Dissonance between the colour presented and the mismatched name interferes with naming the colour. The Stroop Test causes elevated activation in the anterior cingulate cortex, which is involved in detecting the incongruity. The classic Stroop interference task [3] has provided a

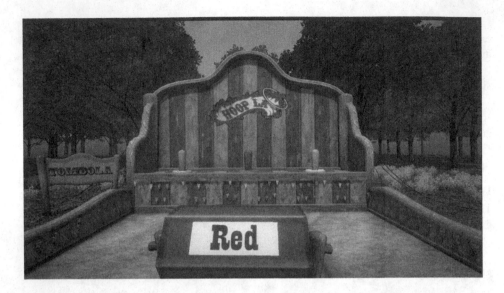

fruitful platform by which to test models of forced-choice decision and response selection under situations where compatible or incompatible components of the stimulus facilitate or impair task performance. In the typical Stroop task, participants are instructed to report the physical colour of a written colour word (e.g., "RED"), while ignoring the semantic meaning of the word. In cases where the physical colour of the presentation is congruent with the semantic meaning of the word, participants are both faster and more accurate at reporting the physical colour. However, when the physical colour differs from the semantic meaning of the word (i.e., is incongruent) participants are slower and more prone to error [2].

Golf

This is game is to help improve spatial memory. The user has to use a golf swing gesture to put the ball into play. They are then shown a view of the fairway with the golf ball displayed. The ball then disappears and a few distractors are displayed. The user then has to remember and select where the golf ball was displayed.

The spatial span task exercises your visuospatial working memory; the component of working memory that allows you to temporarily hold and manipulate information about places. Many everyday activities involve visuospatial working memory, including finding your way around your environment, judging the position of other motorists while you are driving and searching for your keys. According to one very influential cognitive model of working memory [1] visuospatial working memory depends on a specialised sub-component of the working memory system. This is referred to as the "visuospatial sketchpad" and is thought to have a visual "cache", responsible for storing visual form and colour information, and an "inner scribe" which deals with spatial and movement information.

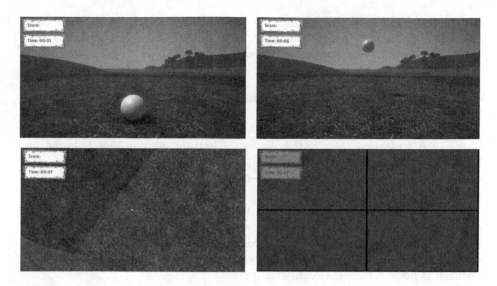

Smiling

This is a social cognition game. The user will see a series of smiling, neutral and frowning faces and they have to select the smiling faces as quickly as possible. The idea is that each time the user drags their attention away from one of the frowning faces in order to find a smiling, accepting face, it helps to build a mental habit. The next time they are reminded of a rejection or criticism from someone else, rather than dwelling on it, they may be able to 'let it go'. This is because the mental habit generalizes beyond the visual domain of disengaging from frowning faces, to apply to disengaging from thoughts and worries about social rejection and criticism.

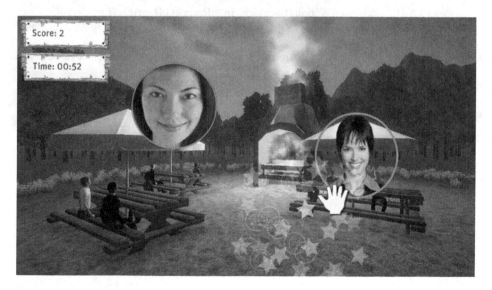

For all of the games we will measure the user reaction times, the accuracy and each game will have a scoring system. This will enable the SafeMove system to track user progress and help to identify a decline in the user's physical and cognitive abilities.

3   Benefits of Conference Participation

The core innovative component of the SafeMove solution is our ability to seamlessly integrate the 3 elements described above into a **holistic solution that is based on clinical research and can provide customized and effective assistance for elderly people, at home and on tour, thus creating a solution that will significantly improve their well-being.**

During the conference, we would like to present the innovative concept of the SafeMove solution and demonstrate key components and features that were already developed, emphasizing the serious games component. We are sure that in the project's present state (2 years out of 3), the knowledge we are able to convey would be beneficial to other participating consortia.

As the representatives of the SafeMove consortium, we look forward to receiving new ideas and best practices concerning technological integration and development of serious games for the elderly population.

Proposed conference Attendees
Mrs. Irit Luft Madar - Senior Consultant at Methodica Effective Learning.

References

1. Baddeley, A.D., Hitch, G.: Working memory. In: Bower, G.H. (ed.) The Psychology of Learning and Motivation: Advances in Research and Theory, vol. 8, pp. 47–89. Academic Press, New York (1974)
2. MacLeod, C.M.: Half a century of research on the Stroop effect: an integrative review. Psychol. Bull. **109**, 163–203 (1991)
3. Stroop, J.R.: Studies of interference in serial verbal reactions. J. Exp. Psychol. **18**, 643–662 (1935)
4. http://baldwinlab.mcgill.ca/labmaterials/materials_BBC.html

HealthyIoT 2014

A Ubiquitous Telehealth System for the Elderly

M.W. Raad[(⊠)], Tarek Sheltami, and Muhammad Deriche

King Fahd University of Petroleum and Minerals (KFUPM),
Box # 1874, Dhahran 31261, Saudi Arabia
{raad,tarek,mderiche}@kfupm.edu.sa

Abstract. Chronic diseases are becoming the world's leading causes of death and disability, and are predicted to account for almost three quarters of all deaths by 2020. A working prototype was built to capture vital signs for the elderly staying at home and deliver prompt care remotely by using wearable ECG wireless sensors. This prototype has been tested to capture data on a 24/7 basis for a number of patients at the KFUPM Medical Center. The developed system includes a suit of signal processing algorithms for the detection of severe cases of arrhythmias in elderly patients. After identifying patients with potential arrhythmia variability, an alarm system sends emergency requests to caregivers for immediate response. Our results were benchmarked against the standard MIT physiobank. The performance of the system was also tested on simulated data with very satisfactory results, and very positive feedback from users and medical practitioners.

Keywords: Telehealth · Ubiquitous · Electrocardiogram · Arrhythmia

1 Introduction

During the last few years we have witnessed an increasing interest in wearable/mobile health monitoring devices, both in research and industry. These devices are particularly important to the world's increasingly aging population, whose health has to be assessed regularly or monitored continuously. Chronic diseases are becoming the world's leading causes of death and disability, and are predicted to account for almost three quarters of all deaths by 2020 [1].

Traditionally, part of the difficulty in achieving equitable access to healthcare has been the required presence of the patient at the Medical Center. Recent advances in information and communication technologies, in addition to wearable computing technologies, have created unprecedented opportunities for overcoming this. This is possible by increasing the number of ways that healthcare can be delivered. Telehealth, the area where medicine, information, and telecommunications technology meet, is probably the part of this revolution with the greatest impact on healthcare delivery. A telehealth system can be defined as the delivery of medical information over a distance by using telecommunication means. Home telehealth, on the other hand involves the use of telehealth techniques in a non-institutional setting such as home, or in an assisted-living facility. In store-and-forward telehealth, vital signs and clinical data are captured and stored, then sent to caregivers for further analysis. Physiological monitoring leads to richer data and therefore to improved decision making [2, 3].

© Institute for Computer Sciences, Social Informatics and Telecommunications Engineering 2015
R. Giaffreda et al. (Eds.): IoT360 2014, Part I, LNICST 150, pp. 159–166, 2015.
DOI: 10.1007/978-3-319-19656-5_23

Recently, there has been a growing awareness of the need for new ways to improve the well-being of older people at home as well as the availability of increasingly affordable technology and computational power. Nevertheless, consumer and clinician adoption and acceptance have been slow. For example, social alarms or personal emergency response systems (PERS) enable a person to call for help in the event of an accident (e.g. fall) or other problem. Services like using a wireless pendant or wearable bracelet connect the older person to a call center, which then notifies ambulance services and family members in the event of an emergency [4]. The usual clinical or hospital monitoring of physiological events such as electrocardiogram or blood pressure provides only a brief window on physiology of a patient. It usually fails to capture rare events during sleep times, while it performs well during daily life activities. Therefore, there is a vast need for acquiring and adopting wearable telehealth solutions for the long run.

The implications of wearable health monitoring technologies are paramount, since they could: (1) enable the detection of early signs of health problems; (2) notify healthcare providers in critical situations; (3) find correlations between lifestyle and health; (4) bring healthcare to remote locations and developing countries, and help doctors and researchers with accessing multi-sourced real-time physiological data [5]. With the advent of advanced telecommunication technology, long-term home care of the elderly or what we call telehealth is becoming a rapidly growing area of healthcare industry. Lately, many researchers have begun investing their time into the research of wireless telehealth systems. Proponents of wireless systems claim that the increased mobility and the lower cost of the systems are highly beneficial to telehealth. Mobility and lower cost healthcare solutions are benefits of new telecommunications technologies. [6]. Telehealth has the potential of improving the quality of delivered health services and reducing total healthcare costs by avoiding unnecessary hospitalisations and ensuring the fast delivery of healthcare. In addition to cost-effective telehealth, remote health monitoring can significantly contribute to the enhancement of disease prevention, early diagnosis, disease management, treatment and home rehabilitation [7, 8]. This paper presents a novel approach to affordable mobile telehealth infrastructure for the purpose of arrhythmia early detection in KFUPM for patients to satisfy the vast need for the telehealth solution in Saudi Arabia . The paper is organized as follows. Section 2 describes the proposed system architecture. Section 3 presents the ECG Graphical user interface used by the elderly. Section 4 presents the Wavelet transform approach or algorithm for arrhythmia analysis.

2 Proposed System Architecture

In the following section, system architecture for telehealth is developed. We propose an architectural telehealth solution for the elderly living at home. The elderly might be handicapped in various ways, as senses and capabilities to remember are not always good. Also relatives, who might be spread all over the world, would like to make sure that loved ones are all right and perhaps keep an eye on them 24/7. The elderly may not able to see a physician anytime they need, because they may be unable to make their way to the clinic or hospital. Therefore, a solution must be developed to allow the elderly to talk to their physicians in a user-friendly manner. The physicians must have a remote-view of the vital signs that they look at, like electrocardiogram (ECG), oxygen saturation, blood pressure, heart rate, etc. In case of emergency, a reliable emergency system must call a physician and ambulance for help. We have integrated a portable ECG sensor with a Bluetooth interface, called Alive ECG, into the proposed Telehealth system. A number of sample ECG data were captured from 30 volunteers between the ages of 20 and 23, in addition to a couple of elderly patients suffering from arrhythmia using the alive ECG sensor and sent through Bluetooth to a PC for further analysis. The ECG data captured is compared on the spot with normal ECG stored in a local database server to detect any abnormalities. The R-R interval in a typical ECG sample is the time taken to conduct electrical discharge spread through different parts of the heart. Any deviation of the R-R interval from its normal range can indicate the onset of arrhythmia and hence requires immediate intervention by specialists. Figure 1 shows an overview of the general layout of the proposed Telehealth monitoring system for the elderly using an IP digital camera and the web, in addition to a GSM modem for sending emergency messages or calls to the physician as well as to the ambulance. The database is used to store the information related to the health status of the elderly to be analyzed by a physician or caregiver. The layout shown in Fig. 1 has been built and tested in the lab for the purpose of using it as a ubiquitous Telehealth solution for home use. It also includes a smart card access control interface for securing access to critical medical information. Changes in an individual's daily routine often signal onset of illness and potentially cognitive decline.

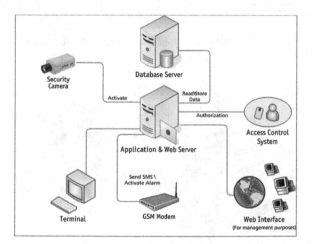

Fig. 1. An overall layout of the elderly monitoring system

The focus in this paper is on a Telehealth monitoring system for the elderly at home, which can also be used to monitor the elderly at the hospital. To make this possible, the biosensors capturing the vital signs are programmed to communicate with a centralized station using Ad hoc network or even wireless infrastructure LAN. The medical wearable sensors capture the vital signs of the elderly and send these vital signs upon request to the physician. The proposed Telehealth system has been successfully tested for sending high and low blood pressure alarms remotely via SMS. The system was tested in the lab for sending blood pressure and pulse rate values to a central database server. Records of the elderly's vital signs measurements, including the ECG (Electrocardiogram) measurements are stored on the local home server for future use. A scenario of how the system is used is that a patient suffering from arrhythmia wears the Bluetooth enabled portable ECG, shown in Fig. 2 and runs his daily life activities for a week or so. If the patient feels unwell, he presses a button and his ECG data is sent immediately to his doctor for examining. While at the clinic, the doctor meets the patient for closer testing. See Fig. 3.

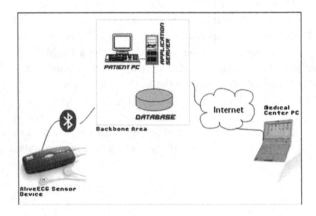

Fig. 2. The layout of a mobile cardiac Telehealth system

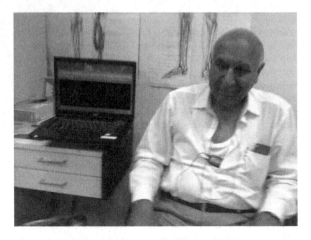

Fig. 3. A snapshot of using the Alive ECG system in KFUPM clinic

3   ECG GUI

The application consists of two main GUI interfaces. One is called ECG SYSTEM and the other is called PATIENT.

The ECG system has the following functions:

- Fetch the data.
- Compare the collected data with the data saved in the server.
- Store the collected data into the SQL server.
- E-mail emergency notifications.

The ECG system captures data generated from MATLAB after specifying the patient ID and presents it on the screen. After that, the program compares the data fetched against some default values to find out the abnormalities. If an abnormality is detected, the application sends a message via OUTLOOK to the medical center specifying the patient ID. See Fig. 4.

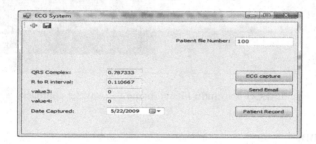

Fig. 4. ECG GUI home alarm system

4   Wavelet Transform Approach

Another effective approach learned from literature was using the wavelet transform approach as follows. Using the LABVIEW ASPT (Advanced Signal processing Toolkit), WA detrend VI, the low frequency trend of the signal can be removed. We used daubechies6 (db06) wavelet which is similar to the real ECG signal for removing the trend.

Prior to the capturing an actual ECG signal, National Instruments software LAB-VIEW was used for the simulation and analysis of the ECG signal. For this purpose, Simulate ECG LABVIEW palette was used as shown below. Using the simulate ECG signal, a lot of parameters could be controlled like the beats per minutes (bpm), P-QRS delay, QRS-T delay, amplitude of ECG, number of samples etc. Also, three different scenarios could be selected from Atrial Tachycardia, Hyperkalemia and normal ECG signal. To this simulated ECG, white Gaussian noise was added programmatically with a controlled signal to noise ratio as seen from the block diagram of the below vi. Finally results were stored in a LABVIEW measurement file for further analysis. See Fig. 5.

See Fig. 6 for using Wavelet algorithm to filter the noisy ECG with LABVIEW.

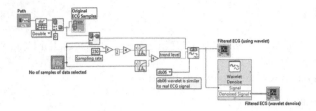

Fig. 5. Simulating the ECG signal with controlled white Gaussian Noise using LABVIEW

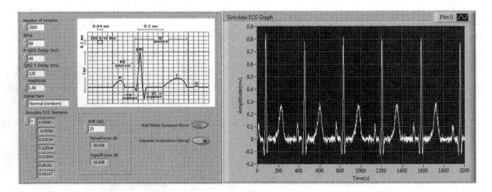

Fig. 6. ECG waveform filtered using the wavelet approach.

5 Discussion

The system will also open new opportunities for further research in the area of biomedical signal and image processing. Rapid development of Telehealth technology will also motivate health centers and hospitals to adopt the infrastructure and necessary skills to provide better & efficient medical treatment for patients to boost the quality of life.

The use of Telehealth will provide higher-quality service and increased efficiency to the practice of medicine. Emergency and critical response professionals can be given immediate access to a wealth of vital information, particularly for the elderly and disabled. It also becomes possible to observe and deliver care to patients while living in their homes, instead of spending months or even years in the hospital. With the development of new products from Telehealth, there is a growing need to develop standards for the field. Standards will improve reliability and allow the interoperability of the various different services being created. The proposed design represents a good approach to research in Telehealth for the elderly, keeping in mind that many things have been generalized to a certain extent and the analysis of the vital sign data captured from the medical sensors is still an on- going research. Certain crucial issues still have to be resolved regarding the user-friendliness of the Telehealth system and how the elderly will interact with all of this complex technology. In addition to that, some measures have to be taken to ensure the privacy of the web enabled solution which physicians use to view the health status of the elderly since the web is vulnerable to hackers. The proposed design has been kept under closed application for a relatively small environment to cut down design cost and simplify the testing methodology. Research is also ongoing to support the automatic self-diagnosis feature of the Telehealth system regarding reliable detection of cardiac diseases symptoms.

6 Conclusion

LABVIEW along with Vernier sensors were used to successfully capture an ECG signal from individuals out of the 30 student's participants, after which ECG signal was filtered using wavelet transform approach. Finally, Heart rate (R-R) and QRS complex of the ECG signal was successfully analyzed from the filtered signal. Further analysis of detecting the p-wave and t-wave is underway which will help us detecting arrhythmia later.

A graphical user interface (GUI) based Telehealth system has been developed using LABVIEW instrumentation software. The purpose of the developed system is real time analysis of the vital signs captured from the elderly suffering from arrhythmia. The MATLAB & LABVIEW simulation results were used to validate the real data captured from volunteers using ECG sensors. The successful implementation and utilization of the wireless ECG system in the KFUPM Medical Center has paved the way for establishing a ubiquitous mobile Telehealth which proved to be a cost effective solution for patients suffering from severe arrhythmia. The deployed system provides big hope for patients with chronic diseases and it could therefore help avoid catastrophic results in the future by providing immediat medical care in the field. The real-time analysis and feature extraction algorithms implemented in LABVIEW, in conjunction with the ALIVE wireless ECG will enable physicians to use the system by delivering better emergency care.

Acknowledgements. The authors would like to acknowledge the support of King Fahd University of Petroleum & Minerals for this research.

References

1. Hung, K., Zhang, Y.T., Tai, B.: Wearable medical devices for tele-home healthcare. In: IEEE Proceedings of the 26th Annual International Conference of Engineering Medicine and Biology Society, vol. 2, pp. 5384–5387 (2004)
2. Wootton, R., Dimmick, S.L., Kvedar, J.C.: Home Telemedicine: Connecting Care within the Community. Royal Society of Medicine Press Ltd, London (2006)
3. Wootton, R., Craig, J., Patterson, V.: Introduction to Telemedicine. Royal Society of Medicine Press, London (2006)
4. Coughlin, J.F, Pope, J.: Innovations in health: wellness, and aging-in-place. In: IEEE Engineering in Medicine and Biology Magazine, vol. 27, pp. 47–52 (2008)
5. Oliver, N., Mangas, F.F.: HealthGear: a real-time wearable system for monitoring and analyzing physiological signals. Technical report MSR-TR-182 (2005)

6. Xiao, Y., Chen, H.: Mobile Telemedicine: A Computing and Networking Perspective. CRC Press, Boca Raton (2008)
7. http://www.suunto.com
8. http://www.bodymedia.com
9. Judi, H.M., Razak, A.A., Sha'ari, N., Mohamed, H.: Feasibility and critical success factors in implementing Telehealth. Inf. Technol. J. **8**, 326–332 (2009)
10. Wangenheim, A.V., Nobre, L.F., Tagnoli, H., Nassar, S.M., Ho, K.: User satisfaction with asynchronous telemedicine: a study of users of santa catarina's system of telemedicine and telehealth. J. Telemedicine e-Health **18**, 339–347 (2012)

Location! Location! Location! The Architect's Contribution to IoT for Healthcare

Steven Rowland[✉]

BIM for Healthcare, White Arkitekter AB, Stockholm, Sweden
steven.rowland@outlook.com

1 Introduction to BIM in the Healthcare Typology

This paper aims to introduce the IoT community of scientists and technical researches to the concepts integral to BIM and the Architectural design process in large scale healthcare projects. In particular, this paper puts forward the potential for BIM database systems to be used as primary sources of building information and locational data for IoT systems, and makes suggestions about further studies.

1.1 The Room as the Architect's Base Product

We generally think of Architects as creators of buildings, but the building is, in fact, a conglomeration of individual rooms, each designed to fulfill a specific function for the users and owners. Architects will often begin healthcare projects with lists of room types that must be designed and detailed.

Rooms have requirements. In the healthcare space, rooms have requirements such as hygiene class, security level, acoustics, radiation shielding etc. Through the work of designing hospitals, Architects will create relationships between room objects, according to functional neighborhoods, or departments such as Acute Care, Operation, or Intensive Care. We group these departments together into user-friendly buildings and wrap it all in a pleasing and functional aesthetic shell. Architects combine art, healing spaces, protection, heating/cooling, logistical flows, people flows, and many other aspects together the final buildings, but we always return to the room.

Healthcare projects, in particular, are amongst the most complex building types for an Architect to design. Hospitals have high information density and complexity of function, logistics, equipment, and staff. To give a sense of scale, a recent large-scale hospital in Stockholm comprises of 300,000 + sq meters of new hospital, including 11,000 + rooms, and over 300,000 pieces of equipment or furnishings. A more typical new hospital may hover around 50,000 sq meters, with over 2,000 rooms and 50,000 distinct facility assets to keep track of. Each object may also have 20 + columns of parametric data to fully identify the instance or type. Add it all up, and we are rapidly approaching big data scale.

To organize this complexity, current Architectural best practice is to use specialized, spatial, relational database systems; the Building Information Model. Popular platforms include Autodesk's Revit and Graphisoft's Archicad, for example. The Building Information Model combines 2-D/3-D visualization, document creation/management,

© Institute for Computer Sciences, Social Informatics and Telecommunications Engineering 2015
R. Giaffreda et al. (Eds.): IoT360 2014, Part I, LNICST 150, pp. 167–171, 2015.
DOI: 10.1007/978-3-319-19656-5_24

information management, object creation/management and design flexibility into a single visual database system, or BIM. In practice, for larger or more complex facilities, Architects will network multiple BIM databases together, each having specific purposes; for example, façade, structure, base-building, mechanical-electrical-plumbing etc. In current best practice we also provision additional custom databases to mediate specific information types across the entire BIM network; for example, change management, room requirements, or equipment/furnishing specifications.

Through it all, Architects always deal with objects, whether those objects are rooms, building parts, doors, MR scanners, or electrical sockets. All objects are uniquely identified via a GUID, or another custom identity code. All objects can thereby be traced through the BIM network for quantity surveying and cost estimation. These objects are all parametric, portable, and reproducible across the BIM network.

The preceding description is to introduce that Architects now design healthcare projects in a data rich environment. Some firms push the state-of-the-art, while others are slowly pulled along by the evolution of the industry.

1.2   So What Happens to All This Information?

Traditionally, the Architectural design is focused on the production, or construction, of the new or improved healthcare facility. Drawings and documents on paper or .pdf are the traditional deliverables to our clients. A subset of the design data is preserved as a record-keeping reference. Despite the dynamic and rich information design environment of BIM, many clients and Architectural firms deliver information as static and barren analogue formats. When the facility or hospital is built, the design documents are put away on dusty shelves.

Increasingly, however, regional healthcare agencies or healthcare developers have adopted a more datacentric model. More complex and high-tech facilities have shifted the production of healthcare facilities away from static documents towards dynamic information structures. Architectural firms by necessity must meet the demands of their evolving clients, and in many cases Architects are leading their clients towards more efficient and useful information management techniques.

The datacentric design is further complemented by the operations and maintenance specialists, structural consultants, plumbing and electrical consultants, security specialist and many others. The design data flows much deeper beyond production and into the life of the healthcare facility. New deliverables include the BIM models, specialized databases, and sharepoints, in addition to the dusty drawings, documents and static.pdfs. Many of these deliverables are used in real-time, and are accessible in mobile formats. See Fig. 1 in the afterword.

There exists, therefore, a rich well of information upon which IoT for Healthcare can draw.

1.3   How to Draw from the Well

Each BIM platform has its own proprietary format which is generally obtuse. The industry standard for sharing BIM data among design professionals is the .ifc format, or Industry Foundation Class, which is maintained and developed by the Building Smart organization. The .ifc is usable across a wide variety of design, analysis, and facilities management software platforms. It is becoming an official International Standard ISO/IS 16739, and the newest version includes a more robust XML interchange ability. The.ifc is an open format, and the complete specifications are available for anyone to view.

Fortunately, the major BIM platforms also have maturing APIs in C#, VB.net, and other supported flavors. Custom and creative tools are built on top of the BIM platform. The trend is to use the BIM platform as the primary tool during the design process, and extract the BIM data to an open database SQL or noSQL for a wider array of non-production uses. The APIs are well supported, and allow flexible and creative management of BIM data and data flows.

1.4   A Word of Caution

As a whole, the construction and development industry moves very slowly towards adopting new technologies. Some of the larger players are leading the way towards exploiting the data density of healthcare projects, but many others are happy to continue with analogue or thin data processes. Forward-looking professionals are able to demonstrate the advantages of managing healthcare design complexity with deeper integration of datacentric methodologies.

1.5   Where Does IoT Come into the Picture?

Let's go back to the room. The room object is a unique entity, comprising of a relative location, a spatial quantity, and a variety of requirements that are described as distinct parameters. Location data can be GPS specific, but is often relative to a regional x,y,z base point. Placing it in a global positioning system, however, is trivial. Spatial quantities can be in terms of volume, areas, and can be measured together into larger grouped volumes and areas. Within and around the room object are building parts, finishes, moveable equipment, fixed furnishings, and people. Furthermore, each room object exists in relation to other room objects, building parts, things, as well as the building or facility as a whole.

Each IoT node is embedded in this web of relationships and the things that comprise and reside therein. Within the finished building, objects are asset-coded and tagged via nfc tags, rfid tags, QR code stickers or bar-codes and referenced back to facilities management systems. Often this is a manual process of identifying, tagging and scanning, but increasingly manufacturers are delivering custom tagged materials, furnishings and equipment according to the BIM data. This is ambient level data, and does not rise to the level of IoT ambitions, however it can be accessed as a data environment via scanning technologies.

As IoT matures in the built environment, the BIM data can be fed to the node and backed by a persistent Building Information data structure. The location and relational information provide a valuable basis for the IoT systems. The information flow from design to living building becomes much more complete and evolved.

1.6   Sounds Great! What's the Catch?

The catch is providing a standardized data and delivery system. The Building Information data structure can and probably should be a cloud-based information store to alleviate the necessity for hospital and building organizations to maintain the IT infrastructure. Collecting and maintaining the design data will need to be organized as a standard building design process. New deliverables will need to be specified and detailed at the beginning of the design process, when healthcare developers are hiring design professionals. Further studies will need to delve into the legal and professional implications of adding new deliverables to the architect's basic services. Return on Investment will need to be studied in detail to motivate healthcare organizations to develop towards IoT applications.

Other complications are more familiar: security, privacy, and maintenance. Security is a serious concern for healthcare facilities. IoT enabled equipment requires a high level of security. Healthcare facilities require very high reliability for all equipment, systems and building components.

- Equipment including cloud and mobile apps, require strong password and permissions.
- Equipment must not collect data that violates patient privacy.
- Equipment must encrypt communications and software updates.
- Equipment requires secure Web interfaces where applicable.
- The Building Information Data must be maintained and updated.

Perhaps the biggest challenge is proving conclusively that IoT for Healthcare provides a compelling advantage for healthcare facilities. The status quo is a powerful force, and healthcare developers and authorities have many bigger priorities; for example, providing a healthy and healing environment for patients. Further studies will need to explore and demonstrate the benefits of IoT for healthcare for various stakeholders and participants; for example doctors, patients, visitors technicians, administrators etc.

2   Pointing Forward

2.1   Afterword and the Datacentric Organisation Model

I am reminded of the early days of the internet, when the web was a barren place. Content creation was a priority, back in the day before everybody had their own blog. IoT for Healthcare has a major advantage, in that the healthcare design process creates a large volume of very useful content. Architects have felt for years that the BIM data was being underutilized and undervalued beyond the building process. IoT is an opportunity to use this content towards its potential.

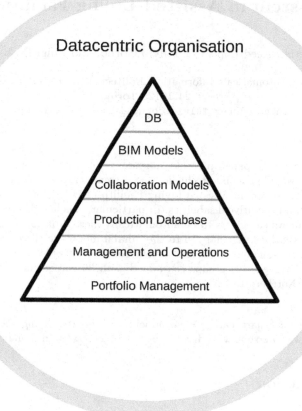

Fig. 1. Datacentric Organisation.

  The Datacentric Organisation shown below is descriptive of the current best practice of healthcare design in major Scandanavian markets. Specialized design databases (DB) sit at the apex, filtering and mediating information through the BIM models. In practice, this tends to be a weblike network, but the hierarchy is generally correct. IoT systems can overlap at several levels, especially in the lower tiers.

IoT Meets Caregivers: A Healthcare Support System in Assisted Living Facilities

Sebastián Aced López[✉], Fulvio Corno, and Luigi De Russis

Dipartimento di Automatica e Informatica ,Politecnico di Torino, Corso Duca Degli Abruzzi, 24, 10129 Torino, Italy
{sebastian.acedlopez,fulvio.corno,luigi.derussis}@polito.it

Abstract. This paper presents a system that exploits the synergy between wearable/mobile technology and smart caring environments to support caregivers in Assisted Living Facilities (ALFs) for persons with physical and cognitive disabilities. In particular, this healthcare support system allows caregivers to be automatically alerted of potentially hazardous situations that happen to the inhabitants while these are alone. The design stemmed from six system requirements derived from the results of three focus groups conducted with 30 caregivers of different ALFs in Northern Italy.

Keywords: Smart caring environments · Assisted living facilities · Caregivers · Persons with disabilities · Ambient assisted living

1 Introduction

Ambient assisted living (AAL) and general healthcare support systems have mainly focused on improving the quality of life for people (especially the elderly) in their own homes and on supporting medical staff in structured environments such as hospitals. From a technical standpoint, the potential of IoT technology to enhance or at least to enrich these systems by sensing physiological signals ubiquitously and unobtrusively, is being increasingly recognized.

However, few studies about IoT-based systems aiming at supporting users different than doctors in hospitals or patients in their homes are available in the literature. In particular, papers that describe systems to support caregivers in ALFs[1] for persons with disabilities are very limited, with some significant exceptions such as WearNET [1] and AMON [2] which are available in the literature for almost a decade now. Another exception, more recent and particularly interesting is presented by Borazio et al. [3], which combines wearable and environmental sensing for sleep studies in a non-structured environment.

---

[1] An assisted living facility is a housing facility for persons with disabilities. ALFs ensure health, safety, and well-being conditions for people in situation of dependency due to cognitive or physical disabilities. In these facilities, unlike in hospitals, there are no full-time nurses nor physicians providing medical treatments.

© Institute for Computer Sciences, Social Informatics and Telecommunications Engineering 2015
R. Giaffreda et al. (Eds.): IoT360 2014, Part I, LNICST 150, pp. 172–177, 2015.
DOI: 10.1007/978-3-319-19656-5_25

The objective of this paper is to present the design and preliminary implementation of an IoT system which combines wearable/mobile technologies with smart caring environments for supporting caregivers that work in ALFs for persons with disabilities. In particular, such a system fulfils six system requirements derived from the results of three focus groups conducted with 30 caregivers of different ALFs in Northern Italy.

2   User Requirements Analysis

At our knowledge, there are no specific design guidelines for healthcare support systems aimed at supporting caregivers that work with persons with disabilities in ALFs. Therefore, the first phase of our study consisted in identifying the needs and concerns that healthcare workers in ALFs have, understanding how they tackle problems and difficulties in their daily work, and how technology can help or support them. To that end, we conducted three 90-min group interviews in the form of focus groups, in three different RAFs (*Residenza Assistenziale Flessibile*, an Italian type of ALF). These group interviews were held in Italian and focused on caregivers' daily activities, common problems and desires. Full audio recordings and photos of particular areas and systems of the three ALFs were collected. We interviewed 30 participants, 22 female and 8 male, with different years of expertise. All of them were professional caregivers, working in three RAFs managed by the Cooperativa Frassati[2]. Two of the structures accommodate people with various degree of mental disorders, while the third one houses people with motor impairments. Each RAF hosts around 10 people and assistance is guaranteed 24/7. All the visited RAFs have a backyard, a fully equipped kitchen, a laundry, an infirmary, a living room, a space used as an office by caregivers and single or shared bedrooms for the inhabitants. Based on such data and on relevant related works such as [4] carried out by Morris et al., we extrapolated the system requirements on which we built the system presented in this paper. Common needs emerge from participants, with some minor differences due to the diverse type of disabilities present in the RAFs. In fact, people with motor disabilities perform most of their activities inside the RAF, while many activities carried on by persons with cognitive disabilities are situated outside the house. During the day, two caregivers are always present in the RAF, performing various activities, such as personal assistance or housework. RAF inhabitants can request the assistance of a caregiver by calling her by voice or using buzzers which are in fixed positions around the house. During the night, only one caregiver is present in the RAF, performing some houseworks and running ward rounds. Each caregiver brings with her a cordless phone, multiple keys and, in some cases, her personal smartphone. RAF inhabitants with mental disabilities, unlike those with motor impairments, do not own any technological tool, such as smartphones, tablets, or computers. Caregivers and inhabitants' parents promote this situation, because of the possibility that such objects might be stolen, broken or forgotten outside the RAF.

---

[2] http://www.coopfrassati.com/ (last visited on July 20, 2014).

3   Discussion and System Requirements

We propose an unobtrusive and ubiquitous IoT system with wearable/mobile components, for effectively tackling the most relevant and frequent problems of caregivers within RAFs, without compromising the privacy or dignity of the RAF inhabitants. The system focus on one important issue that emerged during the focus groups: the modalities to provide and require assistance. Nowadays they have to call caregivers by voice or using a buzzer which is fixed in some locations inside the RAF. However, there are situations where caregivers cannot hear the inhabitants calls, or where the buzzer is not reachable. In fact, inhabitants may be outside the house, away from caregivers (e.g., in the backyard), or they may have fallen out of the wheelchair unable to use the buzzer. These missed calls are a problem that currently is not tackled, but that caregivers perceive as "really important" since they are not able to timely intervene. Another related problem of the RAFs we visited that we tried to address with our system, is how to monitor the inhabitants while they are alone in order to timely assist them, in case of need. Inhabitants with either mental or physical disabilities may need quick assistance, but may not be able to request it, e.g., they may be in the middle of an epileptic seizure. Until now, the problem has been tackled by running overnight ward rounds to constantly check for potentially hazardous situations, while during the day it has not been tackled at all.

The overall system requirements, elicited from the analysis of the focus groups results, are reported below. Some of them can be also found, in similar formulations, in other related works such as [4].

1. *Detection and notification of potentially hazardous situations.* Caregivers should be alerted when an inhabitant is involved in a potentially hazardous situation, without the need of constantly running ward rounds or using privacy invasive methods (e.g., video recording).
2. *Supporting smart assistance.* Provide the inhabitants with a smart way of requiring the caregivers assistance, without using noisy buzzers. Confirm that the assistance requests are addressed properly by at least one caregiver.
3. *Determining inhabitants presence in sensitive areas.* Some places of the RAF may not be suitable for the inhabitants, so caregivers want to know where they are located.
4. *Support for RAF management aspects.* Caregivers require that if some information system has to be implemented, it must support some management aspects of the RAF as well as the inhabitants routines planning.
5. *Unobtrusiveness.* Caregivers do not want more "objects" to carry around or strange "gadgets" to use, even if they give useful functionalities. Therefore, the system must fade in the background of the daily life in an unobtrusive way.
6. *Hands-free operations.* Caregivers require to have their hands free, for being ready to assist inhabitants as soon as possible, without concerning about the "health" of the device (i.e., they must be resistant to water and shocks).

4 System Design

For meeting the requirements reported in the previous section, we designed a system that monitors RAF inhabitants by measuring and interpreting some of their body signals and environmental conditions to notify the caregivers whether and where their assistance is needed. In general, the system first collects data from all the different sources and process it to obtain an overview of the RAF situation. Then, by interpreting such information, it determines if an inhabitant needs assistance. In the case she does, the system is also in charge of notifying it to the caregivers, for her to be assisted. The caregiver that first reaches the inhabitant, has to turn the notification off to prevent his colleagues to come in vain. The system also is in charge of managing notifications regarding the overall RAF management (req. 4).

Sensors. Environmental and wearable sensors are used for measuring the environmental conditions of the RAF and the body signals of its inhabitants, respectively. The former sense ambient light, temperature, and people presence in specific rooms in order to meet the requirement of determining inhabitants presence in "sensitive" areas (req. 3), such as the kitchen or the infirmary. Wearable technology is used because it allows to meet the unobtrusiveness requirement (req. 5). We choose to adopt the wristwatch form factor since watches are ideally located for body sensors [5] and wearable displays. The wearable sensors collect acceleration data that can be processed and analysed for detecting epileptic seizures and falls, which is one of the most important system requirements (req. 1). The wearable devices worn by the inhabitants with adequate cognitive capabilities, have a "call function" that can be used for consciously requesting caregivers' assistance.

Middleware. The middleware is in charge of managing the overall system. It receives the environmental and body measures from the sensors, interprets them and determines if a situation that requires the presence of a caregiver is taking place. The middleware does not aim at assessing exactly what is happening with each RAF inhabitant, but its scope is to point the caregivers attention to "suspicious situations" that *might* require their presence. This means that the middleware is not designed to try to accurately detect potentially hazardous situations, such as epileptic seizures, where the consequences of missing one are very serious and are out of the scope of this kind of support. Caregivers required this type of notification since they are already used to this kind of dynamics in RAFs, given that ward rounds work like this, i.e., by checking on someone even if it is not strictly required. Once the middleware determines that the presence of a caregiver is required somewhere, it sends a proper notification to all the caregivers in the RAF.

Notification Devices. The devices in which caregivers receive the notifications sent by the middleware could be wearable or mobile. Wearable technology is the most suitable for meeting most of the previous requirements. One of those requirements (req. 6) is that caregivers need to have the hands free the most of the time, therefore a smartphone or a tablet are not appropriate for them. As in the case of the inhabitant sensors, the notification devices use a wristwatch form factor that is preferred by the caregivers that do not want *"another gadget to think about"*. Mobile devices can be exploited to satisfy requirement 4. Notification devices should have sound and vibration alerts capable to draw the attention of the caregiver even in noisy environments.

5 Prototype and Preliminary Validation

The designed system was prototyped with reduced functionalities by extending the Dog gateway[3] capabilities to realize the described middleware. We used sensors of presence, temperature, and light intensity for collecting environmental data, and the cost-effective and re-programmable Texas Instruments eZ430-Chronos wristwatch for notifying caregivers and sensing from inhabitants wrists. This smart watch integrates a 96 segment LCD display, a 3-axis accelerometer, sensors of temperature, pressure and a battery voltage, into an affordable device. The only functionality not supported by the eZ430-Chronos is the haptic feedback, so at this stage vibration alerts are not implemented yet. We use a custom firmware extension[4] similar to the one described by De Russis et al. [6]. The interaction between the wearable devices (eZ430-Chronos) and the middleware (Dog) adopts a client-server paradigm. Their communication starts automatically once per minute, or manually when an inhabitant requests the caregiver presence. Each eZ430-Chronos has a unique identifier that is read and stored by the control system to determine with which device is communicating (i.e., who asks for assistance).

The feasibility of the proposed system was verified in the lab and consisted in the deployment of a scaled down version of the overall system. Two volunteers acted like a caregiver and a RAF inhabitant equipped with one eZ430-Chronos wristwatch each. The system encompassed sensors of presence, light and temperature, and the Dog gateway running on a Raspberry Pi[5]. The goal was to verify the correct operation of the notification subsystem either when the assistance is requested from the inhabitants or when it is requested automatically by interpreting sensor data. Two use cases were successfully tried out: *Assistance request from the inhabitant* and *Notification of potentially hazardous situation*. In the first case the volunteer acting as the inhabitant requested the caregiver assistance by tapping on her wristwatch. Dog notified the caregiver providing the name of the inhabitant asking for his help. In the second case, the volunteer acting as the inhabitant moved her arm in such a way that the middleware

---

[3] An open source gateway for home and building automation, based on the OSGi framework which provides interoperability between different IoT devices (http://dog-gateway.github.io).

[4] http://github.com/poelzi/OpenChronos (last visited on July 20, 2014).

[5] A credit-card sized computer with 512 MB of RAM, two USB ports and a 100 Mb Ethernet port.

could interpret that something may be wrong and alerted the caregiver. In both cases the system responded in few seconds and the caregiver turned the assistance request off by reaching the inhabitant and tapping a personal code on the inhabitant's watch.

6 Conclusions

In this paper, we present a system that exploits the synergy between wearable/mobile technology and environmental sensing to support caregivers working in assisted living facilities for people with physical or cognitive disabilities. The system requirements stem directly from three focus groups realized with 30 caregivers in Northern Italy. The system has been prototyped and a preliminary validation has been performed, for verifying its technical feasibility. Future work will be expanding the implemented system to effectively detect potentially hazardous situations by autonomously analysing sensor in real RAFs, and experimenting with other type of wearable/mobile devices.

References

1. Lukowicz, P., Junker, H., Stäger, M., von Büren, T., Tröster, G.: WearNET: a distributed multi-sensor system for context aware wearables. In: Borriello, G., Holmquist, L.E. (eds.) UbiComp 2002. LNCS, vol. 2498, p. 361. Springer, Heidelberg (2002)
2. Anliker, U., Ward, J.A., Lukowicz, P., Troster, G., Dolveck, F., Baer, M., Keita, F., Schenker, E.B., Catarsi, F., Coluccini, L., et al.: Amon: a wearable multiparameter medical monitoring and alert system. IEEE Trans. Inf. Technol. Biomed. 8(4), 415–427 (2004)
3. Borazio,M., Van Laerhoven, K.: Combining wearable and environmental sensing into an unobtrusive tool for long-term sleep studies. In: Proceedings of the 2nd ACM SIGHIT International Health Informatics Symposium, IHI 2012, pp. 71–80. ACM, New York (2012)
4. Morris, M., Lundell, J., Dishman, E., Needham, B.: New perspectives on ubiquitous computing from ethnographic study of elders with cognitive decline. In: Dey, A.K., Schmidt, A., McCarthy, J.F. (eds.) UbiComp 2003. LNCS, vol. 2864, pp. 227–242. Springer, Heidelberg (2003)
5. Maurer, U., Rowe, A., Smailagic, A., Siewiorek, D.: Location and activity recognition using eWatch: a wearable sensor platform. In: Cai, Y., Abascal, J. (eds.) Ambient Intelligence in Everyday Life. LNCS (LNAI), vol. 3864, pp. 86–102. Springer, Heidelberg (2006)
6. De Russis, L., Bonino, D., Corno, F.: The smart home controller on your wrist. In: Proceedings of the 2013 ACM Conference on Pervasive and Ubiquitous Computing Adjunct Publication, UbiComp 2013 Adjunct, pp. 785–792. ACM, New York (2013)

Intelligent Healthcare Services to Support Health Monitoring of Elderly

Mobyen Uddin Ahmed[1][(⊠)], Hadi Banaee[1], Xavier Rafael-Palou[2],
and Amy Loutfi[1]

[1] Center for Applied Autonomous Sensor Systems, Örebro University,
Fakultetsg. 1, 70182 Örebro, Sweden
{mobyen.ahmed,hadi.banaee,amy.loutfi}@oru.se
[2] Barcelona Digital Technology Centre,
C/RocBoronat, 11, 08018 Barcelona, Spain
xrafael@bdigital.org

Abstract. This paper proposed an approach of intelligent healthcare services to support health monitoring of old people through the project named SAAPHO. Here, definition and architecture of the proposed healthcare services are presented considering six different health parameters such as: (1) physical activity, (2) blood pressure, (3) glucose, (4) medication compliance, (5) pulse monitoring and (6) weight monitoring. The outcome of the proposed services is evaluated in a case study where total 201 subjects from Spain and Slovenia are involved for user requirements analysis considering (1) end users, (2) clinicians, and (3) field study analysis perspectives. The result shows the potentiality and competence of the proposed healthcare services for the users.

1 Introduction

According to WHO, healthy ageing is vital for countries' economic development because of it is one of the three pillars of active ageing [1]. Around two billion people i.e., one out of every four will be older than 60 years in the year 2050 according to [2]. As a consequence there is a need to provide efficient healthcare services to the elderlies. Here, the term 'Healthcare' means diagnosis, treatment and prevention of diseases and illnesses of human beings. Traditionally, a healthcare service is mainly focusing on primary care located at a local community where physician consultations take place for all patients as the 1st visit [3]. However, today, the healthcare services are not limited to take place in primary care facilities simply due to deployment of mobile devices and/or wireless communication. The result is a provision of service that could be accessible to anyone at any time and in anywhere with a good quality [4]. Research also shows that several projects like eCAALYX and HELP are on-going which provide home healthcare for elderly [5]. Similarly, due to the need to have ICT and globalization, several web sites or online based healthcare service providers are available in the market which provide possibilities to monitor health parameters such as blood pressure, blood glucose [9, 10], and activity [16, 17].

© Institute for Computer Sciences, Social Informatics and Telecommunications Engineering 2015
R. Giaffreda et al. (Eds.): IoT360 2014, Part I, LNICST 150, pp. 178–186, 2015.
DOI: 10.1007/978-3-319-19656-5_26

This paper presents the definition and architecture of healthcare service to support a health monitoring of elderly based on several health parameters through a project called SAAPHO.[1] In SAAPHO, six different health parameters have been considered: (1) physical activity, (2) blood pressure, (3) glucose, (4) medication compliance, (5) pulse monitoring and (6) weight monitoring. The project is offering intelligent, intuitive and user-friendly tools using a mobile tactile interface (android based tablet) and wireless sensor devices that will allow and facilitate the home monitoring. The sensor devices for these parameters are wearable and have Bluetooth communication to send raw data measurements in the cloud (i.e. Health Intelligent Server) for further processing. Data transfer is done using https and SOAP web services from the sensors to the cloud and cloud to user-interface. The proposed approach identified and constructed three different kinds of healthcare services for each parameter: (1) *real time feedback generation service*, (2) *historical summary calculation service* and (3) *recommendation generation sDevices_Not_Usedervice*. The *1st* service applies a rule-based reasoning technique on each measurement to generate a text based feedback message. The *2nd* service serve a daily/weekly wise historical summary based on raw measurements and store them into a MySQL database for offline access by the user. The *3rd* service generates reminder, alarm and necessary recommendation provided on a weekly basis. A comparison between a case study of user requirements and the proposed approach is presented where the user requirements are conducted by considering three perspectives namely (1) end users, (2) clinicians, and (3) field study analysis.

2 Definitions and Architecture of the Healthcare Services

The main objective of the healthcare services in SAAPHO is to monitor health parameters of elderly and warn them in time in order to increase their personal independence. Moreover, it also provides recommendations to take necessary steps such as when they should go to healthcare provider or do any physical exercises. For instance, considering a scenario of a healthy user, one might have a blood pressure machine or blood glucose measuring device at home and he/she might use the devices in his/her daily lives. However, the devices only provide some values i.e. 122/82 or 5.7 mmol/L [9] and if someone is technically sound they might have the possibility to use internet and Google and try to interpret the measurement values or need to ask to the health provider directly. At the same time, as soon as someone diagnosed with heart disease or diabetes, a clinician might want to see a historical measurement for a week or a month before they start to use any medication. For example, a diabetes patient often asked by the healthcare provider to use a log book or diary where they can write all the measurements they have taken [10]. Moreover, depending on patient's historical measurements a doctor provides his/her recommendation on food, medication or when they should meet again. Thus, the proposed approach has identified the healthcare services

---

[1] http://www.saapho-aal.eu/.

with three different kinds of facilities for each parameter, (1) *real time feedback generation service*, (2) *historical summary calculation service* and (3) *recommendation generation service*.

The goal of the *Real Time Feedback Generation Service* is to provide a feedback message based on sensor readings in real time. Here, a rule-based classification method is applied to classify the measurements. For example, a blood pressure measurement 142/92 mmHg could be classified as "High blood pressure" and/or BMI 26.1 by measuring user's weight[2] could be classified "Overweighed". A set of rules used in the classification method are mainly collected from the literature study [6–9, 11, 12, 15] which is further validated through healthcare practitioners. For example, rules for blood pressure and medication compliance are presented in Table 1. The rule-based classification scheme is developed in an *Intelligent Health Gateway* (see Sect. 2.1 architecture), where as soon as the gateway receives the measurements it classifies them.

Table 1. Rules are used to generate real time feedback for Blood Pressure and, medication compliance Systolic/Diastolic as mmHg.

Health parameters	Rules to generate real time feedback
Blood pressure (BP)	1. If Systolic < 90 or Diastolic < 60 then BP_class = "*Low*"
	2. If Systolic is 90 to 119 and Diastolic is 60 to 79 then BP_class = "*Normal*"
	3. If Systolic is 120 to 139 or Diastolic is 80 to 89 then BP_class = "*Pre-High*"
	4. If Systolic > 140 or Diastolic > 90 then BP_class = "*High*"
Medication	1. If current_device_info ! = stored_device_info then message = "*wrong pills*"
	2. If current_device_info = = stored_device_info and interval_time < 60 then message = "*already taken the pill*"

It is crucial to keep and store all measurements especially if someone has diabetes or high blood pressure since this kind of diseases need a proper management in order to keep a healthy lifestyle. A weekly or monthly diary book is often used to keep track of blood glucose measurements and this helps to adjust medicine and food nutrition for a diabetes patient [9] as an example. A similar concept is proposed here in the *Historical Summary Calculation Service*, which means the service will calculate historical summary on a daily and weekly basis. This historical summary information is calculated automatically and stored into the *Health Intelligent Server (HIS)* as presented in Sect. 2.1 architecture. A user has a possibility to see a summary in a graph for a specific range of dates. In order to calculate the summary, the service uses raw data measurements and the classification. This service mainly considers frequency of each classes and the number of total measurements. For example, in order to monitor medication compliance it calculates "total number of medication is taken", "total number of medications", and "total number of medications are skipped". The historical

---

[2] http://wserver.flc.losrios.edu/~willson/fitns304/handouts/bodyComposition html.

summary calculation service collects the measurements for each individual parameter for user from MySQL health database and starts historical summary calculation on a daily and weekly basis. The automatic scripts for calculating daily and weekly based historical summary are developed using PHP programming language where the script for daily-wise historical summary runs every day at 23:59 and the script for weekly-wise historical summary runs on every Saturday at 23:59 (once a week). After calculating the summary, the information is again saved and stored into the MySQL health database for further use.

The main objective of the *Recommendation Generation Service* is to generate a recommendation including reminder and alarm based on user's historical summary and raw data measurements.

1. *Devices_Not_Used:* a reminder message is generated if there is no measurement received over one week duration i.e. the sensor device is not used for a week.
2. *Medications_Skipped:* an alarm message is generated if the number of medications skipped and the number of medication that should be taken in a day is equal, i.e. the patient totally skipped taking his/her medication for that day.
3. *Out_Of_Normal_Range:* considering a week, if 70 % of the measurements classes are outside the normal range, a recommendation message is generated to "Visit a healthcare provider".
4. *Fluctuation:* if the measurements over a week show fluctuation in more than 70 % of the cases, a recommendation message is generated to "Go to a doctor".
5. *Weight_Loss:* the current weight will be compared with the previous weight (3 months ago) and the recommendation is generate "Visit your doctor" while the difference is more than 3 kg.
6. *Weight_Increased/Weight_Decreased:* considering one month measurements, a slope value will be calculated. Based on positive/negative slope value the weight increased/decreased recommendation is generated.
7. *Activity_Increased/Activity_Decreased:* considering one week measurements, a slope value will be calculated. Based on positive/negative slope value the activity increased/decreased recommendation is generated.
8. A monthly summary is generated based on the raw measurements where statistical features i.e. maximum, minimum, standard deviation, and average for each week is calculated. This information together with the date will be sent to the user via email.

The automatic script for recommendation generation is developed in the *Health Intelligent Server (HIS)* using PHP programming language and they run once in a week, i.e. every Saturday at 23:59. The generated messages are sent to the user according their priority value calculated based on user's age, health parameters and the classification. The monthly summary information and recommendation are also generated automatically once in a month and provide the information to the user's email.

2.1   Architecture of the Healthcare Services

In order to provide an intelligent healthcare service through SAAPHO, several components are considered and integrated. Figure 1 presents all the components related to

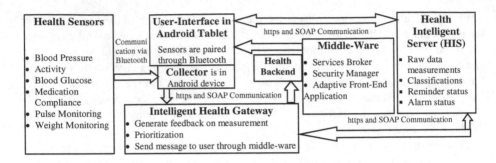

Fig. 1. Communication and components related to the healthcare

the healthcare service and communications between the components. The main components are: (1) sensor devices for healthcare (2) android based user-interface and collector (3) intelligent health gateway (4) health backend including middle-ware and (5) health intelligent server. The *sensor unit* contains six health related sensor devices and the devices are run by battery and communicate via Bluetooth communication. The sensor devices are paired with a Tablet where android operating system is installed. Some sensor devices are just bought from the market and integrated into the system, for example, the blood pressure and weight monitoring devices are collected from a third party vendor OMRON[3] and BeneCheck[4] and others are in-house products provided by the work package partner IZM[5] which are under development. The sensor is sending the data sets via Bluetooth Classic and Bluetooth Low Energy (BTLE) to the collector.

In the Tablet, *user-interface and collector* are running, where the collector receives health measurements using Bluetooth communication from the sensor devices upon user request through the user-interface. The Collector is based on native Java source code, which is in general the main programming language for Android devices. As soon as the collector receives the measurements it transfers them to the *intelligent health gateway* through https protocol and SOAP web service communication. The measurements are sent as a zip file including timestamps, battery and some other related information. The user interface is developed using JAVA programming language so that it can run in Android 4.0 operating system considering the *Google Nexus 10* device. The *Intelligent Health Gateway* mainly conveys the message among the collector, HIS and middle-ware. It classifies the measurements, calculates priority, asks for message id to the *Health Intelligent Server (HIS)* and finally forwards them to the middle-ware through health backend. The *middle-ware* is a module collected from AAL (Ambient Assisted Living) architecture[6] which includes services broker, security manager, adaptive front-end application and etc. The *health backend* is the entry point of the *middle-ware*, where SessionID and UUID are for each user is generated in

---

[3] http://www.healthcare.omron.co.jp/bt/english/.

[4] http://www.glbiotech.com.tw/productdesc.php?pdtid=11.

[5] http://www.izm.fraunhofer.de/en.html.

[6] http://universaal.org/index.php/es/about/about-project-description.

security manager. Adaptive Front-End Application (AFEA), is a module in the user's device, which is in charge of handling the interaction of the user with the User Interface and of presenting the information in the way indicated by the AAL architecture. Services Broker (SB) hosts a registry of descriptions of the services inside the AAL architecture but also of services out of it that could be useful for the users [14]. Middle-ware also stores all the service URLs and user ids and communicates with other components using health backend. Middle-ware receives the measurements and generates a textual feedback message based on the measurements and their classification. Finally, the textual message is sent to the user in SAAPHO user-interface. The *health intelligent server (HIS)* stores all the raw measurements and generates message id for the communication. It also calculates daily and weekly historical summary and store them in a MySQL database. The user has a direct access to the HIS to see the historical summary through the user-interface. HIS also generates recommendation in weekly basis based on historical summary and raw data measurements. The generated recommendations are sent to the user through health gateway, health backend and middle-ware.

3 Evaluations

During the SAAPHO's system design, a *questionnaire* is used to collect the users' needs and preferences. Here, the main goal was to collect the users' requirements to select the technology, devices, to design the components that the system should have, and to define the functionality. Regarding the questionnaires, participants were asked about general requirements for SAAPHO system. Participants also indicated their needs and preferences in monitoring their health (medication, activity and blood pressure). For example: 'How would you like to monitor your medication compliance – e.g. buzzer light...-?'; 'Would you be interested in monitoring your daily physical activity?'. The user requirements presented here considering three perspectives and they are (1) end users, (2) clinicians, and (3) field study analysis. The user requirements have been gathered via a field study conducted in Spain and Slovenia which included a questionnaire with 201 participants followed by 2 focus groups [13]. Below the paper compares the requirements and users viewpoints about the proposed approach i.e. the healthcare services to provide remote health monitoring of elderlies.

According to *end user perspective*, the activity monitoring device should monitor 1st the movement of a user in time stamped and classified them as none, low, medium or high level. 2nd it can also calculate the calorie consumption based on number of step counts and present information in a trending graph on calories/step counts. The blood glucose monitoring could measure blood sugar several times a day and in the case of diagnosed Diabetes it could provide the real time feedback. The blood sugar value could be stored with a time stamp which would then be analyzed to detect the status of diagnosed diabetes. It is important to monitor blood pressure for the elderly, moreover in the case of people who have already experienced high blood pressure. Forgetfulness is one of the leading reasons for medication non-compliance, which could be solved through a reminder system. The medication monitoring tool could track the drug regime and be able to raise alarms when not being followed properly and/or also reminding if the medicine was taken. Using the pulse monitoring tool, one could know whether the intensity of the physical activity was too high, exceeding the threshold value (especially with more strenuous exercises, like walking uphill, running, cycling). Regularly weight monitoring is also interesting and could be used once in a week and some recommendation is necessary when the weight is lost. Moreover and very important is the ease of use, affordability and ease of carrying the device on a person's body. The users would prefer a wearable sensor during training and read results later at home.

According to *clinical perspective*, glucose monitoring should be used by the individuals diagnosed from Type 2 Diabetes to monitor their blood glucose and typically these types of patients measure their blood glucose at least once a day. Activity monitoring could promote physical activity and enhance healthy ageing. Considering the pulse monitoring, it could be useful to detect heart rate during exercise as proxy of exercise intensity and provide information if the intensity of exercise they do is right or too demanding for them. In medication monitoring, the treatment plan of medication should be adjusted on a weekly basis mainly by the patients themselves and a formal or informal career. Depending on specified times (i.e. morning, midday, night, before sleep) a reminder could be generated and presented. Blood pressure is very important to measure for the older persons who are diagnosed with Hypertension (high blood pressure), as they typically need frequent monitoring. Similarly, checking weight is also valuable; it will help to adjust daily meal. Moreover, all the monitoring systems could facilitate self-management and communication with health professionals. That means the results could be presented very clearly and could display the trends and comparison with reference values. In order to facilitate communication with healthcare professionals, data could be transferred to the healthcare center and be read by clinicians, but also the older person could present them personally in his/her smartphone or tablet PC to the healthcare provider (if no e-health system is available).

According to the *field study analysis and results*, the activity monitoring should calculate both the step count and calorie burn and be presented in trending graphs (calorie, weight, step counts). Presenting data graphically could be done using some summary bar graph where the accumulated (weekly or monthly) duration of non-walking activities are shown together with bars for the step count and calories for the same period. Concerning the blood glucose monitoring, the diabetes patients require a direct feedback on glucose value both when at home and on the go. Regarding the blood pressure monitoring, users would typically take a reading once a week and add comments to blood pressure readings like, "gym", "measured when feeling unwell" etc. to facilitate interpretation in the context. The user would like to have reminders for their medication however, the length of the so called "reminder cancel window" has to be adjustable as it depends on the type of medication. On the sensor side, the reminder signal should be both buzzer and light, the reminder function should continue as long as the cap is left off. Considering the pulse monitoring, the sensor should alarm in real-time during training especially when the pulse is too high.

4   Conclusions

This paper has provided a description of the definition of the healthcare services and their design in the context of the SAAPHO project. Specific emphasis has been placed on detailing the different type of services and health parameters that will be used in the project. The paper has also provided a comparison of these services against the perspective of the end-users and the healthcare professionals. The aim of this paper has been to share the design of the healthcare services so that other similar efforts can take part in the specific values and rules that have been used within the context of the project. Future work will evaluate this first version of the services in a controlled field trial.

Acknowledgments. This work has been supported by the project named SAAPHO (aal-2010-3-035) is funded by Vinnova Sweden's Innovation Funding Agency and by the Call AAL (Ambient Assisted Living) within the Call 3, ICT-based solutions for advancement of older persons' independence and participation in the self-serve society.

References

1. WHO: Healthy ageing is vital for development - prevention of non-communicable diseases throughout the life course is key says new who policy roadmap (2002). http://www.who.int/mediacentre/news/releases/release24/en/. Accessed 30 June 2014
2. Connecting and caring: innovations for healthy ageing. http://www.who.int/bulletin/volumes/90/3/12-020312/en/index.html. Accessed 30 June 2014
3. Jennifer, L.S., David, O.W., Barbara, P.Y., Debra, J.J., Michaela, E.M., Joshua, J.P., Joseph, M., Véronique, L.R., Jon, O.E., Walter, A.R.: Why do patients visit their doctors? Assessing the most prevalent conditions in a defined US population. US National Library of Medicine National Institutes of Health (2014)
4. Varshney, U.: Pervasive healthcare and wireless health monitoring. J. Mobile Netw. Appl. Arch. **12**(2–3), 113–127 (2007)
5. Catalogue of Projects, Ambient Assisted Living Joint Programme (AAL JP) (2011). http://www.aal-europe.eu/wp-content/uploads/2012/04/AALCatalogue_onlineV4.pdf.   Accessed 30 June 2014
6. Medication Compliance Monitoring System (MCMS), Cybernet Medical. http://www.cybernetmedical.com/index.php/mcms. Accessed 30 June 2014
7. eCAP monitor for bottled medications, Information Mediary Corporation (IMC). http://informationmediary.com/ecap. Accessed 30 June 2014
8. Culhane, K.M., O'Connor, M., Lyons, D., Lyons, G.M.: Accelerometers in rehabilitation medicine for older adults. Acad. J. Age Ageing **34**(6), 556–560 (2005)
9. Alberti, K.G.M.M., Zimmet, P.Z.: Definition, diagnosis and classification of diabetes mellitus and its complications. Part 1: Diagnosis and classification of diabetes mellitus. Provisional report of a WHO Consultation. J. Diabetes Med. **15**(7), 539–553 (1998)
10. Strowig, S.M., Raskin, P.: Improved glycemic control in intensively treated type 1 diabetic patients using blood glucose meters with storage capability and computer-assisted analysis. J. Diabetes Care **21**, 1694–1698 (1998)

11. Understanding blood pressure readings. American Heart Association (2011). http://www.heart.org/HEARTORG/Conditions/HighBloodPressure/AboutHighBloodPressure/Understanding-Blood-Pressure-Readings_UCM_301764_Article.jsp. Accessed 30 June 2014

12. Why exercise with a Heart Rate Monitor. https://zsig.com/content/why_exercise_with_a_heart_rate_monitor_/. Accessed 30 June 2014

13. Domenech, S., Rivero, J., Coll-Planas, L., Sainz, F.J., Reissner, A., Miralles, F.: Involving older people in the design of an innovative information and communication technologies system promoting active aging: the saapho project. J. Accessibility Des. All **3**(1), 13–27 (2013)

14. Sala, P., Tazari, S., Farshchian, B., Furfari, F.: The universAAL Reference Architecture. universAAL Deliverable D1.3 – E (2013)

15. Deurenberg, P., Weststrate, J.A., Seidell, J.C.: Body mass index as a measure of body fatness: age- and sex-specific prediction formulas. Br. J. Nutr. **65**(2), 105–114 (1991)

16. Ahmed, M.U., Banaee, H., Loutfi, A.: Health monitoring for elderly: an application using case-based reasoning and cluster analysis. ISRN Artif. Intell. **2013**, 11 (2013). 380239

17. Ahmed, M.U., Loutfi, A.: Physical activity identification using supervised machine learning and based on pulse rate. Adv. Comput. Sci. Appl. **4**, 209–217 (2013)

Real-Time Monitoring Using Finite State-Machine Algorithms

Sebastian Fuicu$^{(\boxtimes)}$, Andrei Avramescu, Diana Lascu,
Roxana Padurariu, and Marius Marcu

Politehnica University of Timisoara, Timişoara, Romania
{sebastian.fuicu,marius.marcu}@cs.upt.ro,
{andrei.avramescu,diana.lascu,
roxana.padurari}@student.upt.ro

Abstract. This paper presents the architecture of a medical platform for chronic diseases sufferers that enables specialist physicians to have a permanent overview of the patient's health. The proposed system, HChecked, integrates the monitoring of vital parameters, reception of notification in case of any exceeding of the pre-defined limits of these parameters and prediction of the evolution of the current disease or of the possibility of occurrence of another disease. The software system follows the idea of trading systems that offers efficient prediction with a high level of security. This concept is based on a particular implementation of finite state-machine algorithms, which enable physicians to run complex rules against particular health information of a certain patient to predict the evolution of the current diseases or the appearance of others. Although the system allows many points of view, this paper is oriented towards the specific way in which complex rules are created.

Keywords: Finite state machine algorithms · e-health · Chronic diseases · Patient monitoring · Permanent watch · Medical complex rules

1 Introduction

The potential for pervasive computing is evident in almost every aspect of our lives including the hospital, emergency and critical situations, industry or education. The use of this technology in the field of health and wellness is known as pervasive health care. Mobile computing describes a new class of mobile computing devices which are becoming omnipresent in everyday life [1].

A significant proportion of the human population suffers from various medical conditions, including chronic ailments and medical emergencies due to sudden injuries. In absence of continuous medical care, many chronic ailments prove to be fatal. On the other hand, in various medical emergency scenarios, timeliness of medical attention is even more important [2]. Today, chronic diseases represent the major share of the burden of disease in Europe and are responsible for 86 % of all deaths. They affect more than 80 % of people aged over 65 and represent a major challenge for health and social systems [3].

© Institute for Computer Sciences, Social Informatics and Telecommunications Engineering 2015
R. Giaffreda et al. (Eds.): IoT360 2014, Part I, LNICST 150, pp. 187–192, 2015.
DOI: 10.1007/978-3-319-19656-5_27

One of the main challenges in the management of chronic diseases is the efficient and continuous monitoring of the patient's health by the health professionals. In that sense, the patient-doctor interaction is preferred to not happen in a monthly basis scheme, but it can be continuous by using monitoring systems [4]. Although this statement may seem obvious, the continuous care they should be provided is often overlooked. The use of a history of a patient's evolution may be helpful not only for that particular individual, but also for those suffering of similar symptoms. The help they need should not come only in case of an emergency, prevention being an important factor to take into consideration when speaking about chronic disease sufferers. We propose a system that is able to record and monitor a patient's health parameters by creating and distributing notifications when the received data exceeds the limits of the complex conditions that are pre-defined by the specialist physicians.

This paper is structured as follows: Sect. 2 describes the system from the hardware and software point of view, also presenting the applications the specialist physician and patient can use. Section 3 presents the finite state machine algorithm that is used to analyze the patient's data. Section 4 gives an example of how this algorithm can be used to create complex rules for a patient.

2 System Overview

Recent advances in biomedical engineering, wireless network and computer technologies have enabled the possibility of remote patient monitoring. Based on these technologies, it is possible to improve patient care, chronic disease management, and promote lifelong health and wellbeing [5].

Data mining in the medical context can be seen very challenging from the specialist's physician point of view which does not possess technical skills to write and execute complex algorithms to analyze patient health data. Moreover, adding real-time analyzing and large data sets of medical information to the equation makes the problem seem unsolvable for the end-user.

We propose as a solution a medical platform capable to abstract the problem of real-time big data analyzing, including an interface that offers the possibility to create complex equations on patient data defined as finite state-machine algorithms.

In this section we look at the complex e-health platform, taking into consideration the way the data flow is structured. This project represented Romania in the Worldwide Final of the Imagine Cup competition 2013. This is the reason why the main software technologies used in the current system are Microsoft based.

To enable the continuous care a chronic disease patient needs, the platform offers the doctors various applications that work on different devices. The smartphone/tablet application for physician helps the doctors to be up to date with the health state of the patient and can receive notifications. The desktop application for physician produces the environment where the doctors can create complex rules. The smartphone application for patient collects medical data from the sensors and sends them forward to be analyzed (Fig. 1).

The data acquisition system that we used as a development kit contained different types of sensors (electrocardiogram, glucometer, pulse and oxygen in blood, galvanic

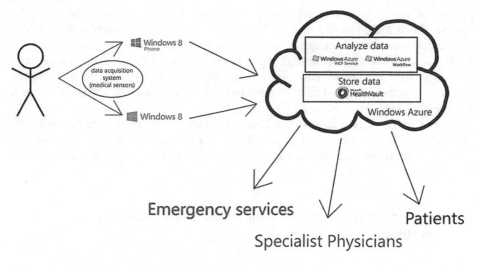

Fig. 1. Overview of the system

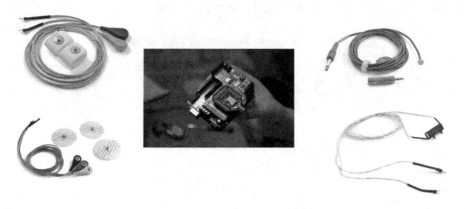

Fig. 2. Sensors

skin response, blood pressure, body temperature, patient position, airflow) depending on the diseases that we wished to be monitored (see Fig. 2).

From the software point of view, this system offers accurate predictions, but also a high level of security. After creating complex rules that will be described in the next section, the specialist physician will receive notifications at certain moments.

These notifications can be classified into two categories: General Notifications and Emergency Notifications. When a doctor receives a General Notification it means that the limits that he has enforced have been overcome. In such cases, the treatment should be checked or further investigations should be considered. If an Emergency Notification has been sent, physicians enrolled in the community who are in the vicinity and the ambulance are announced. For the physicians to be correctly localized, the system uses the GPS, feature that is used also for localizing the patient in need. Using these two points, the system is able to generate a map, which the doctor follows to get to the patient. When the physician reaches the patient, he is provided with a small health profile that gives him the necessary clues to know in which way he should act.

If the system were to collect all the data received from the sensors, storing them would represent a problem. However, because the limits in which we should find the health information are pre-defined, the system stores the data in the cloud only after it has been filtered.

Although the system comes in use for every individual patient in the community, the collected information, after approval and anonymization, can be also used in research projects and statistics. In this way, medical and pharmaceutical institutions can use these results for further research.

3   Analyzing Patient Data Using Finite State Machine Algorithms

We modeled the complex-rules part of the system using finite state machine algorithms because they can be easily comprehended by any specialist physician without any technical background or programming knowledge (Fig. 3).

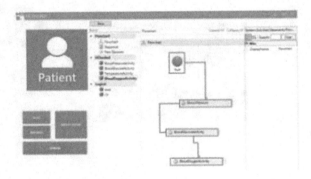

Fig. 3. Desktop application - screenshot.

We introduce the concept of operator, which is a component of a state of the finite state-machine algorithm. Each of them can be seen as a template of simple, pre-defined equations that can be combined in any way to create a complex rule to be verified against patient data. In the first version of the system we introduce four categories of operators:

Data operators (= , < , > , ≤ , ≥). These are the simplest operators that can be used directly with the patient data. For example, the doctor can set the heart rate to be greater than 80.

Time operators (time interval, minimum period, maximum period).These operators can be used only if they are correlated with data operators. Basically, continuing the same example as above, we are able to define the heart rate to be greater than 80 for seven days (or for minimum seven days or for maximum seven days).

Number of occurrences (minimum, maximum, equal). These operators can be used with any other type, having different behavior based on the correlation that has been made. If we refer to the data operators, we verify that a patient health data respects the rule for a number of times; if we combine them with time operators we check if the occurrences happen in a certain period of time; finally if we combine them with notification operators, that will be described, there will be a number of notifications equal to the number of occurrences. It will also be included in the meta-data of the online version.

4   Use Case Example

For a better understanding of how the proposed platform can be used and how simple it is for patients to be monitored we will take a particular case of a patient suffering of both diabetes and heart disease. Diabetes by itself is now regarded as the strongest risk factor for heart disease [6]. Cardiovascular disease (CVD) is a major complication of diabetes and the leading cause of early death among people with diabetes – about 65 % of people with diabetes die from heart disease and stroke. Intensive glucose control reduces the risk of any CVD event by 42 % and the risk of heart attack, stroke, or death from CVD by 57 % [7].

Based on the data acquisition system that we currently use we will take into consideration that the patient is wearing sensors for blood glucose, heart rate and blood pressure. An example of a complex rule created by specialist physicians is presented in Fig. 4.

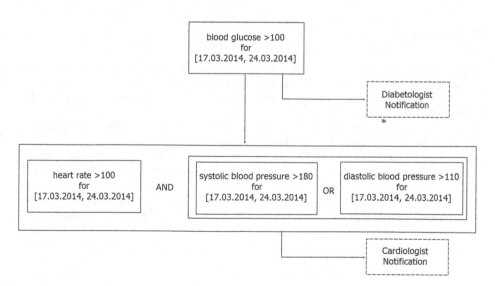

Fig. 4. Example of complex rule.

This complex rule is aimed to keep under control the blood glucose and the parameters regarding the heart disease and has two stages: first stage verifies the blood glucose of the patient for one week and the second stage checks if the heart rate and blood pressure exceed the limits pre-defined by the physician.

As seen in Fig. 4, if the patient's blood glucose is greater than 100 for one week, the diabetologist will receive a notification and then and only then the system will analyze the history data for the heart rate and blood pressure. If these parameters overcome the limits set by the cardiologist, he will be announced.

5 Conclusions

In this paper we have described an e-health platform created especially for chronic disease patients, focusing upon the way finite state machine algorithms are used to enable the physicians to create complex rules in an easy-to-use environment. While designing our system, our team consistently took into consideration the advice of medical professionals in order to identify their points of interest. The specific element of the system is the possibility to create individualized operators using basic operators, which were also previously described. This paper includes also a use case example to offer an idea about how the finite state machine algorithm is used for designing rules.

Acknowledgement. This work was partially supported by the research grant CHIST-ERA/1/ 01.10.2012 – "GEMSCLAIM: GreenEr Mobile Systems by Cross LAyer Integrated energy Management".

References

1. Shahriyar, R., Faizul, M.F., Kundu, G., Ahamed, S.I., Akbar, M.M.: Intelligent mobile health monitoring system (IMHMS). Int. J. Control Autom. **2**(3), 13–28 (2009)
2. Chakravorty, R.: Mobicare: a programmable service architecture for mobile medical care. In: Proceedings of UbiCare (2006)
3. The 2014 EU Summit on Chronic Diseases, Brussels (2014). http://ec.europa.eu/health/ major_chronic_diseases/docs/ev_20140403_mi_en.pdf
4. Kouris, I., Koutsouris, D.: Application of data mining techniques to efficiently monitor chronic diseases using wireless body area networks and smartphones. Univ. J. Biomed. Eng. **1** (2), 23–31 (2013)
5. Kańtoch, E., Jaworek, J., Augustyniak, P.: Design of a wearable sensor network for home monitoring system. In: Proceedings of the Federated Conference on Computer Science and Information Systems, pp. 401–403
6. Diabetes and Heart Disease — An Intimate Connection. http://www.joslin.org/info/diabetes_ and_heart_disease_an_intimate_connection.html
7. The Link Between Diabetes and Cardiovascular Disease. http://www.ndep.nih.gov/media/ CVD_FactSheet.pdf

Development of a Remote Monitoring System for Respiratory Analysis

Atena Roshan Fekr[✉], Majid Janidarmian, Katarzyna Radecka,
and Zeljko Zilic

Department of Electrical and Computer Engineering,
McGill University, Montreal, QC, Canada
{atena.roshanfekr,majid.janidarmian}@mail.mcgill.ca,
{katarzyna.radecka,zeljko.zilic}@mcgill.ca

Abstract. In order to prevent the lack of appropriate respiratory ventilation which causes brain damage and critical problems, it is required to continuously monitor the breathing signal of a patient. There are different conventional methods for capturing respiration signal, such as polysomnography and spirometer. In spite of their accuracy, these methods are expensive and could not be integrated in a body sensor network. In this work, we present a real-time cloud-based respiration monitoring platform which allows the patient to continue treatment and diagnosis from different places such as home. These remote services are designed for patients who suffer from breathing problems or sleep disorders. Our system includes calibrated accelerometer sensor, Bluetooth Low Energy (BLE) and cloud database. Based on the high correlation between spirometer and accelerometer signals, the Detrended Fluctuation Analysis (DFA) has been applied on respiration signals. The obtained results show that DFA can be used as an efficient feature while classifying the healthy people from patients suffering from breath abnormalities.

Keywords: Breath analysis · Detrended fluctuation analysis · Accelerometer sensor

1 Introduction

Recently, there are different studies and reports which show the importance of monitoring and analyzing the respiration signals in many fields such as medicine and physiology [1–4]. Today about 7 % of the population of developed countries suffer from Chronic Obstructive Pulmonary Disease (COPD), and it is a growing problem in developing countries. For example, an estimated of 3.7 million people live with COPD in UK, predicted to increase by one-third by 2030, costing the NHS £1.2 billion/yr [3]. Moreover, professionals in breathing and sleep centers are demanded to assist people with shortness of breath, cardiovascular problems, such as hypertension, atherosclerosis, stroke, heart failure, cardiac arrhythmias, and sudden infant death syndrome (SISD). Therefore, a real-time monitoring of the respiration rhythm plays an important role in both diagnosis and treatment of different disorders. Remote monitoring also helps in prevention and early diagnosis of adult diseases, such as obesity, diabetic ketoacidosis

© Institute for Computer Sciences, Social Informatics and Telecommunications Engineering 2015
R. Giaffreda et al. (Eds.): IoT360 2014, Part I, LNICST 150, pp. 193–202, 2015.
DOI: 10.1007/978-3-319-19656-5_28

(DKA), brain disorders as well as abnormal breathing of newborns at home. There are different conventional methods for respiration waveform measurement, such as spirometry, nasal thermocouples, impedance plethysmography, inductance pneumography strain gauge measurements of thoracic circumference, whole-body plethysmography [4], pneumatic respiration transducers, the fiber-optic sensor method [4, 5], the Doppler radar [5, 6], and electrocardiogram (ECG)-based derived respiration measurements [7–9]. However, in spite of their accuracies, these methods are expensive and inflexible which may bring discomfort to the patients and physicians. One recent area of interest is applying motion sensors to detect the small movements of the chest wall that occur during expansion and contraction of the lungs. In preliminary trials on hospital patients, it has been shown that [10] with proper signal processing, this method can produce results that closely match with measurements of nasal cannula pressure [10]. A validation of respiratory signal derived from suprasternal, notch acceleration has been investigated by [11] for different body positions. Their data storage and processing is performed on a computer with their custom build LabVIEW Virtual Instrument. The main objective of this study is to provide a new cloud-based tool for monitoring and analyzing the respiration patterns with accelerometer sensor. The previous approaches are primarily based on the use of offline data loggers and on-board signal processing. However, in our system we use cloud database which can offer significant advantages over traditional methods, including increased on-line accessibility, scalability, automatic failover and fast automated recovery from failures. The accelerometer data is transmitted via Bluetooth Low Energy (BLE) to PC/iPhone and then it is sent to the cloud to be processed and saved, immediately. Therefore, the physicians can track the patients wherever they are with devices such as an iPhone, iPad or the web regardless of their proximity to the patients. Moreover the fluctuation analysis of the signals for each patient is investigated as an effective feature to distinguish breath problems.

In Sect. 2, the signal processing procedures applied on accelerometer signal are explained. In Sect. 3, the Detrended Fluctuation Analysis (DFA) has been applied on respiration signals derived from the accelerometer to help distinguishing between normal and abnormal respiration patterns. Experimental results are presented and discussed in Sect. 4. Finally Sect. 5 concludes the paper.

2   Data Preprocessing

We mounted the sensor on the chest where is more comfortable compared to suprasternal notch position used in [11]. In order to make sure that the sensors' readings are accurate enough to be processed, we calibrate our accelerometer sensor using linear least square method proposed by [12]. Due to inherent deficiency or aging problems in cyber-biological systems, sensors calibration is suggested. Calibration, which is defined as the process of mapping raw sensor readings into corrected values, can be used to compensate the systematic offset and gain [13]. Generally, calibration of sensors requires experience and special accurate tools; however, a straightforward method to calibrate an accelerometer is performed at 6 stationary positions. We need to collect a few seconds of accelerometer raw data at each position. Then the least square method is applied to obtain the 12 accelerometer calibration parameters. The calibration procedure is simple, and needs to be executed once. The calibration procedure can be briefly explained as:

$$[a_{x'}a_{y'}a_{z'}] = [a_x\, a_y\, a_z\, 1] \cdot \begin{bmatrix} acc_{11}\ acc_{21}\ acc_{31} \\ acc_{12}\ acc_{22}\ acc_{32} \\ acc_{13}\ acc_{23}\ acc_{33} \\ acc_{10}\ acc_{20}\ acc_{30} \end{bmatrix}, \qquad y = w.X$$

where:

- Vector w is accelerator sensor raw data collected at 6 stationary positions.
- Vector y is the known normalized Earth gravity vector.
- Matrix X is the 12 calibration parameters that is determined as below:

$$X = \left[w^T.w\right]^{-1}.w^T.y$$

Based on the fixed sensor position, the data processing and analysis are performed on z-axis of the accelerometer. The accelerometer data is filtered through a 10th order Butterworth low pass filter with cutoff frequency 1 Hz. In the next part we are going to analyze the fluctuation of different breathing patterns resulted from five types of respiration disorders.

3   Detrended Fluctuation Analysis (DFA)

Detrended Fluctuation Analysis (DFA) quantifies fractal like auto-correlation properties of the signals [14]. It is generally accepted that the significant complexity of biological signals is due to two main factors [15] i.e. high complexity of systems and their susceptibility to environmental factors [14]. Biological signals are difficult to analyze because they are mostly non-stationary and from a wide range of physiological phenomena possess a scale invariant structure [16, 17]. Indeed, they have a scale invariant structure when the structure repeats itself on subintervals of the signal [17].

The validation of accelerometer driven respiration signal is investigated in [18] and the mean correlation of 0.84 which shows a very close correspondence of the accelerometer sensor and spirometer data is obtained. Therefore, here we make use of this result and DFA effectiveness is analyzed to discriminate healthy from pathological accelerometer driven respiration patterns.

DFA was first introduced by Peng et al. [19]; and Acharya et al. [20] uses DFA for disease classification in ECG studies. In many cases the DFA scaling exponent can be used to distinguish healthy and unhealthy data [21]. Indeed, DFA is a scaling analysis method that provides a simple quantitative parameter to represent the autocorrelation properties of a signal [19]. Thus, it could be a good feature to be utilized in the classification techniques. Figure 1, briefly summarized the proposed procedures.

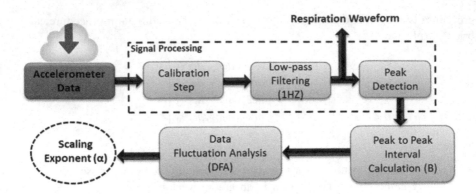

Fig. 1. Signal processing flowchart

3.1 DFA Algorithm

In the application of DFA to our extracted respiration signal, parameter B is the peak to peak *(P_P)* interval of breathing signal. We applied a peak detector algorithm which defined a customized threshold to decide whether each peak is significantly larger than the local data and then the peak intervals are calculated. B is first integrated in Eq. (1) to calculate the sum of the differences between the i_{th} P_P interval $B(i)$ and the mean P_P interval B_{ave}.

$$y(k) = \sum_{i=1}^{k} |B(i) - B_{ave}| \tag{1}$$

Next, as is shown in Fig. 2 for respiration signal, the integrated series $y(k)$ is divided into boxes of equal length n. Each box is subsequently detrended by subtracting a least square linear fit, denoted as $y_n(k)$. Then the Root Mean Square (RMS) of this integrated and detrended time series is obtained by:

$$F(n) = \sqrt{\frac{\sum_{k=1}^{N} [y(k) - y_n(k)]^2}{N}}$$

In the example in Fig. 2, n is equal to 3. The linear dependence indicates the presence of self-fluctuations and the slope of the line determines the scaling exponent α [17, 22]:

$$F(n) \sim n^{\alpha}$$

The parameter α (scaling exponent, autocorrelation exponent, self-similarity parameter) shows the autocorrelation properties of the signal [20, 23]:

1. $\alpha < 0.5$ anti-correlated signal
2. $\alpha = 0.5$ uncorrelated signal (white noise)
3. $\alpha > 0.5$ positive autocorrelation in the signal

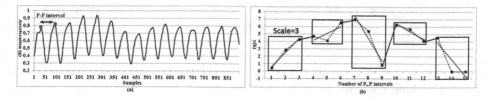

Fig. 2. (a) Original signal, (b) Integrated signal with trends

4. α = 1 Pink noise or 1/f noise
5. α = 1.5 Brownian noise or random walk.

Gifani et al. [14] claims that using scaling exponent α, one can completely describe the significant autocorrelation properties of the bio-medical signals. In this study, we use scaling exponent α of normal breathing as well as five different diseases.

4 Experimental Results

In our experiments, the acceleration signal was acquired with MEMS, KXTJ9, 3-axis low-power accelerometer with 12-bit resolution and sampling rate 50 HZ (Fig. 3(a)). The data is transmitted via CC2541 BLE, a new standard that allows Bluetooth equipment to run for long time on a single coin cell battery. It is worth noting that our node is fully radio type approved for US, Europe, Japan and Canada. The received sensors data are stored in the cloud in order to real-time or further analysis.

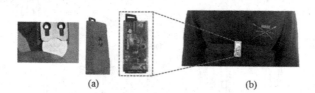

Fig. 3. (a) Sensory node, (b) Hardware module being worn

4.1 Test Setup

The participants of this study were five males and six females aged 4 to 48 with Mean ± SD, 26.54 ± 11.9026. They were instructed how to perform each breath exercise before their recording sessions. The experimental trials lasted for about 50 min per subject. We asked the subjects to perform Normal (N1), Bradapnea, Tachypnea, and Cheyn-stokes patterns, each for 2 min (6000 samples) and the other two types for 1 min with a 3 min rest interval. For simulating apnea in Cheyn-stokes and Biot's breathing exercises, we requested the participants to pause breathing for at least 3 s. Besides, for DFA analysis we asked our subjects to repeat normal breathing for another 1 min (N2). The sensor was mounted on the subject's chest in the middle of sternum region (Fig. 3(b)) and secured by a soft and elastic strap which is easy to attach and comfortable to wear. In the trial session, the subjects were in the lying position; however, the rest positions or activities in which rib cage is stationary could be considered.

4.2   Breathing Patterns

In our test, the subjects are asked to perform six breathing patterns i.e., Normal, Bradapnea, Tachypnea, Cheyn-stokes, Kaussmal, and Biot's. Bradapnea is regular in rhythm but slower than normal in rate. Tachypnea is the condition of rapid breathing, with respiration rate higher than 20 respirations per minute (rpm). Tachypnea may occur due to physiological or pathological problems [24]. Cheyn-stokes breathing pattern is determined by gradually increasing, then decreasing the lung volume with a period of apnea. People suffering from central sleep apnea syndrome (CSAS) have the same breathing pattern at sleep [25]. Kussmaul which is defined as a rapid, deep and labored breathing type usually occurs in diabetics in diabetic ketoacidosis [26]. Biot's breathing is characterized by periods of rapid respirations followed by regular periods of apnea. There are different reasons which causes Biot's breathing, such as damage to the medulla oblongata by stroke (CVA) or trauma, or pressure on the medulla due to uncal or tentorial herniation and prolonged opioid abuse [26]. Figure 4 shows samples of all normalized patterns extracted from accelerometer sensor.

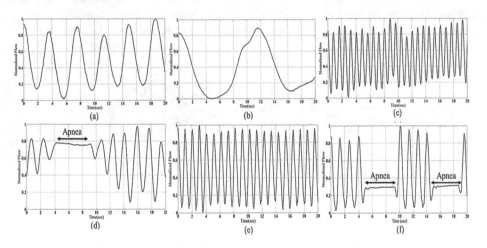

Fig. 4.   (a) Normal (b) Bradapnea, (c) Tachypnea, (d) Cheyn-stokes, (e) Kussmaul and (f) Biot's breathing patterns extracted from accelerometer sensor.

4.3   DFA Analysis

In this section the respiration data are successfully analyzed using the DFA algorithm. Short-term data of 1-min duration for periods of normal and abnormal breathings and five scales 3, 4, 5, 6, and 7 are considered. The average fluctuations versus box-size are plotted in Fig. 5.

The graphs in Fig. 5 are for one of our subjects. It was observed that, each subject has its own signal characteristics based on the fluctuation analysis. It is worth noting that for all subjects, there is a difference in the average scaling exponent α of normal and abnormal respirations which helps us to use DFA as one of the effective features for healthy and unhealthy classification. This difference is various for different types of disorders and in some cases we can see the higher diverse which results in more reliable distinction. As a sample in Fig. 5, the blue and red lines are two normal patterns which obviously resulted in parallel lines (equal slope) while the black lines depict the specific disorders with different slopes. Table 1 shows the obtained scaling exponent for the whole population and patterns. Considering object 1, her normal respiration signal based on α is an anti-correlated signal shown in Fig. 5(a).

According to the obtained results in Fig. 5, the Kaussmal and Biot's respiration signals are close to white noise while for Bradapnea and Cheyn-stokes breathing models, the signals are included in positive autocorrelation category. Her Tachypnea breathing is close to Pink noise in which the power spectral density is inversely proportional to the frequency of the signal. The absolute differences of scaling exponents of N2 and abnormal patterns with respect to N1 are presented in Fig. 6(a).

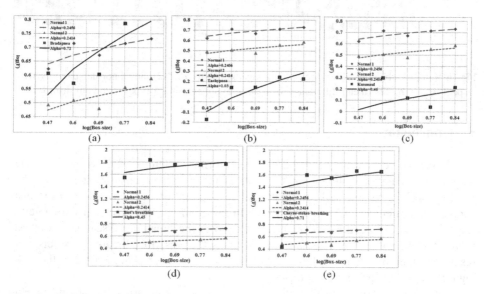

Fig. 5. Scaling exponents for (a) two Normal breathing and Bradapnea, (b) Tachypnea, (c) Kaussmaul, (d) Biot's and (e) Cheyn-stokes breathing patterns

It can be also seen in Fig. 6(b) that for all subjects, the greater mean differences are belong to the abnormal patterns while the differences of the second normal breathing are very close to zero. If we consider all subjects and breath patterns, α differences of abnormal breathings and N2 with regard to N1 are 0.51 ± 0.19 and 0.05 ± 0.04, respectively. Therefore, we conclude that DFA on respiration signals is a good and simple criterion to be used as an important feature in breath disorders detection.

Table 1. Scaling exponent (Alpha) for all subjects and different patterns

Subjects ID	Gender/ Age	Normal 1(N1)	Normal 2(N2)	Bradapnea	Tachypnea	Kussmaul	Biot's	Cheyn- stokes
1	M/48	0.24	0.24	0.72	1.03	0.46	0.45	0.71
2	F/37	0.96	1.05	0.44	0.17	1.19	0.82	1.71
3	M/30	0.39	0.32	0.61	0.82	1.02	0.86	0.83
4	M/29	1.30	1.29	2.61	0.14	1.19	0.10	0.94
5	F/28	0.22	0.15	0.36	0.70	0.64	0.35	0.07
6	F/28	0.60	0.60	0.34	0.83	0.84	0.39	0.70
7	F/28	1.22	1.15	1.50	0.82	1.42	1.40	2.74
8	F/27	1.37	1.46	0.53	0.76	1.09	2.38	0.66
9	F/24	0.82	0.75	0.30	0.45	1.010	1.00	2.15

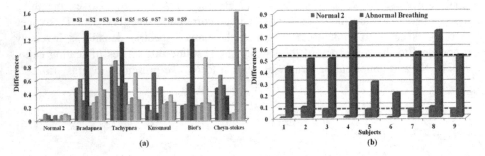

(a)   (b)

Fig. 6 (a) The absolute differences of scaling exponents of N2 and abnormal patterns with respect to N1 (b) The mean differences of scaling exponents (all 5 types of breath disorders)

5   Conclusion

In this paper, we presented a respiration monitoring system as well as applying the detrended fluctuation analysis on the accelerometer driven respiration signal. The results revealed the potential of remote diagnosis based on accelerometer sensor as a simple, convenience and low-cost method. In this platform, the physicians are able to share information together and precisely diagnosis the breathing diseases as well as monitoring the patient's progressing in performing the prescribed breathing exercises in respiratory therapy wherever they are with devices such as an iPhone, iPad or the web regardless of their proximity to the patients.

Therefore, early identification through this portable monitoring system and timely treatment of exacerbations can decrease the hospital admissions and slow deterioration while reducing early mortality and disease costs [27].

References

1. Bannister, R., Cunningham, D.: The effects on the respiration and performance during exercise of adding oxygen to the inspired air. J. Physiol. **125**, 118–137 (1954)

2. Zhu, X., Chen, W., Nemoto, T., Kanemitsu, Y., Kitamura, K., Yamakoshi, K., Wei, D.: Real-time monitoring of respiration rhythm and pulse rate during sleep. IEEE Trans. Biomed. Eng. **53**, 2553–2563 (2006)

3. Mann, J., Rabinovich, R., Bates, A., Giavedoni, S., MacNee, W., Arvind, D.K.: Simultaneous activity and respiratory monitoring using an accelerometer. In: International Conference on Body Sensor Networks (BSN), pp. 139–143, May 2011

4. Neuman, M.R., Watson, H., Mendenhall, R.S., Zoldak, J.T., Di Fiore, J.M., Peucker, M., Baird, T.M., Crowell, D.H., Hoppenbrouwers, T.T., Hufford, D., Hunt, C.E., Corwin, M.J., Tinsley, L.R., Weese-Mayer, D.E., Sackner, M.A.: Cardiopulmonary monitoring at home: the CHIME monitor. Physiol. Meas. **22**(2), 267–286 (2001)

5. Lindberg, L.G., Ugnell, H., Oberg, P.A.: Monitoring of respiratory and heart rates using a fibre-optic sensor. Med. Biol. Eng. Comput. **30**(5), 533–537 (1992)

6. Matthews, G., Sudduth, B., Burrow, M.: A noncontact vital signs monitor. Crit. Rev. Biomed. Eng. **28**(1–2), 173–178 (2000)

7. Moody, G.B., Mark, R.G., Zoccola, A., Mantero, S.: Derivation of respiratory signals from multi-lead ECGs. Proc. Comput. Cardiol. **12**, 113–116 (1985)

8. de Chazal, P., Heneghan, C., Sheridan, E., Reilly, R., Nolan, P., O'Malley, M.: Automated processing of the single-lead electrocardiogram for the detection of obstructive sleep apnoea. IEEE Trans. Biomed. Eng. **50**(6), 686–696 (2003)

9. Dobrev, D., Daskalov, I.: Two-electrode telemetric instrument for infant heart rate and apnea monitoring. Med. Eng. Phys. **20**(10), 729–734 (1998)

10. Bates, A., Ling, M., Geng, C., Turk, A., Arvind, D.K.: Accelerometer-based respiratory measurement during speech. In: International Conference on Body Sensor Networks (BSN), pp. 95–100, May 2011

11. Dehkordi, P.K., Marzencki, M., Tavakolian, K., Kaminska, M., Kaminska, B.: Validation of respiratory signal derived from suprasternal notch acceleration for sleep apnea detection. In: International Conference of the IEEE on Engineering in Medicine and Biology Society EMBC, pp. 3824–3827 (2011)

12. Tilt measurement using a low-g 3-axis accelerometer, Application note, STMicroelectronics group of companies (2010)

13. Fekr, A.R., Janidarmian, M., Sarbishei, O., Nahill, B., Radecka, K., Zilic, Z.: MSE minimization and fault-tolerant data fusion for multi-sensor systems. In: IEEE 30th International Conference on Computer Design (ICCD), pp. 445–452 (2012)

14. Gifani, P., Rabiee, H.R., Hashemi, M.H.: Optimal fractal-scaling analysis of human EEG dynamic for depth of anesthesia quantification. J. Franklin Inst. **344**, 212–229 (2007)

15. Kushida, C.A., Littner, M.R., Morgenthaler, T., Alessi, C.A., Bailey, D., Coleman, J., Friedman, L., Hirshkowitz, M., Kapen, S., Kramer, M., Lee-Chiong, T., Loube, D.L., Owens, J., Pancer, J.P., Wise, M.: Practice parameters for the indications for polysomnography and related procedures: an update for 2005. Sleep **28**(4), 499–521 (2005)

16. Gifani, P., Rabiee, H.R., Hashemi, M.H.: Optimal fractal-scaling analysis of human EEG dynamic for depth of anesthesia quantification. J. Franklin Inst. **344**, 212–229 (2007)

17. Lee, J.M., Kim, D.J., Kim, I.Y.: Detrended fluctuation analysis of EEG in sleep apnea using MIT/BIH polysomnography data. Comput. Biol. Med. **32**, 37–47 (2002)

18. Fekr, A.R., Janidarmian, M., Radecka, K., Zilic, Z.: A medical cloud-based platform for respiration rate measurement and hierarchical classification of breath disorders. Sensors **14**(6), 11204–11224 (2014)

19. Peng, C.K., Havlin, S., Stanley, H.E., Goldberger, A.L.: Quantification of scaling exponents and crossover phenomena in nonstationary heartbeat time series. Chaos **5**, 82–87 (1995)

20. Acharya, R.U., Lim, C.M., Joseph, P.: Heart rate variability analysis using correlation dimension and detrended fluctuation analysis. ITBM-RBM **23**(6), 333–339 (2002)

21. Rodriguez, E., Echeverria, J.C., Alvarez-Ramirez, J.: Detrended fluctuation analysis of heart intrabeat dynamics. Phys. A **384**, 429–438 (2007)
22. Ihlen, E.A.F.: Introduction to multifractal detrended fluctuation analysis in matlab. Front Physiol. **3**(141) 4 June 2012
23. Wilkinson, T.M.A., Donaldson, G.C., Hurst, J.R., Seemungal, T.A.R., Wedzicha, J.A.: Early therapy improves outcomes of exacerbations of chronic obstructive pulmonary disease. Am. J. Respir. Crit. Care Med. **169**(12), 1298–1303 (2004)
24. William, H., Myron, L., Robin, D., Mark, A.: Current Diagnosis and Treatment in Pediatrics. 21 edn., McGraw-Hill Professional, New York City, p. 989
25. Kumar, P., Clark, M.: "13". In: Clinical Medicine, 6 edn., p. 733. Elsevier Saunders, Philadelphia (2005). ISBN 0-7020-2763-4
26. Farney, R.J., Walker, J.M., Boyle, K.M., Cloward, T.V., Shilling, K.C.: Adaptive servoventilation (ASV) in patients with sleep disordered breathing associated with chronic opioid medications for non-malignant pain. J. Clin. Sleep Med. **4**(4), 311–319 (2008). PMC 2542501. PMID 18763421
27. Wilkinson, T.M.A., Donaldson, G.C., Hurst, J.R., Seemungal, T.A.R., Wedzicha, J.A.: Early therapy improves outcomes of exacerbations of chronic obstructive pulmonary disease. Am. J. Respir. Crit. Care Med. **169**(12), 1298–1303 (2004)

HeartSense: Estimating Heart Rate from Smartphone Photoplethysmogram Using Adaptive Filter and Interpolation

Anirban Dutta Choudhury, Aditi Misra, Arpan Pal, Rohan Banerjee$^{(\boxtimes)}$,
Avik Ghose, and Aishwarya Visvanathan

Innovation Lab, Tata Consultancy Services Ltd., Kolkata, India
{anirban.duttachoudhury,aditi.misra,arpan.pal,rohan.banerjee,
avik.ghose,aishwarya.visvanathan}@tcs.com

Abstract. In recent days, physiological sensing using smartphones is gaining attention everywhere for preventive health-care. In this paper, we propose a 2-stage approach for robust heart rate (HR) calculation from photoplethysmogram (PPG) signal, captured using smartphones. Firstly, Normalized Least Mean Square (NLMS) based adaptive filter is used to clean up the noisy PPG signal. Then, heart rate is calculated from the frequency spectrum, which is further fine-tuned using different interpolation techniques. Experimental results, show that the overall HR calculation improves significantly due to the proposed 2-stage approach.

Keywords: Photoplethysmography · Heart rate · Adaptive filtering · Noise removal · Interpolation

1 Introduction

Personal healthcare and wellness have emerged as a powerful market segment and has empowered active research in that domain. Several approaches have been used to measure physiological parameters and record them for further study by healthcare professionals and care-givers. Early devices came with connectivity to personal computers which allowed data logging and display. This was replaced with Bluetooth and Zigbee enabled devices that can transmit wireless data to gateway devices or the user's mobile phone for local logging or remote logging via server connectivity.

Although the above model brought in ease of use for both the user as well as the care-givers and physicians, the cost of ownership and maintenance of such devices lies largely with the users, preventing their mass penetration especially in developing countries.

The above problems created the need for alternative approaches. One such approach is to use smartphone sensors for monitoring physiological parameters [3]. Though such readings may not be used for diagnostic purposes, they can provide indicative value to the user. Since in developing countries, the patient to doctor ratio is highly skewed, and the cost of owning multiple devices is relatively high, such approaches are more viable.

© Institute for Computer Sciences, Social Informatics and Telecommunications Engineering 2015
R. Giaffreda et al. (Eds.): IoT360 2014, Part I, LNICST 150, pp. 203–209, 2015.
DOI: 10.1007/978-3-319-19656-5_29

The sensors available on a smartphone platform that can be used for physiological sensing includes accelerometer, microphone and camera where the camera can be used for capturing photoplethysmography (PPG) signal unobtrusively.

PPG is defined as the volumetric measurement of blood flow in body organs [1]. In principle the volume of blood flowing at a capillary is a function of the rate at which the heart pumps blood to the body. Hence, the PPG signal over time reflects the heart-rate value of a person. Equipped with camera and flash, smartphones are able to capture fingertip PPG signal [7]. Although this is true in theory, the mobile camera based PPG suffers from several practical issues. Firstly, most mobile phones have a camera that can capture video at a maximum rate of 30 frames per second (fps), yielding a very low sampling-rate data, compared to medical grade PPG (100 Hz[1]). Secondly, since the mobile PPG technology works on reflected light rather than transmitted light, oftentimes the signal quality is poor [6]. Thirdly, user movement and pressure variance causes artifacts, which adds to the noise, resulting into inaccurate heart-rate detection. Finally, turning on the LED flash continuously for longer period increases the temperature of the region surrounding the camera, causing thermal noise in captured video. In this paper, we demonstrate the behavior of Normalized Least Mean Square (NLMS) filter and it's effects of noise cleaning on noisy phone PPG signals. In addition, we have also explored different interpolation techniques to fine-tune peak detection in frequency domain analysis for improved HR calculation.

2   Extraction of Smartphone PPG

There are many techniques available in the literature to extract PPG signal in reflective mode using smartphones. Most of them include capturing of a video stream by placing the fingertip of the user on the smartphone camera with flash on. PPG signal is extracted as a time series data, by analyzing the change in intensity of 'RED' component in each frame of the captured video. Three such methods have been used in the current context for comparative studies.

2.1   Method 1 (PPG_{avg})

This method, proposed by Pal et al. [7] selects a region of $m \times m$ pixels from the center of each frame of captured video. The value of PPG signal for l^{th} frame is represented by the mean value of all the 'Red' pixels in that selected region.

2.2   Method 2 (PPG_{area})

Kurylyak et al. calculates a person specific threshold (T) for each video by analyzing the first few frames as in [6]. The value of PPG signal for l^{th} frame is calculated by

$$PPG_{area}[l] = \frac{number\ of\ Red\ pixels > T}{total\ number\ of\ Red\ pixels} \qquad (1)$$

---

[1] http://itee.uq.edu.au/~davel/uqvitalsignsdataset/download.html.

2.3   Method 3 (PPG_{rad})

Extending Method 2, Kurylyak et al. [6] proposed a newer methodology to extract better PPG signal that fits a circle in the region of each video frame, where the pixel values cross the threshold. The value of the PPG signal of that frame is represented by the radius of the circle.

3   Filtering and Interpolation for Cleaner PPG Signal

As mentioned earlier, smartphone PPG signals get corrupted by several noise sources. In this section, we propose a 2-stage approach to clean up the noise for better HR estimation. Firstly, we investigate the usage of adaptive filter to enhance the Signal to Noise Ratio (SNR) in time domain, followed by different interpolation techniques to further fine-tune HR estimation in frequency domain.

3.1   Normalized LMS Based Filtering

LMS (Least Mean Square) filters encompass a class of adaptive filters, which tries to match a desired filter, by calculating the filter coefficients which leads to least mean squares of the error signal.

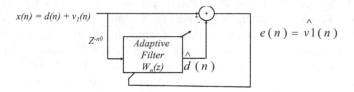

Fig. 1. Normalized Least Mean Square Filter

However, LMS filter has one inherent difficulty in estimating the step size μ. To mitigate this issue, Hayes et al. [4] presented the concept of normalized LMS (NLMS) where β, a normalized step size, typically within the range $\{0,2\}$ is introduced. As shown in Fig. 1, $x(n)$ is the noisy raw PPG signal, i.e. the *desired signal* $d(n)$ corrupted by noise $v_1(n)$. A delay z^{-n_0} is introduced to the input signal to obtain a reference signal, which is applied to the adaptive filter to get the *estimated signal* $\hat{d}(n)$ close to $d(n)$.

3.2   Interpolation

Heart rate is calculated by searching the dominant peak in the frequency spectrum of the signal. For frequency domain peak estimation, it's often common to have a coarse estimation of the dominant peak, followed by fine search around that to get the accurate peak location using interpolation. In this paper, we have explored two interpolation techniques.

1. *Linear Interpolation:* A simple linear interpolation was employed to fine tune the frequency domain resolution of PPG signal. This can serve as an ultra-light reconstruction technique, while porting HeartSense to smartphones.
2. *Jacobsen Interpolation:* Jacobsen et al. presented the following interpolation technique for fine resolution frequency estimation in DFT domain [5].

$$\hat{\delta} = Real[\frac{(R_{k-1} - R_{k+1})}{(2 * R_k - R_{k-1} - R_{k+1})}] \tag{2}$$

Later Candan [2] proposed a finer version of Jacobsen Intepolation technique as follows.

$$\hat{\delta} = \frac{\tan(\pi/N)}{\pi/N} * Real[\frac{(R_{k-1} - R_{k+1})}{(2 * R_k - R_{k-1} - R_{k+1})}] \tag{3}$$

However, in our approach, we chose N=512^2, which makes $\frac{tan(\pi/N)}{\pi/N} \rightarrow 1$. Hence we have limited our experimentation to Jacobsen interpolation.

4   Experimental Setup

A total of 11 subjects having male to female ratio of 7:4, with an age distribution of 22-40 years volunteered in our experimentation. During data capture, the subjects were asked to be in rest position, seating on a chair in an air-conditioned room for half a minute at the beginning. Later they were asked to make some light but predefined body movements while seating to add artifacts in their PPG signal for another half a minute, making the data collection duration of one minute per subject. Ground truth heart rate for all the subjects was recorded using a CMS 50D+ digital pulse-oximeter[3] from their right hand middle finger. Smartphone video for every individual was also collected simultaneously from the index finger of the same hand, while keeping the LED flash on. Videos were collected using the native camera app of iPhone4, iOS 6. All the videos are recorded in the highest resolution i.e. 1280×720 at 30 fps. A total of 11 videos were collected from 11 subjects. All the 3 algorithms (PPG_{avg}, PPG_{area} and PPG_{rad}) were applied to extract 3 sets of PPG signals per video file.

5   Results

Our experimental results are broadly classified into two major sections, 1) Effects of NLMS filtering on raw phone captured PPG data and 2) Effects of interpolation techniques in estimating HR on NLMS filtered data.

---

[2] At 30 Hz, 512 samples amount to 17 sec video.
[3] www.pulseoximeter.org/cms50d.html.

5.1   Effects of NLMS Filtering on Raw Phone Captured PPG Data

The delay parameter plays an important role in the NLMS filter. As the delay increases, the correlation of the *noise in actual signal* with the *noise in the delayed signal* drops, resulting in increasing SNR. As shown in Fig. 2, SNR of the filtered PPG signal is improving along with an increase in delay till a *delay of 12 data points*.

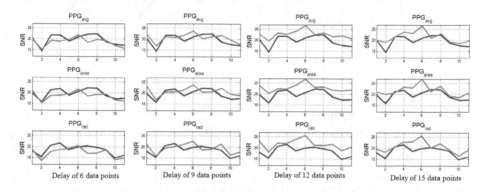

Fig. 2. SNR for Different Delay Parameters for 11 Subjects and 3 PPG Extraction Algorithms(the *darker* and *lighter* line represents *unfiltered* and *filtered* PPG respectively)

However, as the delay becomes comparable to the time period of signal, the signal also tends to become uncorrelated. Hence the SNR starts to deteriorate. In our case, the drop in SNR is visible for a delay of 15 data points. So we fixed a delay of 12 data points for the rest of our experimentation. Given our data rate of 30 Hz, a delay of 12 data points would correspond to 40 %-80 % cycle period, for a heart range of 60-120 respectively.

The effect of NLMS filtering on a typical noisy PPG signal is shown in Fig. 3(a). It is evident that the peaks and troughs in the filtered signal is far more prominent in the filtered signal. So for the rest of the experiment, we incorporate NLMS filtering on the raw PPG signal first and then investigate the effect of different interpolation techniques.

5.2   Effects of Interpolation Techniques in Calculating Heart Rate

Interpolation techniques are used to fine tune the dominant peak location in the frequency response. We have explored 2 different interpolation techniques (linear and Jacobsen interpolation) against 3 PPG extraction methods. As shown in Fig. 3(b), HR estimation improves when interpolation is applied. However, it can also be observed that the performance of Jacobsen interpolation technique outperforms others.

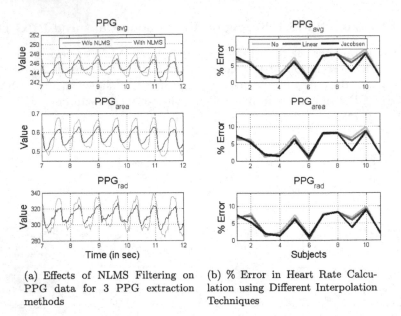

(a) Effects of NLMS Filtering on PPG data for 3 PPG extraction methods

(b) % Error in Heart Rate Calculation using Different Interpolation Techniques

Fig. 3. Effect of NLMS filtering and Interpolation

6   Conclusion and Future Work

In this paper, we have demonstrated a two-stage approach, i.e. noise cleaning in time domain and peak frequency estimation in frequency domain by applying NLMS filtering and different interpolation techniques respectively. Jacobsen interpolation technique has outperformed 'No Interpolation' and 'Linear Interpolation' techniques. Hence, according to our experimentation, irrespective of various smartphone PPG extraction procedures, NLMS filtering followed by Jacobsen interpolation is the most optimum method to find HR from smartphone PPG. Our future work includes analyzing the effects of NLMS filtering on PPG signal captured using other smartphone models. We also aim to explore extraction of other physiological parameters, e.g. respiratory rate, blood oxygen content (SpO_2) and blood pressure from the clean PPG signal obtained using the proposed methodology.

References

1. Allen, J.: Photoplethysmography and its application in clinical physiological measurement. Physiol. Meas. **28**, R1–R39 (2007)
2. Candan, C.: A method for fine resolution frequency estimation from three dft samples. IEEE Signal Process. Lett. **18**(6), 351–354 (2011)
3. Ghose, A., Sinha, P., Bhaumik, C., Sinha, A., Agrawal, A., Choudhury, A.D.: Ubiheld: ubiquitous healthcare monitoring system for elderly and chronic patients. In: Proceedings of the 2013 ACM conference on Pervasive and Ubiquitous Computing Adjunct Publication, pp. 1255–1264, ACM (2013)

4. Hayes, M.H.: Statistical Digital Signal Processing and Modeling. John Wiley & Sons, New York (2009)
5. Jacobsen, E., Kootsookos, P.: Fast, accurate frequency estimators. IEEE Signal Process. Mag. **24**(3), 123–125 (2007)
6. Kurylyak, Y., Lamonaca, F., Grimaldi, D.: Smartphone Based Photoplethysmogram Measurement. River Publishers, Aalborg (2012)
7. Pal, A., Sinha, A., Choudhury, A., Chattopadhyay, T., Visvanathan, A.: A robust heart rate detection using smart-phone video. In: MobileHealth Workshop in Mobi-Hoc (2013)

An Innovative Approach for the Protection of Healthcare Information Through the End-to-End Pseudo-Anonymization of End-Users

Panagiotis Gouvas, Anastasios Zafeiropoulos,
Konstantinos Perakis[✉], and Thanasis Bouras

UBITECH Research, Athens, Greece
{pgouvas,azafeiropoulos,kperakis,bouras}@ubitech.eu

Abstract. Protection of data privacy and anonymity in the healthcare domain is of crucial importance and imposes many challenges since it regards a multi-fold and multidimensional process that needs to be safeguarded on multiple levels. Data protection has to be safeguarded at application and context layer, at session layer and at network layer. Taking into account the existing challenges, the scope of the current paper is to present the approach and conceptual architecture of SHIELD, an innovative methodological approach and network architecture- deployed within the framework of the FI-STAR project- targeting at the protection of healthcare information through the pseudo-anonymization of end-users. SHIELD aspires to provide value added services that could complement the service offering of the FI-STAR project in particular for the target sector of health care, and strengthen its technology basis.

Keywords: Data integrity · Data protection · Medical data management · Privacy · Pseudonymisation · Security

1 Introduction

The European Union is very sensitive with regards to the protection and integrity of personal healthcare information since processing of and access to healthcare data imposes severe legal and ethical issues, and has thus issued a plethora of guidelines and recommendations that need to be met in order to safeguard that the personal information of European patients is not forged, tampered with, or retrieved by unauthorised users in any way, as well as that the processing of information stored in clinical sites and healthcare facilities does not allow back tracking to patients, at least not without their informed consent [1, 2].

Privacy protection however is a multi-fold and multidimensional process that needs to be safeguarded on multiple levels. To comply with the aforementioned regulatory requirements, everything - the hardware, the software, the network, even the data itself - must be secured [3, 4]. As such, data protection in the healthcare domain needs to be safeguarded at (1) application and context layer, deterring phishing and impersonation attempts that may allow access to a (healthcare) information system where

© Institute for Computer Sciences, Social Informatics and Telecommunications Engineering 2015
R. Giaffreda et al. (Eds.): IoT360 2014, Part I, LNICST 150, pp. 210–216, 2015.
DOI: 10.1007/978-3-319-19656-5_30

personal information is stored, which an unauthorised user may retrieve and/or alter, allowing access to such a system and to the information it encloses only to authorised and verified users, (2) at session layer, deterring data flow manipulation, malicious attacks, interception and tampering attempts, that may allow the eavesdropping and/or tampering with the exchanged information during an open session between two non-authenticated parties, and allow end-users of a (healthcare) information system (e.g. a patient) to securely exchange information with this system over the internet throughout the period during which a session is active between the involved parties [5], and (3) at network layer, deterring real-time sniffing of network packets and network level traceability, protecting the end-users by preventing third-parties from monitoring the end-users' Internet connection, and retrieving the end-users' physical location which may in turn be used for malicious acts.

The scope of the current paper is to present the approach and conceptual architecture of SHIELD, an innovative methodological approach and network architecture for the protection of healthcare information through the pseudo-anonymization of end-users. The SHIELD platform approach was submitted at the Future Internet Social Technological Alignment in Healthcare (FI-STAR) Open Call for additional Project Partners and included in the FI-STAR project consortium. Towards this end, SHIELD aspires to provide value added services that could complement the service offering of the FI-STAR project in particular for the target sector of health care, and strengthen its technology basis.

2 Methodology

SHIELD will deliver a methodology, network architecture and software infrastructure by which the end-user adopts a new artificial identity, called pseudonym, pseudo-identity or pseudo-profile, provided by the proposed trusted and secure mechanism, inheriting and including all features and credentials needed by the existing Identity Management Generic Enabler of FI-WARE [6].

The proposed SHIELD Platform consists of three (3) sets of software components, facilitating end-users to preserve their anonymity while interacting with the FI-STAR healthcare applications and services, without restricting their privileges and benefits raised from their actual profile:

(1) The Pseudo-anonymization Networking Infrastructure, which guarantees the anonymity of end-users and the protection of the personal data, at network and session level, incorporating two main software artifacts: (a) the Pseudonimity Network Client that operates on-top of a standard TOR-client and is responsible for anonymizing the communication at IP-level, and (b) the Opportunistic & Ephemeral Negotiator that establishes a mutual agreement between the negotiating parties, i.e. the end-user pseudonymity client and the SHIELD server, with regard to the utilization of a symmetric key for encrypting the communication among them;

(2) The Pseudo-anonymization Application Layer, which guarantees the anonymity of end-users in the course of their interaction with given applications provided

though the FI-WARE platform, including two main software components: (a) the Pseudonymizer that facilitates the generation of discrete pseudonyms and pseudo-profiles for each end user (Pseudonym Generator), ensures that no reference to these pseudo-profiles exists from any profile publicly available on social networks (Social Clearance), issues a digital certificate for each pseudo-profile (Digital Certificates Creator) that will be used for the user's interaction with the provided applications and services, and stores the associations among real users and pseudonyms in an Encrypted Database; and (b) the Virtual Proxy that acts as an intermediary for requests from end-users seeking resources from the deployed technical implementations of the FI-WARE Identity Management General Enabler (Fig. 1).

(3) The Context Aware Services, which allows the preservation of the context coherence as well as the secure logging and monitoring of all access to personal data, including (a) an Activities Monitoring service that gathers all data related with the activities of a pseudonym, (b) a Secure Logging and Audit Trail Service, and (c) an Authorized Pseudonym Resolution Service that allows authorized third-parties to resolve the association between the pseudonym and the real identity of the end-user.

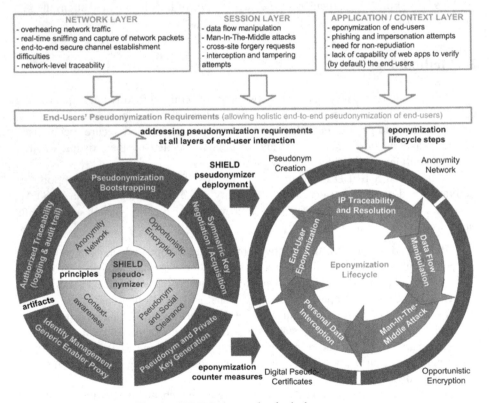

Fig. 1. SHIELD key technological concepts.

2.1 SHIELD Pseudo-Anonymization Networking Infrastructure

The SHIELD Pseudo-anonymization Networking Infrastructure will be based on the establishment and operation of a TOR network combined with the development of the SHIELD pseudonymity network client [7]. The pseudo-anonymization process begins with the installation and initiation of a Pseudonimity Network Client at the typical Web browser of the end-user. The Pseudonimity Network Client constitutes a JAVA-based client component that is able to be installed and executed on all major operating systems and encapsulates all the pseudonym acquisition business logic. This acquisition business logic is realized through a concrete interaction with the SHIELD Server. The network client will be used by the end-users of the provided services in order to join the TOR network and handle all the networking communication activities of the client, ensuring its anonymity in the IP network.

By joining the SHIELD TOR network, connections among network nodes will be based on the dynamic creation of virtual tunnels. Network flows within the virtual tunnels will follow random pathways through several relays. The path from the source to the destination node will be created on the fly and each relay node will be aware of only the predecessor relay. Network flows data will be encrypted multiple times while each relay node will be able to decrypt the "layer" of encryption that permits him to be aware of the successor relay. The negotiation of the per network flow set of encryption keys for each hop will be done by the SHIELD network client. Thus, the complete end-to-end path among the SHIELD end-users and the application servers will be unknown to all the relays in the network. Since the routing scheme followed for the establishment of communication among the SHIELD nodes of the TOR network will not follow any specific rules, traffic analysis from malicious users will be very hard to be achieved [8].

By ensuring the anonymity of the SHIELD users at network level, the SHIELD Opportunistic & Ephemeral Negotiator will be used for establishing a mutual agreement between the end-user clients and the SHIELD server. Through the exchange of a mutually-agreed symmetric key between the end-user and the SHIELD server through a 1-way SSL secure communication channel, end-to-end encryption between the sender and the recipient is supported. The key agreement takes place on top of a completely un-trusted network (although TOR provides anonymity, the risk of packet overhearing from a third-party still exists). In order to achieve a shared key agreement the principles of ephemeral Diffie–Hellman keys will be employed [9].

2.2 SHIELD Pseudo-Anonymization Application Layer

The Pseudo-anonymization Application Layer builds upon the functionality provided by the operation of the Pseudo-anonymization Networking Infrastructure and is responsible for the generation of discrete pseudonyms and pseudo-profiles and the deployment of the Virtual Proxy for the interconnection to the FI-WARE Identity Management General Enabler. Since a shared-key is already selected based on the Diffie–Hellman key exchange method, a secure channel based on 2-way SSL is going to be established over which the communication of the Pseudonimity Network Client with the SHIELD Pseudonymizer will be realized.

In order to support pseydonymization of end-users, the generation of the discrete pseudonyms and pseudo-profiles for each end user is required. These pseudonyms and profiles consist the unique identifiers of the users that are used later on for the generation of digital certificates. In order to create these pseudonyms, a combination of proper parameters has to be defined, ensuring that the correlation that arises does not correspond to any profile that is publicly available on existing social or other type of community networks. By creating such pseudonyms by the SHIELD Pseudonymizer, it is ensured that the de-pseudonymization cannot lead to identification of the end-user. Untraceable pseudonymization is validated through the Social Clearance Component of the SHIELD Server that will be based on existing state of the art tools, such as Maltego.

In case the evaluation of the produced pseudonym is successful, the SHIELD PKI can be used in order to create, manage and distribute a digital certificate for the pseudonymized user. The digital certificate is communicated and installed to the end users' PC/browser while it is also used in order to store the associations among the real users and pseudonyms in an Encrypted Database.

Upon the successful installation of the certificate, the end user is able to access the SHIELD server. Since this server acts as an intermediary Virtual Proxy for requests from end-users seeking resources from the deployed technical implementations of the FI-WARE Identity Management General Enabler, access is provided to the FI-WARE Identity Management (IM) services. User identification is achieved through the two-way SSL communication and the produced pseudonym of the end user.

One critical issue that has to be tackled regarding the Virtual-Proxying of FI-WARE Identity Management services is the fact that many authentication and authorization implementations check the end-user's IP. Since in our approach the IP is continuously changing (because of the TOR anonymity), the Pseudonimity Network Client will be responsible to configure the user's browser in order to use a predefined HTTP proxy, which is bundled with the SHIELD Server and provides the end-user with a predefined validated IP address.

2.3   Context Aware Services

In addition to the services that are directly provided from existing implementations within FI-WARE, access will be given to an additional set of context-aware services. Part of these services regard personalized services targeted at the end-user associated with a specific pseudonym and include access to personal data, view of statistics as well as monitoring of the daily end-user activities. Another set of context-aware services will be provided to authorized third-parties that will be able to resolve the established association between the created pseudonyms and the end users.

3   Discussion

SHIELD suggests a new network and software architecture targeting at the provision of high quality pseudonymized context-aware services. SHIELD will provide a holistic framework for the provision of pseudonymized services in the healthcare domain, based on: (1) the design of the networking architecture that guarantees the anonymity of end-users and the protection of their personal data, (2) the dynamic creation of unique pseudonyms for the SHIELD end users based on the design and development of the SHIELD Pseudonymizer and (3) the deployment and operation of a PKI and issuance of digital certificates per pseudonymized end user.

By combining and integrating the abovementioned technologies, and coupling them with properly designed testing pilots, business planning and targeted dissemination, SHIELD will provide end-users with value-added services including: (1) preventing non-authorized third-parties to trace the IP or the physical location of the user, to intercept the personal data and the real identity of the end-user during his first interaction with the platform, and to trace back the association of the pseudonym to the end-user; (2) preserving application and context coherence implementing secure logging, audit trail and monitoring of all access to healthcare applications and services,; (3) preserving the non-repudiation security requirement allowing authorized parties to resolve the association between the pseudonym and the real identity.

SHIELD architecture and software paradigm can be used for the provision of advanced pseudonymized services within the FI-STAR and FI-WARE platforms, thus widening the opportunities to deploy new innovative services in the healthcare domain by exploiting the provided extensions in these platforms.

Acknowledgments. SHIELD is funded within the context of FI-STAR from the European Union's FP7 under grant agreement No. 318389.

References

1. EU Directive 95/46/EC of the European Parliament and the Council of 24 October 1995 on the protection of individuals with regard to the processing of personal data and on the free movement of such data. Official J. EC L **281**, 31–50 (1995)
2. Callens, S.: The EU legal framework on e-health. In: Mossialos, E., Permanand, G., Baeten, R., Hervey, T.K. (eds.) Health Systems Governance in Europe: The Role of EU Law and Policy, pp. 561–588. Cambridge University Press, Cambridge (2010). ISBN 978-0-521-76138-3
3. Riedl, B.; Grascher, V.: Assuring integrity and confidentiality for pseudonymized health data. In: International Conference on Electrical Engineering/Electronics Computer Telecommunications and Information Technology, pp. 473–477 (2010)
4. Neubauer, T.; Kolb, M.: Technologies for the pseudonymization of medical data: a legal evaluation. In: 4th International Conference on Systems, ICONS 2009, pp. 7–12 (2009)
5. Jovanovic, D.; Mladenovic, D.; Blagojevic, D.: Implementation of ZRTP protocol for protection multimedia session. In: 19th Telecommunications Forum (TELFOR), pp. 246–249 (2011)
6. FIWARE Architecture Description, Open Specification, Security, Identity Management Generic Enabler. http://forge.fi-ware.eu/plugins/mediawiki/wiki/fiware/index.php/FIWARE. ArchitectureDescription.Identity_Management_Generic_Enabler
7. Chaabane, A.; Manils, P.; Kaafar, M.-A.: Digging into anonymous traffic: a deep analysis of the Tor anonymizing network. In: 4th International Conference on Network and System Security (NSS), pp. 167–174 (2010). doi:10.1109/NSS.2010.47

8. Kelly, D., Raines, R., Baldwin, R., Grimaila, M., Mullins, B.: Exploring extant and emerging issues in anonymous networks: a taxonomy and survey of protocols and metrics. IEEE Comm. Surv. Tutorials **14**(2), 579–606 (2012)
9. Diffie, W., Hellman, M.E.: New directions in cryptography. IEEE Trans. Inf. Theor. **22**(6), 644–654 (1976). doi:10.1109/TIT.1976.1055638

A Trustworthy Mobile Solution for Healthcare Based on Internet of Things

Kai Kang[1,2(✉)] and Cong Wang[1,2]

[1] School of Software Engineering, Beijing University of Posts
and Telecommunications, Beijing 100876, China
onefish@126.com
[2] Key Laboratory of Trustworthy Distributed Computing and Service (BUPT),
Ministry of Education, Beijing 100876, China

Abstract. Healthcare services based on the Internet of Things (Health-IoT) has great potential. The popularity of intelligent mobile medical devices, wearable bio-medical sensor devices, cloud computing and big data analysis have dramatically changed the usage pattern and business rule of Health-IoT. The rapid development of mobile solutions towards Health-IoT contains the risk of security and privacy. In this paper, a comprehensive trustworthy mobile solution based on architecture modeling with fuzzy-set theory towards Health-IoT is proposed. In particular, the solution is an semantics-based and fuzzy set theory mechanism to calculate trustworthiness for every stakeholders in mobility ecosystem for Health-IoT. An analytic methodology is presented backed with theoretical metrics and evaluated experimentally. The feasibility of the implemented about trustworthy mobile solution Health-IoT has been partly proven in field trials.

Keywords: Internet of things · Fuzzy set · Trustworthy · Mobile · Healthcare

1 Introduction

The rapid development of modern Information and Communication Technologies (ICTs) has led to a new circumstance of the social environment. The Internet of Things (IoT) is heterogeneous Internet-based information architecture in the wave of development [1]. The IoT connects all the ordinary physical objects to the Internet through kinds of information perception devices. The perception devices in IoT are able to exchange information with each other, and ultimately achieve the goal of intelligent recognition, locating, tracking, monitoring and management [2].

The mobile device based on IoT has been widely used as a pervasive healthcare gateway that collects data from the medical devices. Several connected healthcare devices like body fat analyzer, blood pressure monitor, ECG and etc., have been used

---

Kai Kang, he is with School of Software Engineering, Beijing University of Posts and Telecommunications; Key Laboratory of Trustworthy Distributed Computing and Service (BUPT), Beijing, China (e-mail:onefish@126.com).

© Institute for Computer Sciences, Social Informatics and Telecommunications Engineering 2015
R. Giaffreda et al. (Eds.): IoT360 2014, Part I, LNICST 150, pp. 217–222, 2015.
DOI: 10.1007/978-3-319-19656-5_31

in conjunction with the mobile gateway of IoT [3–5]. Plenty of the mobile applications afford constant monitoring service of patient's symptoms and needs, enabling physicians to diagnose and monitor health problems wherever the patient is, either at home or outdoors.

Mobile solution for healthcare on the basis of IoT (mHealth-IoT) offers a unique opportunity to tailor and customize care services for individual patients health needs and behavioral attributes. With the convenience of mHealth-IoT, rapidly increasing demands of daily monitoring would be satisfied. However, the security and privacy risk is increasing rapidly due to its armature. In order to develop and integrate effective ubiquitous sensing for healthcare, trustworthiness as an important design goals should be taken into account in future mHealth-IoT [6].

In this paper, to tackle with the risk of security and privacy emerging in mHealth-IoT, a trustworthy mobile solution is proposed. Trustworthy fuzzy set theory evaluates trustworthiness of stakeholders in ecosystem are discussed.

The rest of this paper is organized as follow: some related works are summarized in Sect. 2, theoretical method for evaluation of stakeholders is presented in Sect. 3, and conclusion and future work are discussed in Sect. 4.

2   Related Works

Generally, an IoT system could be decomposed into three layers, which are sensor (recognition) layer, network (transformation) layer and application (services) layer. Traditional strategies, such as access control, are no longer suit for resolving security and privacy issues of distributed system because of their centre-dependence and poor scalability.

Trust is a multidimensional, multidisciplinary, and multifaceted concept. Common to these definitions are the notions of confidence, belief, and expectation on the reliability, integrity, ability, or characters of an entity. To reduce and solve the risk, a number of literature articles in terms of trust management in IoT domain were published. A trustworthy IoT system or service relies on not only reliable cooperation among layers, but also the performance of the whole system and each system layer with regard to security, privacy and other trust-related properties. Ensuring the trustworthiness of one IoT layer (e.g., network layer) does not imply that the trust of the whole system can be achieved.

Trust management (TM) plays an important role in IoT [7]. It enhances user privacy and information security, and improves quality of services. A trustworthy mHealth-IoT should consist of reliable mobile devices, provides secure communications, and preserves users' privacy, part or all of the ways to gain user trust. In this paper, a trustworthy mHealth-IoT is present in order to illustrate what trust properties should be enhanced in order to achieve holistic trust management.

A number of studies pay special attention to TM in IoT. The main issues focus on the following aspects: Secure framework and architecture [8, 9]; Secure data transmission and communication [10, 11]; Privacy preservation [12, 13].Yan et al. [14] reviews and summaries the existing work as eight taxonomies: Trust Evaluation, Trust Framework, Data Perception Trust, Identity Trust and Privacy Preservation,

Transmission and communication Trust, Secure Multi-Party Computation, User Trust and Application Trust. In the domain of Health-IoT, Pang et al. [15–17] establishes special ecosystem for Health-IoT, and design a trustworthy in-home medication management solution. Yang et al. [18] upgrades the solution above and implements a comprehensive intelligent home-based platform for iHome Health-IoT. Kang et al. [18] proposes a security and privacy mechanism for rural areas in China towards Health-IoT. Their works do not attach importance to the capability of mobile devices in Health-IoT. In another word, mobility of "things" (e.g. mobile medical devices and mobile terminals) is not the kernel part of Health-IoT. Kang et al. [20] proposes an innovative ecosystem and model for Health-IoT. In his study, a mobile application market ecosystem is described, notion of application trustworthiness is defined, case study and experiment is implemented. He depicts a fundamental solution for mHealth-IoT in the view of security and privacy. However, the role of mobile terminal has not illuminates clearly; theoretical method and measurement for trustworthiness is difficult to utilize in mHealth-IoT. With advantage of his study, considering stakeholders, a trustworthy mHealth-IoT is proposed in next section, which focuses on the evaluation for stakeholders.

3 Trustworthy mHealth-IoT

A trustworthy mHealth-IoT should be operating in particular ecosystem, which consists of trustworthy devices and trustworthy services. In the ecosystem, many roles in different society domains are involved. The theory of ecosystem was introduced: *"Products and services mainly flow from means providers, through service providers, to end users. Payments (obligatory or optional, depending on different cases) flow back from end users, through financial sources, to the means providers and service providers. Thus a close-loop is established. It is exactly the "close-loop" feature that makes the ecosystem economically sustainable. Win-win cooperation is enabled only if every stakeholder's benefit is guaranteed"* [21]. In the ecosystem, many roles in different society domains are involved. The major stakeholders in the ecosystem as following: Healthcare mobile service providers; Healthcare financial sources; Content providers; Telecom operators; Mobile devices providers; Mobile medical devices providers; Mobile application broker and etc. [18, 21]. In this section, a trustworthiness evaluation for every stakeholder is proposed based on Sugeno Integral of fuzzy set theory.

3.1 Trustworthiness Evaluation for Stakeholders

In the view of TM, traditional solutions for Health-IoT, spend much effort to solve problems at some points, such as recognition, transformation, storage, processing and etc. All the key points belong to different stakeholders in ecosystem. Evaluating the trustworthiness of stakeholders in ecosystem is a direct way for build up a trustworthy mHealth-IoT. Stakeholder is abstract concept; it is difficult to calculate its trustworthiness directly. Sugeno Integral [22] always is used for evaluating reputation and trustworthiness in TM. Hence, it helps us to solve the problem about trustworthiness evaluation for stakeholders.

Definition 1. Assume measurable space (X, Ω), $h : X \to [0, 1]$ satisfying the following conditions:

(1) $m(\emptyset) = 0, m(X) = 1$;
(2) $A \subseteq B \Rightarrow m(A) \leq m(B)$;
(3) $h_\lambda = \{x \in X : h(x) \geq \lambda\}$, whenever $\lambda \in [0, 1]$.

h is measure function.

Definition 2. Assume that the (X, Ω, m) is a fuzzy measurable space, $A \in \Omega, X = \{x_1, x_2, \cdots, x_n\}, h : X \to [0, 1]$

The Sugeno integral for h is:

$$\int_A h \circ m = \sup_{A \in [0,1]} \min\{\lambda, m(A \cap h_\lambda)\} \tag{1}$$

whenever satisfying the condition: $h(x_i) \leq h(x_{i+1}), 1 \leq i \leq n - 1$.
    The Sugeno integral for h is:

$$\int_A h \circ m = \max_{i \in \{1,2,\cdots,n\}} \min\{h(x_i), m(A \cap X_i)\} \tag{2}$$

Attributes for stakeholder should be mapping to X in measurable space (X, Ω). x stands for attribute in X. $m(A \cap X_i)$ denotes as measure. Different people or institutions can describe degree of importance for each attribute denotes as $h(x)$. In this paper, the result of Sugeno Integral with attributes and measurements is equivalent to the trustworthiness of stakeholders. Trustworthiness evaluation for mobile medical device provider as an example is explained.

To simplify the condition, four attributes are mentioned for mobile medical device provider. The formula description is shown as following:

$$\begin{array}{c} x_1(product\_quality), \\ x_2(research\_ability), \\ x_3(enterprise\_scale), \\ x_4(enterprise\_reputation) \end{array} \tag{3}$$

The value of them is calculated by questionnaire survey.
    If someone evaluates mobile medical device provider for each attributes, the result should be:

$$h(x_i), \quad i = 1, 2, 3, 4 \tag{4}$$

The trustworthiness for mobile medical device provider is shown as following:

$$\int_A h \circ m = \max \left\{ \begin{array}{l} \min\{h(x_1), m(X)\}, \\ \min\{h(x_2), m(\{x_2, x_3, x_4\})\}, \\ \min\{h(x_3), m(\{x_3, x_4\})\}, \\ \min\{h(x_4), m(\{x_4\})\} \end{array} \right\}$$

t is short for trustworthiness for every stakeholders, and w represents weights. The trustworthiness for mHealth-IoT is:

$$T = \frac{\sum_n t \cdot w}{n} \tag{5}$$

4 Conclusions and Future Works

A trustworthy mobile solution based on architecture modeling with fuzzy-set theory towards Health-IoT is proposed. Fuzzy set theory and mechanism help people to calculate and evaluate trustworthiness of stakeholders. A trustworthy mobile solution for Health-IoT is still on trial, the details and experiments is taken into consideration in future works.

Acknowledgments. This work is supported by the National Key Technology R&D Program of the Ministry of Science and Technology of China (2012BAJ18B07-05).

References

1. Xu, L., He, W., Li, S.: Internet of things in industries: a survey. IEEE Trans. Ind. Inf. **10**(4), 2233–2243 (2014)
2. Li, T., Liu, Y., Tian, Y., Shen, S., Mao, W.:A storage solution for massive iot data based on nosql. In: 2012 IEEE International Conference on Green Computing and Communications (GreenCom), pp. 50–57 (2012)
3. Ghose, A., Bhaumik, C., Das, D., Agrawal, A.K.: Mobile healthcare infrastructure for home and small clinic. In: Proceedings of the 2nd ACM International Workshop on Pervasive Wireless Healthcare, Hilton Head, South Carolina, USA, (2012)
4. Paschou, M., Sakkopoulos, E., Sourla, E., Tsakalidis, A.: Health internet of things: metrics and methods for efficient data transfer. J. Simul. Model. Pract. Theory **34**, 186–199 (2013)
5. Sama, P.R., Eapen, Z.J., Weinfurt, K.P., Shah, B.R., Schulman, K.A.: An evaluation of mobile health application tools. JMIR mHealth and uHealth **2**(2), e19 (2014)
6. Zhang, Y., Sun, L., Song, H., Cao, X.: Ubiquitous WSN for healthcare: recent advances and future prospects. IEEE J. Internet Things **1**, 497–507 (2014)
7. Gu, L., Wang, J., Sun, B.: Trust management mechanism for internet of things. China Commun. **11**(2), 148–156 (2014)
8. Ning, H., Liu, H., Yang, L.T.: Cyberentity security in the internet of things. J. Comput. **46** (4), 0046–0053 (2013)

9. Li, X., Xuan, Z., Wen, L.: Research on the architecture of trusted security system based on the internet of things. In: 2011 International Conference on Intelligent Computation Technology and Automation (ICICTA), vol. 2, pp. 1172–1175 (2011)

10. Isa, M.A.M., Mohamed, N.N., Hashim, H., Adnan, S.F.S., Manan, J.A., Mahmod, R.: A lightweight and secure TFTP protocol for smart environment. In: 2012 IEEE Symposium on Computer Applications and Industrial Electronics (ISCAIE), pp. 302–306 (2012)

11. Heer, T., Garcia-Morchon, O., Hummen, R., Keoh, S.L., Kumar, S.S., Wehrle, K.: Security challenges in the IP-based internet of things. J. Wirel. Pers. Communic. 61(3), 527–542 (2011)

12. Køien, G.M.: Reflections on trust in devices: an informal survey of human trust in an internet-of-things context. J. Wirel. Pers. Commun. 61(3), 495–510 (2011)

13. Thoma, C., Cui, T., Franchetti, F.: Secure multiparty computation based privacy preserving smart metering system. In: North American Power Symposium (NAPS), pp. 1–6 (2012)

14. Yan, Z., Zhang, P., Vasilakos, A.V.: A survey on trust management for internet of things. J. Netw. Comput. Appl. 42, 120–134 (2014)

15. Pang, Z., Tian, J.: Ecosystem-driven design of in-home terminals based on open platform for the internet-of-things. In: International Conference on Advanced Communication Technology (ICACT), pp. 369–377 (2014)

16. Pang, Z., Chen, Q., Zheng, L., Dubrova, E.: An in-home medication management solution based on intelligent packaging and ubiquitous sensing. In: 15th International Conference on Advanced Communication Technology (ICACT), pp. 545–550 (2013)

17. Pang, Z., Zheng, L., Tian, J., Kao-Walter, S., Dubrova, E., Chen, Q.:Design of a terminal solution for integration of in-home health care devices and services towards the internet-of-things. Enterprise Information Systems, (ahead-of-print), pp.1–31. (2013)

18. Yang, G., Xie, L., Mantysalo, M., Zhou, X., Pang, Z., Xu, L., Kao-Walter, S.,Chen, Q., Zheng, L.: A health-IoT platform based on the integration of intelligent packaging, unobtrusive bio-sensor and intelligent medicine box. IEEE Trans. Ind. Inf. 10(4), 2180–2191 (2014)

19. Kang, K., Pang, Z.B., Wang, C.: Security and privacy mechanism for health internet of things. J. China Univ. Posts Telecommun. 20, 64–68 (2013)

20. Kang, K., Pang, Z., Ma, L., Wang, C.: An interactive trust model for application market of the internet of things. IEEE Trans. Ind. Inf. 10(2), 1516–1526 (2014)

21. Pang, Z., Chen, Q., Tian, J., Zheng, L., Dubrova, E. :Ecosystem analysis in the design of open platform-based in-home healthcare terminals towards the internet-of-things. In: 15th International Conference on Advanced Communication Technology (ICACT), pp. 529–534 (2013)

22. Sugeno, M.: Theory of fuzzy integrals and its applications. Tokyo Institute of Technology. (1974)

Security and Privacy Issues in Wireless Sensor Networks for Healthcare

Vivek Agrawal[✉]

Norwegian Information Security Laboratory (NISLab), Gjøvik Univeristy College,
Gjøvik, Norway
vivek.agrawal@hig.no

Abstract. *Background* –The design and development of wearable sensors enable user to monitor physiological data using wireless sensor networks (WSNs) in healthcare. *Problem* –healthcare applications based on WSNs are not addressing security and privacy issues. *Effect* –A healthcare system using a sensor network can subject to the privacy breach of the patients as the sensitive data may be exposed to a malicious party. Serious security threats might compromise the healthcare service, disabling patients to avail healthcare facilities. *Contribution* –(a) An overview of the status of security requirements in various WSNs healthcare application. (b) An overview of potential security and privacy threats that can compromise the normal functionality of a WSNs healthcare system. (c) We also present a study on the existing security mechanisms to safeguard WSNs healthcare system.

Keywords: Healthcare applications · Patient privacy issues · Security threats · Security mechanism · Wireless sensor network

1 Introduction

The main components of a healthcare monitoring system are –Hardware, software, System Interfaces, Data, services and people. The sensor data being collected by the WSNs contains information about the health status of the patient and stored in a database. Health status data commonly include information of blood pressure, heart rate, distance traveled through walking/ running, playing activities, and surroundings (e.g. room temperature). We are mainly focusing on the medical data as an important asset in this report. The security requirements, threats and mechanism are proposed in the context of protecting Health data. This review report addresses the security challenges in WSNs for healthcare systems. Section 2 discusses major security requirements to protect user's health related data in the most important and widely employed wearable system to monitor physiological data of the user. Section 3 presents a list of possible threats on the security and privacy of user's data. Section 4 proposes various mechanism to counter security threats identified in the Sect. 3. Section 5 offers some concluding thoughts and reflection on the findings of this study.

© Institute for Computer Sciences, Social Informatics and Telecommunications Engineering 2015
R. Giaffreda et al. (Eds.): IoT360 2014, Part I, LNICST 150, pp. 223–228, 2015.
DOI: 10.1007/978-3-319-19656-5_32

2   Security Requirements in a WSNs Healthcare System

Data Confidentiality: The health data should be confidential and available only to the authorized doctors or other caregivers. A sensor network should not leak sensor readings to neighboring networks. **Data Integrity:** It must be ensured that content of the messages must remain unchanged throughout the process of data recording to data storage and manipulation. **Data Availability:** In many sensor network deployments, keeping the network available for its intended use is essential. **Data Authentication:** In WSNs healthcare applications, authentication is a must for every medical sensor and the base-station to verify that the data were sent by a trusted sensor or not. **Data Freshness:** Data freshness implies that the patient physiological signs are captured in recent time, and thus, an adversary has not replayed the old messages. **Consent & Privacy:** A User's consent/ permission is needed when a healthcare provider is sharing his/ her health records to another healthcare consultant. Health information should not be distributed without patient authorization. Persons are entitled to access and amend their health records.

We considered some well-known wireless sensing healthcare applications to analyze the status of security and privacy. It can be seen in the Table 1 that there is low awareness of security and privacy in the wireless healthcare application. **UbiMon, LifeGuard** not even raised the issue of privacy violation while developing their system. Authors did not consider any security requirements for this application. They did not even address the importance of security or their intention to implement any in the future. **CodeBlue** and **AUBADE** discussed the importance of data privacy but didn't mention any mechanism to ensure it. Authors of **SATIRE** made a weak assumption that the use of internet can guarantee proper availability without any adoption of secure mechanism. Authors of **AMON** project [1] claimed to implement a mechanism to secure confidentiality, integrity, authentication and privacy in their system. However, the technical report does not mention anything explicitly about the security measures. The entries in the Table 1 consist of: NA: the requirement is not acknowledged in the report, NI: no mechanism is enforced to implement the security requirement, I: a mechanism is used to implement security requirement, A: the requirement is acknowledged in the report as a current/ future work.

Table 1. An overview of the status of security requirements in healthcare applications

Projects	Confidentiality	Integrity	Availability	Authentication	Consent &Privacy	Freshness
UbiMon [2]	NA-NI	NA-NI	NA-NI	NA-NI	NA-NI	NA-NI
LifeGuard [3]	NA-NI	NA-NI	NA-NI	NA-NI	NA-NI	NA-NI
AMON [1]	A-I	A-I	A-NI	A-I	A-I	NA-NI
CodeBlue [4]	A-NI	A-NI	NA-NI	A-NI	A-NI	NA-NI
AUBADE [5]	A-NI	A-NI	A-NI	NA-NI	A-NI	NA-NI
SATIRE [6]	A-NI	A-NI	A-I	A-NI	A-I	NA-NI

3   Security and Privacy Threats

This section describes potential security and privacy issues associated to a WSNs healthcare application. These issues may impose severe threats in the absence of proper security counter-measure. Private information of the user/ patient can be leaked to the malicious party.

Eavesdropping or Snooping: This is a passive form of security attack, suggesting simply that some entity is listening to (or reading) communications or browsing files or system information. **LifeGuard** project uses 802.11b (IEEE wireless local area network standard) over the internet to a central server. 802.11 provides no protection against attacks that passively observe traffic [7]. Frame headers of the traffic messages are sent without any encryption and visible to everybody with a wireless network analyzer. **CodeBlue** Technical report does not mention whether the framework employs some cryptographic methods in the upper layers of network.

Routing Attack: Kambourakis et al. [8] mentioned that **CodeBlue** is prone to Sybil attack when it is operated in ad-hoc mode. In the case of *Sybil* attack [9], a single node duplicates itself and presented in the multiple locations. The attacking node acting as a publisher could advertise through its multiple false identities that he has medical data to send. In the case of **CodeBlue**, an attacker can alter the header of the ADMR packets changing one or more of the address fields (senderAddr, destAddr, originAddr, groupAddr).

Masquerading or Spoofing: Masquerading is an impersonation of one entity by another. **AUBADE** uses IEEE 802.11b for transmitting all the bio-signals obtained from the sensors of the wearable. AUDABE system can be a subject to spoofing as 802.11 networks do no authenticate frames. Attacker can modify the sender address in ADMR packets in **CodeBlue** devices and camouflage its device to make the others believe that s/he is someone else. A proper implementation of 'authentication services' counter this threat.

Denial-of-Service (DoS) Threats: Denial of Service is some occasion that diminishes or eliminates a network's capacity to execute its expected function. In the physical layer the DoS attacks could be network-jamming and node-tampering. At link layer, collision, exhaustion can be executed to produce DoS attack. Similarly, Network layer can be affected with misdirection, black holes. This attack can jam the network in **LifeGuard**, **CodeBlue**, etc. and disrupt the normal service of the system.

Privacy Issues: The definition of privacy, which is adopted in this report, is defined by North Carolina Healthcare Information and Communication Alliance, Inc. It defines privacy as *"'An individual's right to control the acquiring, use or release of his or her personal health information"'* [10]. **CodeBlue, AUBADE, LifeGuard, UbiMon** neither address not implement any mechanism to protect the privacy of the user. Authors in [11] discussed several questions related to privacy of medical data. The questions raised in [11] are (a) Who has the authority to delete, add and edit information to health data? (b) What type of data, and how much data, should be stored? (c) Where should the health data be stored? (d) Who can view a patient's medical record? (e) To whom should this information be disclosed to without the patient's consent?

As we have seen in the above section, there are potential security and privacy threats exist in healthcare system. Each and every healthcare application is to security and privacy threats. It is obvious that extensive security and privacy research is needed in wireless healthcare application, which can fill the security gaps that we have discussed in the above section.

4   Security Mechanism

A wireless sensor network consists of a large number of tiny sensor nodes deployed over a geographical area. These nodes have *limited processing* capability, *low-storage* capacity and *constrained communication* bandwidth. Therefore, a set of appropriate security mechanisms is proposed and analyzed by many researchers in order to suit the requirements of medical WSNs. Consequently, the security gap between the above security measures are still needs to be explored for healthcare applications.

Encryption: Encryption can be used to ensure the confidentiality of the data and prevent eavesdropping/ snooping. In sensor networks, **TinySec** [12] is proposed as a solution to achieve link-layer encryption and authentication of data. Authors of **SATIRE** project [6] indicated the use of TinySec to ensure security and privacy in their system.

Secure Routing: Karlof & Wagner [9] argued that sensor network routing protocols are not designed with security as a goal. Ferng et al. [13] proposed an energy-efficient secure routing protocol for WSNs. Their protocol addresses issues of delivery rate, energy balancing, and routing efficiency. It also includes authentication and encryption mechanism in the data delivery. The μTESLA (Timed Efficient Stream Loss-tolerant Authentication) protocol [14] can be used for the authentication of broadcast messages with minimal packet overhead. μTESLA is a routing protocol which provides authenticated broadcast for severe resource-constrained environments.

Secure Authentication: Authentication mechanism can be used to ensure the data/ requests are coming from the valid entity it is claiming to be. Guo et al. [15] has proposed a certificate-less authentication scheme without bilinear pairing while providing patient anonymity. Yu et al. [16] proposed password-based user authentication scheme for the wireless healthcare system. The proposed scheme consists of four phases, namely the registration phase, the pre-computing phase, the authentication phase and the password change phase.

Freshness Protection: Perrig et al. proposed **SPINS** protocol [14] to ensure data freshness in a WSN. Their protocol achieves both weak freshness –required by sensor measurements, and strong freshness –is useful for time synchronization within the network. SPINS uses nonce to achieve message freshness.

Regulation and Laws: United States law mandates that medical devices meet the privacy requirements of the 1996 Health Insurance Portability and

Table 2. Security risks and corresponding security requirements

Security Threats	Security Requirements	Security Solutions
Eavesdropping/ Snooping	Data Confidentiality	Data Encryption
Routing attacks	Data Confidentiality, data integrity, data availability	Secure Routing
Masquerading/ spoofing	Data Authentication	Secure Authentication
Privacy	User's Consent	Law & Regulation
Data Replay	Data Freshness	Freshness protection
Denial-of-service	Data availability	Secure routing

Accountability Act, **HIPAA**. The rule gives patient's rights over their health information, including rights to examine and obtain a copy of their records, and to request corrections. The European Union Directive **2002/58/EC** [17] taking care of the privacy of sensitive medical and health data. It mandates to erase traffic data or to make such data anonymous when it is no longer in use.

5   Discussion and Conclusion

The potential of Wireless sensor networks has been widely accepted in the healthcare system. However, advantages of sensor applications can be exploited effectively if the desired level of security and privacy can be ensured. It is found in our study that almost all the WSNs healthcare applications lack a measure to counter security and privacy challenges. Researchers are either ignoring the security aspects or keeping it aside for the future works. This has created a major security gaps in the existing healthcare solution. We presented a list of potential threats to manifest the importance of proper acknowledgment of security and privacy issues in the healthcare system. We also discussed possible mechanisms to counter threats and ensure privacy of user's data. The relationship among various security requirements, attacks and countermeasures, discussed in this study, can be presented using Table 2. This table serves as a guideline to understand the associated security requirement with each security threats and how can it be mitigated using a security mechanism. Consequently, general public awareness is a vital mechanism that must be given proper importance to address various security and privacy issues. It can be extremely useful if people are educated regarding security, privacy issues, existing laws and regulations.

References

1. Anliker, U., Ward, J., Lukowicz, P., Troster, G., Dolveck, F., Baer, M., Keita, F., Schenker, E., Catarsi, F., Coluccini, L., Belardinelli, A., Shklarski, D., Alon, M., Hirt, E., Schmid, R., Vuskovic, M.: Amon: a wearable multiparameter medical monitoring and alert system. IEEE Trans. Inf. Technol. Biomed. **8**(4), 415–427 (2004)

2. Ng, J.W.P., Lo, B.P.L., Wells, O., Sloman, M., Peters, N., Darzi, A., Toumazou, C., Yang, G.Z.: Ubiquitous monitoring environment for wearable and implantable sensors (UbiMon). In: UbiComp 2004 - The Sixth International Conference on Ubiquitous Computing, Poster Proceedings. UbiComp 2004 (2004)

3. Mundt, C., Montgomery, K., Udoh, U., Barker, V., Thonier, G., Tellier, A., Ricks, R., Darling, B., Cagle, Y., Cabrol, N., Ruoss, S., Swain, J., Hines, J., Kovacs, G.T.A.: A multiparameter wearable physiologic monitoring system for space and terrestrial applications. IEEE Trans. Inf. Technol. Biomed. 9(3), 382–391 (2005)

4. Shnayder, V., Chen, B.r., Lorincz, K., Jones, T.R.F.F., Welsh, M.: Sensor networks for medical care. In: Proceedings of the 3rd International Conference on Embedded Networked Sensor Systems SenSys 2005, pp. 314–314. ACM, NY, USA (2005)

5. Katsis, C., Ganiatsas, G., Fotiadis, D.: An integrated telemedicine platform for the assessment of affective physiological states. Diagn. Pathol. 1(1) (2006)

6. Ganti, R.K., Jayachandran, P., Abdelzaher, T.F., Stankovic, J.A.: Satire: A software architecture for smart attire. In: Proceedings of the 4th International Conference on Mobile Systems, Applications and Services. MobiSys 2006, pp. 110–123, ACM, NY, USA (2006)

7. Gast, M.: The Top Seven Security Problems of 802.11 Wireless. Technical report, May 2002

8. Kambourakis, G., Klaoudatou, E., Gritzalis, S.: Securing medical sensor environments: the codeblue framework case. In: ARES 2007 The Second International Conference on Availability, Reliability and Security, pp. 637–643, April 2007

9. Karlof, C., Wagner, D.: Secure routing in wireless sensor networks: attacks and countermeasures. Elsevier's AdHoc Netw. J. 1(2–3), 293–315 (2003). Special Issue Sensor Network Applications Protocols

10. Information, N.C.H., Communication Alliance, I.: Glossary of Top 45 Security & Privacy Terms June 2014

11. Meingast, M., Roosta, T., Sastry, S.: Security and privacy issues with health care information technology. In: EMBS 2006, 28th Annual International Conference of the IEEE, Engineering in Medicine and Biology Society, pp. 5453–5458, August 2006

12. Karlof, C., Sastry, N., Wagner, D.: Tinysec: A link layer security architecture for wireless sensor networks. In: Proceedings of the 2nd International Conference on Embedded Networked Sensor Systems. SenSys 2004, pp. 162–175. ACM, NY, USA (2004)

13. Ferng, H.W., Rachmarini, D.: A secure routing protocol for wireless sensor networks with consideration of energy efficiency. In: Network Operations and Management Symposium (NOMS), pp. 105–112. IEEE, April 2012

14. Perrig, A., Szewczyk, R., Tygar, J.D., Wen, V., Culler, D.E.: Spins: security protocols for sensor networks. Wirel. Netw. 8(5), 521–534 (2002)

15. Guo, R., Wen, Q., Shi, H., Jin, Z., Zhang, H.: An efficient and provably-secure certificateless public key encryption scheme for telecare medicine information systems. J. Med. Syst. 37(5), 1–11 (2013)

16. Wu, Z.Y., Lee, Y.C., Lai, F., Lee, H.C., Chung, Y.: A secure authentication scheme for telecare medicine information systems. J. Med. Syst. 36(3), 1529–1535 (2012)

17. Directive 2002/58/ec concerning the processing of personal data and the protection of privacy in the electronic communications sector (2002)

Multilingual Voice Control for Endoscopic Procedures

Simão Afonso, Isabel Laranjo, Joel Braga, Victor Alves$^{(\boxtimes)}$,
and José Neves

CCTC - Computer Science and Technology Center, University of Minho,
Braga, Portugal
{simaopoafonso, joeltelesbraga}@gmail.com,
{isabel, valves, jneves}@di.uminho.pt

Abstract. In this paper it is present a solution to improve the current endoscopic exams' workflow. These exams require complex procedures, such as using both hands to manipulate buttons and pressing a foot pedal at the same time, to perform simple tasks like capturing frames for posterior analysis. In addition to this downside, the act of capturing frames freezes the video. The developed software module was integrated with the *MIVbox* device, a device for the acquisition, processing and storage of the endoscopic results It uses libraries developed by the PocketSphinx project to recognize a small amount of commands. The module was fine-tuned for the Portuguese language which presents some specific difficulties with speech recognition. It was obtained a Word Error Rate (WER) of 23.3 % for the English model and 29.1 % for the Portuguese one.

Keywords: Automatic speech recognition · Hidden Markov Models · Pocketsphinx · Sphinxtrain · Endoscopic procedures

1 Introduction

Nowadays it is accepted by most healthcare professionals that information technologies and informatics are crucial tools to enable a better healthcare practice. The Pew Health Professions Commission (PHPC) recommended that all healthcare professionals should be able to use information technologies in their workout [1]. Indeed the technological evolution has led to an enormous increase in the production of diagnostic tests [2].

EsophagoGastroDuodenoscopy (EGD) and Colonoscopy occupy relevant positions amongst diagnostic tests, since they combine low cost and good medical results. The current endoscopic systems do not fully utilize the current advances in technology, and require a multi-step process to perform simple tasks such as video acquisition and frame capturing. A gastroenterologists needs to press a programmable button on the endoscope to freeze the image and then press the pedal to capture and save the displayed image [3]. These procedures are not optimal and raise several issues, such as limiting the range of possible movements of everyone involved and distracting the gastroenterologist from the objective of the exam: diagnosing anomalies. A possible solution to this problem could consist in adding a voice recognition module to the

© Institute for Computer Sciences, Social Informatics and Telecommunications Engineering 2015
R. Giaffreda et al. (Eds.): IoT360 2014, Part I, LNICST 150, pp. 229–235, 2015.
DOI: 10.1007/978-3-319-19656-5_33

video acquisition system, providing hands-free control. This module, named *MIV-control*, will be integrated into the device named *MIVbox*.

The module should be speaker-independent and have a very low error rate, even in noisy environments, and it should be able to capture audio from a microphone continuously, so that it can run in the background unattended, without human intervention. This requires automatic word segmentation to make recognition possible. *Barnett* et al. [4] confirmed that not every language can be recognized with the same accuracy. Although no definitive theory is provided, they present data that confirms the claims. Some possible reasons for some languages being harder to recognize than other include increased frequency of smaller words, language-specific phonemes, and lack of training data [4].

2 Speech Recognition

Automatic Speech Recognition (ASR) is a process by which a computer processes human speech, creating a textual representation of the spoken words [5]. *Aymen* et al. presented the theoretical foundation of Hidden Markov Models (HMM) for automatic speech recognition that underpin most recent implementations [6]. There are several HMM accomplishments, but the most mature ones are the Hidden Markov Model Toolkit (HTK) [7] and the CMU Sphinx system [8]. HTK is a set of libraries used for research in automatic speech recognition, implemented using HMM. Its last release was launched in 2009 and since then it has been largely abandoned [7]. The CMU Sphinx project started on 1990 and already produced 4 (four) versions of its recognizer [8–11]. *Vertanen* [12] tested both the HTK and the Sphinx systems with the Wall Street Journal (WSJ) *corpus* and found no significant differences in error rate and speed which is corroborated by independent researchers [13]. *Huggins-Daines* et al. [14] optimized SPHINX-II for embedded systems, primarily for those with ARM architecture. This work has led to the creation of the PocketSphinx project, a Large Vocabulary Continuous Speech Recognition system developed at the CMU University as an open source initiative [14]. The PocketSphinx project has been used for many different idioms, from Native American and Roma [15], Mexican Spanish [16], Mandarin [17], Arabic [18], and Swedish [19]. These examples show that the PocketSphinx system is flexible enough so that it is relatively easy for people with phonetics training to extend it to other languages, with acceptable results. *Harvey* et al. [5] focused on the creation of models and general optimization tasks, and managed to create a multilingual system that has a 2-s processing time on embedded systems, with error rates below 30 % [5]. *Kirchhoff* et al. suggested other methods to improve the ASR systems' performance, such as including non-acoustic data [20].

3 Voice-Controlled Endoscopic Exams Acquisition

MyEndoscopy is a web-based system developed to link different entities and standardize the patient's clinical process management, in order to promote sharing of information between different entities [21]. It acts like a private cloud, with several devices providing and using services via common protocols. As more health institutions need this kind of services, it can be useful to pool users in common clouds, with costs shared between all the institutions, increasing the scale at which services are provided, to lower individual costs [21].

The *MIVbox* device is part of that system, and was developed to tackle the problems that healthcare professionals face when performing endoscopic procedures, including replacing the current analogue video acquisition with a more up-to-date integrated digital system [21]. Currently, gastroenterologists use a pedal to capture relevant frames. The main goal of the *MIVcontrol* module is to replace the pedal with voice commands collected from a microphone that interact with the *MIVacquisition* module. As presented on Fig. 1, the *MIVacquisition* module receives the video that is feed directly from the endoscopic tower and provides it to all the other *MIVbox* devices [22]. By integrating the *MIVcontrol* module on the gastroenterologist's workflow, the system can perform frame capturing and video control on the fly, without the need for any extra buttons. In addition, it is much easier to extend it to accept new functionalities, which stand for new commands.

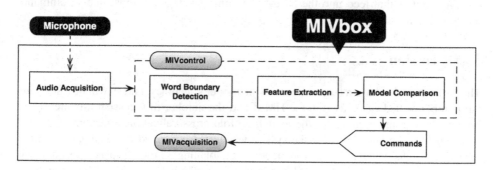

Fig. 1. *MIVcontrol* global architecture

4 Implementation

The creation of the speech model used in the *MIVcontrol* module requires annotated audio and consists of two phases: creating the text model and creating the acoustic model. The language model is a high-level description of all valid phrases (*i.e.* combination of words) in a certain language. It may be classified either as statistical models [23] or as Context-Free Grammars [24]. SphinxBase requires the grammar to be defined in Java Speech Grammar Format (JSGF) [25]. The statistical language model is automatically created based on the command list. The dictionary is a map between each command and the phonemes it contains. A phoneme is defined as the basic unit of phonology, which can be combined to form words. Since the list of required commands is small, all the dictionaries were created manually. It is presented on Fig. 2 as **LmCreate**. The acoustic model is trained using SphinxTrain and maps audio features to the phonemes they represent, for those included in the dictionary.

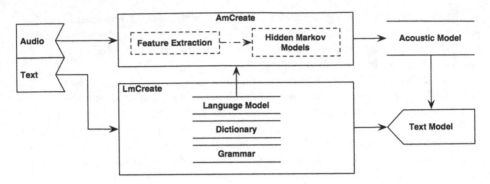

Fig. 2. *MIVcontrol* model training procedure

The training performed by SphinxTrain requires previous knowledge of the dictionary and a transcription for each utterance, in order to map each utterance to its corresponding phonetic information. It is presented on Fig. 2 as **AmCreate**. The audio is split into utterances by tracking silent periods between them, and processed to create a set of features that feed into the HMM. The final result is the most likely command contained in its dictionary.

5 Discussion

The parameters that have a larger impact on the model's accuracy, and so will be tested, are the number of tied states used in the HMM and the number of Gaussian mixture distributions. To test the accuracy of the model, 10-fold cross-validation is performed on the data. The audio corpus in which the system was tested contained two languages, Portuguese and English, with a total of 1405 recordings, totalling 25 min of speech, recorded by 5 female and 7 male speakers, recorded in both noisy and quiet conditions. The vocabulary used was chosen so that it would be useful for direct application is the context of endoscopic procedures. The results are presented as precision-recall matrices. The OTHER label consists of unrecognizable commands or out-of-vocabulary predictions.

To the English model, the best results were obtained for 100 Gaussian mixture distribution and 8 tied states (Table 1). This model has a Total Error Rate of 23.27 %, corresponding to 128 errors in 550 commands.

Table 1. Confusion Matrix for the English model, for 100 Gaussian mixtures and 8 tied states

	"continue"	"end"	"hold"	"start"	"take picture"	OTHER	RECALL
"continue"	69	8	3	2	21	7	62.73 %
"end"	3	74	3	17	9	4	67.27 %
"hold"	0	4	89	8	0	9	80.91 %
"start"	0	7	4	95	0	4	86.36 %
"take picture"	1	4	2	2	95	6	86.36 %
OTHER	0	0	0	0	0	0	0
PRECISION	94.52 %	76.29 %	88.12 %	76.61 %	76.00 %	30	550

For the Portuguese (pt-PT) model, the best results were obtained for 150 Gaussian mixture distributions and 8 tied states (Table 2). This model has a Total Error Rate is 29.1 %, corresponding to 249 errors in 855 commands. The difference can be explained by the fact that the similarity among the Portuguese commands is superior, and some sounds might not be detected by the recognizer.

Table 2. Confusion Matrix for the pt-PT model, for 150 Gaussian mixtures and 8 tied states

	"acaba"	"começa"	"continua"	"pausa"	"tira imagem"	OTHER	RECALL
"acaba"	**160**	1	0	0	0	10	**93.57 %**
"começa"	22	**87**	2	2	41	17	**50.88 %**
"continua"	19	2	**110**	0	13	27	**64.33 %**
"pausa"	44	2	0	**102**	2	21	**59.65 %**
"tira imagem"	14	2	3	0	**147**	5	**85.96 %**
OTHER	0	0	0	0	0	**0**	*0*
PRECISION	**61.78 %**	**92.55 %**	**95.65 %**	**98.08 %**	**72.41 %**	*80*	*855*

6 Conclusions

This paper presents a voice recognizer for a very small vocabulary to be used as a command and control system, integrated on the *MyEndoscopy* system, leveraging the capabilities of the CMU Sphinx project, particularly the PocketSphinx libraries. It was created to respond to issues with the current solutions reported by gastroenterologists, and can be presented as an alternative to cloud-based solutions, such as Google Speech API. In a medical environment, cloud-based solutions pose certain challenges that might degrade their desirability, such as security and privacy issues. Legal reasons on systems that deal with sensitive data also have to be accounted with. Having a system that can be installed inside the healthcare institutions' network without external dependencies is a plus for the reasons presented above. The results obtained required an extensive tuning to the PocketSphinx parameters, particularly for the Portuguese model. This tuning is necessary because the system was not designed to recognize Romance languages like Portuguese one. Future work may involve the creation of models adapted to each specific user, instead of the one-size-fits-all approach followed in this work.

Acknowledgments. This work is funded by ERDF - European Regional Development Fund through the COMPETE Programme (operational programme for competitiveness) and by National Funds through the FCT - *Fundação para a Ciência e a Tecnologia* (Portuguese Foundation for Science and Technology) within project PEst-OE/EEI/UI0752/2014.

References

1. O'Neil, E.H.: Recreating Health Professional Practice For A New Century, p. 106. Pew Health, San Francisco (1998)
2. Summerton, N.: Positive and negative factors in defensive medicine: a questionnaire study of general practitioners. BMJ **310**, 27–29 (1995)

3. Canard, J.M., Létard, J.-C., Palazzo, L., et al.: Gastrointestinal Endoscopy in Practice. 1st ed., p. 492. Churchill Livingstone, Paris (2011)
4. Barnett, J., Corrada, A., Gao G., et al.: Multilingual speech recognition at dragon systems. In: Proceeding Fourth International Conference on Spoken Language Process, ICSLP 1996, pp. 2191–2194. IEEE (1996)
5. Harvey, A.P., McCrindle, R.J., Lundqvist, K., Parslow, P.: Automatic speech recognition for assistive technology devices. In: Proceedings Of The 8th International Conference On Disability Virtual Reality And Associated Technologies. Valparaíso, pp 273–282 (2010)
6. Aymen, M., Abdelaziz, A., Halim, S., Maaref, H.: Hidden Markov Models for automatic speech recognition. In: 2011 International Conference on Communications, Computing and Control Applications, pp. 1–6. IEEE (2011)
7. Young, S., Evermann, G., Kershaw, D., et al.: HTK speech recognition toolkit. http://htk. eng.cam.ac.uk/. Accessed 3 February 2014
8. Lee, K.-F., Hon, H.-W., Reddy, R.: An overview of the SPHINX speech recognition system. IEEE Trans. Acoust. **38**, 35–45 (1990)
9. Huang, X., Alleva, F., Hon, H.-W., et al.: The SPHINX-II speech recognition system: an overview. Comput. Speech Lang. **7**, 137–148 (1993)
10. Seltzer, M.: SPHINX III signal processing front end specification, vol. 31, pp. 1–4 (1999)
11. Lamere, P., Kwok, P., Gouvea, E., et al.: The CMU SPHINX-4 speech recognition system. In: IEEE International Conference on Acoustics, Speech, and Signal Processing (ICASSP 2003). Hong Kong, pp. 2–5 (2003)
12. Vertanen, K.: Baseline WSJ Acoustic Models for HTK and Sphinx: training recipes and recognition experiments. Cavendish Laboratory University, Cambridge (2006)
13. Ma, G., Zhou, W., Zheng, J., et al.: A comparison between HTK and SPHINX on chinese mandarin. In: IJCAI International Joint Conference on Artificial Intelligence, pp. 394–397 (2009)
14. Huggins-Daines, D., Kumar, M., Chan, A., et al.: Pocketsphinx: a free, real-time continuous speech recognition system for hand-held devices. In: 2006 IEEE International Conference on Acoustics, Speech, and Signal Processing, vol. 1, pp. I-185–I-188 (2006)
15. John, V.: Phonetic decomposition for speech recognition of lesser-studied languages. In: Proceedings of 2009 International Conference on Intercultural Collaboration, p. 253. ACM Press, New York (2009)
16. Varela, A., Cuayáhuitl, H., Nolazco-Flores, J.A.: Creating a Mexican Spanish version of the cmu sphinx-iii speech recognition system. In: Sanfeliu, A., Ruiz-Shulcloper, J. (eds.) CIARP 2003. LNCS, vol. 2905, pp. 251–258. Springer, Heidelberg (2003)
17. Wang, Y., Zhang, X.: Realization of Mandarin continuous digits speech recognition system using sphinx. In: 2010 International Symposium on Computer, Communication, Control and Automation, pp. 378–380 (2010)
18. Hyassat, H., Abu Zitar, R.: Arabic speech recognition using SPHINX engine. Int. J. Speech Technol. **9**, 133–150 (2008)
19. Salvi, G.: Developing Acoustic Models For Automatic Speech Recognition (1998)
20. Kirchhoff, K., Fink, G.A., Sagerer, G.: Combining acoustic and articulatory feature information for robust speech recognition. Speech Commun. **37**, 303–319 (2002)
21. Laranjo, I., Braga, J., Assunção, D., Silva, A., Rolanda, C., Lopes, L., Correia-Pinto, J., Alves, V.: Web-based solution for acquisition, processing, archiving and diffusion of endoscopy studies. In: Omatu, S., Neves, J., Corchado Rodriguez, J.M., Paz Santana, J.F., Gonzalez, S.R. (eds.) Distributed Computing and Artificial Intelligence. AISC 217, pp. 317–324. Springer, Heidelberg (2013)
22. Braga, J., Laranjo, I., Assunção, D., et al.: Endoscopic imaging results: web based solution with video diffusion. Procedia Technol. **9**, 1123–1131 (2013)

23. Clarkson, P., Rosenfeld, R.: Statistical language modeling using the CMU-cambridge toolkit. In: 5th European Conference on Speech Communication and Technology, ISCA Archive, Rhodes, Greece, pp. 2707–2710 (1997)
24. Bundy, A., Wallen, L.: Context-free grammar. In: Bundy, A., Wallen, L. (eds.) Catalogue of Artificial Intelligence Tools, pp. 22–23. Springer, Heidelberg (1984)
25. Hunt, A.: JSpeech Grammar Format (2000)

Recognition of Low Amplitude Body Vibrations via Inertial Sensors for Wearable Computing

Marian Haescher[1(✉)], Gerald Bieber[1], John Trimpop[1], Bodo Urban[1],
Thomas Kirste[2], and Ralf Salomon[2]

[1] Fraunhofer IGD, Joachim-Jungius-Straße 11, 18059 Rostock, Germany
{marian.haescher,gerald.bieber,john.trimpop,
bodo.urban}@igd-r.fraunhofer.de
[2] University of Rostock, Universitätsplatz 1, 18055 Rostock, Germany
{thomas.kirste,ralf.salomon}@uni-rostock.de

Abstract. Pathological shaking of the body or extremities is widely known and might occur at chronic diseases e.g. Parkinson. The rhythmical shaking, also known as tremor, can be such intense that extremities are flapping. Under certain circumstances, healthy people also show a shivering and shaking of their body. For example, humans start to shiver whenever it is too cold or if feelings such as stress or fear become dominant. Some wearable devices that are in direct contact to the body, such as smartwatches or smartglasses, provide a sensing functionality of acceleration force that is sufficient to detect the tremor of the wearer. The tremor varies in frequency and intensity and can be identified, by applying detection algorithms and signal filtering. Former works figured that all endotherms show muscle vibrations. These vibrations occur in the condition of sleeping as well as when being awake, or in unconsciousness. Furthermore, the vibrations are also present when subjects are physically active, emotionally stressed, or absolutely relaxed. The vibration itself varies in structure, amplitude, and frequency. This paper shows that these muscle vibrations are measureable by acceleration sensors attached to the user, and provides an outlook to new applications in the future. It also proves that custom mobile devices are able to detect body and muscle vibration and should motivate designers to develop new applications and treatment opportunities.

Keywords: Activity monitoring · Inactivity · Acceleration · Sensor · Recognition · Wrist · Watch · Smart · Sleep

1 Introduction

Muscle activity is important for a variety of processes that take place in human organism. For instance, shivering is an unconscious movement of muscles to increase the core temperature for compensating heat loss. Other examples for body-controlled muscle contractions and vibrations would be the support of blood and liquid exchange in the vessels and cells. This influence of vibrations and oscillations was addressed by former work [1]. The effect of autonomous muscle activity is mainly visible at patients

© Institute for Computer Sciences, Social Informatics and Telecommunications Engineering 2015
R. Giaffreda et al. (Eds.): IoT360 2014, Part I, LNICST 150, pp. 236–241, 2015.
DOI: 10.1007/978-3-319-19656-5_34

with disorders of the muscle function, e.g., Parkinson disease or cerebral palsy patients. Current technology in signal processing and sensor technics is able to detect pathological muscle activity that is not even visible to the human eye. Moreover, it is possible to measure that every muscle is vibrating, even if the person is calm or sleeping [2]. This paper proposes new approaches for detecting microvibrations in a mobile context for providing services in Wearable Computing, which are not only applicable for patients but also for healthy people. Therefore, new interaction concepts are presented as well as new measurement methods and hardware requirements are being discussed. Future work is then outlined as a motivation for researchers to explore the influences and dependencies of microvibrations on healthcare and other areas of application.

2 Related Work

In 1944, Rohracher [2] explored very low amplitude muscular vibrations in endotherm organisms. He was the first scientist to refer to these small amplitude oscillations as microvibrations. Rohracher used piezo-electric pick-ups to detect the muscular activity. With these also known as phonograph needle sensors, he detected vibrations that where present even in complete relaxation or sleep. Rohracher's research has shown that all endotherms generate these so-called microvibrations. Moreover, the vibrations could also be measured even one hour after the dead of the organism. Rohracher also measured variations in frequency and amplitude for different conditions, such as temperature variations. He pointed out that low temperature leads to an increasing frequency of vibrations. Marko [3] made microvibrations visible by magnifying them 400 times with a microscope. Pacela [4] evaluated five sensor technologies for the measurement of human body surface vibrations. Pacela used besides a non-contacting capacitance sensor a seismic (velocity) sensor, linear-variable-differential transformer sensors and a miniature accelerometer. A second kind of body vibration is the so-called tremor. Many works in the field of vibration measurement mostly refer to this as a pathologic body movement. However, Rohracher [2] has recommended differentiating between microvibrations and macroscopic tremors. He has pointed out that in case of healthy subjects, tremor only occurs in certain stimulus situations, such as excitement and coldness, whereas microvibrations occur constantly. Furthermore, he has pointed out that macroscopic tremor, that occurrs on patients with Parkinson's disease, disappears while sleeping or being in anesthesia.

Microvibrations in Current Research

Currently there are very few papers working on this topic. Recently, Bieber et al. [5] identified sensor requirements for measuring biometric data with accelerometers. They identified that accelerometers build in custom off-the-shelf hardware are able to measure data, such as heart rate. In this research a smartwatch was placed on the chest of a lying or sitting user and captured data for short periods of time (15–30 s). The resulting accelerometer data contained suitable heart rate information. The attempt of measuring the pulse frequency in absolute rest showed frequencies in the Fourier spectrum that where located clearly over pulse or breathing thresholds. These frequencies where identified as small vibrations that occurred even in total relaxation. The authors expect commercial smart devices (mobile devices with inertial sensors) to be capable to measure microvibrations.

Characteristics of microvibrations presented by Rohracher [2]:

- Frequency between 7 Hz and 11 Hz
- Amplitude in total relaxation between 1 to 5 micro meter
- During muscle contraction the amplitude increases to ten times the rest value
- During psychological tension and bodily strain, the amplitude increases
- During fever or hyperthyreoses the frequency increases up to 14 Hz
- While sleeping the amplitude decreases about half of its value in wakefulness
- Medication can lower the amplitude
- Even up to 60 min after death, microvibrations are still measureable
- Can be measured at any body-part
- Only present in endotherm organisms
- Constantly measureable

3   Example Implementation

This section proposes three ways of detecting microvibrations using gyroscopes or accelerometers. Therefore, three different positions had been chosen: (1) head placement, (2) arm placement, and (3) leg placement. To perform the measurements, the Invensense IMU-3000 gyroscope, which is built into the SensorTag from Texas Instruments [7], and the Kionix KXTi9 accelerometer of the TI MetaWatch Strata were used [8]. The gyroscope collects data with a resolution of 7-bit and a sampling rate of 100 Hz. The accelerometer was set to a 13-bit resolution with a sampling rate of 32 Hz. Both sensor boards are light and relatively small. After dismantling the MetaWatch board off its wristband, both devices could be placed at different body positions as illustrated in Fig. 1. For measurement at the head, the devices were simply attached to a pair of glasses. To perform the measurement at arm and leg, both devices were simply laid down, thus not being affected by static fixations (Fig. 2).

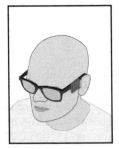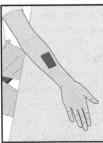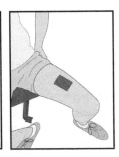

Fig. 1. Sensor positions for vibration measurement. The placement is directly on the muscle and without adjustment (except the head placement). Placement positions were: (1) head placement, (2) arm placement, (3) leg placement.

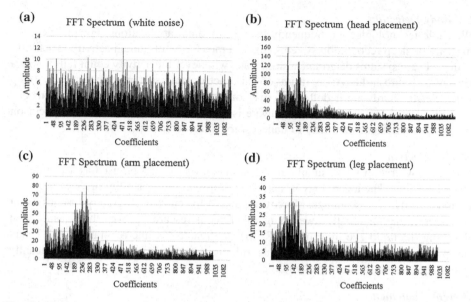

Fig. 2. Frequency spectrum of the gyroscope sensor data. Subfigure (**a**) shows a white noise. In this measurement setup the sensor was lying on a table. Subfigure (**b**) shows the frequency spectrum for a head placement. Subfigure (**c**) shows the frequency spectrum for an arm placement. Subfigure (**d**) shows the frequency for a leg placement.

To collect the sensor data, the devices were connected via Bluetooth to an Android smartphone. For this purpose a rudimentary app was implemented, which simply reads out sensor data and saves it into a CSV file. After that, the analysis of the raw data could be comfortably done. When the app was recording, the subjects were instructed to sit down, while being as calm as possible. To obtain the signal information and to calculate the frequency of each signal, a Fast Fourier Transformation (FFT) was performed on each sensor axis with 2048 samples. The signals provide different frequencies roughly between 4–11 Hz. The direct position of the body parts did not play a significant role. Nevertheless, the frequencies of the head are slightly lower than those of the other parts. After more tests, it could be shown that the head data was very similar, even by varying the recording setting, e.g., by lying down on the ground or by bracing the head onto the arm on a table.

4   New Applications

This section discusses new ways on how to integrate the recognition and assessment of microvibrations into new applications. The aim of these approaches is to measure microvibrations with off-the-shelf hardware such as smartwatches, to provide services to the user, which is derived off the vibration information.

On-Body-Detection

Wearable technologies are frequently used in medical applications. For instance, actigraphy or sleep recognition systems enable a measuring of human activity in activity-counts. These systems determine a sleep state, whenever the activity count falls below a pre-defined threshold. As a result of this, actigraphy systems often detect sleep whenever the hardware is doffed. To overcome this shortcoming, microvibrations can be utilized to detect whether the hardware is worn or doffed. Similar effects occur on fall detection systems and lead to unnecessary false detections.

Sleep Detection

Low microvibration signal amplitudes - in relaxation - could be used as a feature for sleep detection. The technology is suitable to improve the capability of detecting short periods of nightly awakenings. Moreover, most of the current actigraphy systems suffer of underestimating nightly awakening [6]. Recent research proves the feasibility of detecting the rapid eye movements (REM) sleep state via microvibrations [9]. Using our proposed system to improve the algorithmic detection of sleep could significantly gain better results in sleep recognition.

Weight Abatement

Fitness applications or other technologies try to motivate the user to lose weight. Physical activity is a major aspect in a successful therapy for patients for adiposity. Microvibrations are also a kind of muscle activity, and deliver valuable information on energy consumption. The progress in current technologies suggests that the inclusion of relevant features of the muscle microvibration could improve, or support a therapy for obese or overweight people.

Individual Medication

Microvibrations are depending on many parameters. However, current data gives rise to the expectation that monitoring these vibrations would possibly provide essential information on individual patients' drug dosage.

Anomaly Detection

Based on the knowledge of microvibrations, varying amplitudes in the state of unconsciousness possibly concludes to a better prediction of an anomaly for epilepsy patients or patients with narcolepsy. Therefore, wearable devices could be used to detect vibration amplitudes in a daily context for recognition of anomalies in sleep-like situations.

5   Conclusions and Future Work

Currently, microvibrations are known in the field of medical diseases, but not in the field of human physical activity recognition. It might be expected that new analyzing features and algorithms combine the area of unconsciously movements and deliberately movement to create new application fields and new scientific findings. The advantages of measuring microvibrations with wearable technologies lie in the wide area of application fields (e.g. sleep detection, anomaly detection etc.). Most of the results presented in previous research where achieved by using stationary devices (e.g., [2, 4, 9]), and therefore is not applicable to most real world scenarios. The aim of this paper was to prove that microvibrations are measureable with mobile inertial sensors. Preliminary measurements, presented here, with mobile CE (Customer Electronics) devices, namely MetaWatch Strata and TI SensorTag, showed promising results for detecting microvibrations. These results are consistent and are matching with the findings of Pacela [4] in terms of sensor accuracy and technology as well as measured frequency. However, for future wearable application scenarios, the quality of recognition for microvibrations has to be further evaluated. Therefore, the results of previous research on non-inertial sensors (e.g. conducted by Rohracher [2]) have to be validated with a reconstructed study with off-the-shelf wearable devices. This way, a comparison and evaluation of both detection techniques would be possible. In addition, the connection between microvibration and sleep (or even diseases such as diabetes) are worthy to be investigated. This could possibly lead to more insight on nightly hyperglycemia. Another field of interest that requires further research is the detection of stress or tension.

References

1. Nyborg, W.L., Miller, D.L., Gershoy, A.: Physical consequences of ultrasound in plant tissues and other bio-systems. Fundam. Appl. Aspects Nonionizing Radiat. **236**(5), 192–201 (1975)
2. von Rohracher, H.: Permanente rhythmische Mikrobewegungen des Warmblüter-Organismus ("Mikrovibrationen"). Die Naturwiss. **49**(7), 145–150 (1962)
3. Marko, A.R.: Optisch-mikroskopische Registrierung der Mikrovibration des menschlichen Koerpers. Mikroskopie **14**(1), 102–105 (1959)
4. Pacela, A.F.: Measurement of the body surface physiologic tremor or "microvibration". Behav. Res. Meth. Instru. **1**(2), 60–70 (1968)
5. Bieber, G., Haescher, M., Vahl, M.: Sensor requirements for activity recognition on smart watches. In: Proceedings of the 6th International Conference on Pervasive Technologies Related to Assistive Enviroments, ACM (2013)
6. Cole, R., Kripke, D., Gruen, W., Mullaney, D., Gillin, J.: Automatic sleep/wake identification from wrist activity. Sleep **15**(5), 461–469 (1992)
7. Texas Instruments: SensorTag User Guide. Processors.wiki.ti.com. http://processors.wiki.ti.com/index.php/SensorTag_User_Guide. Accessed 26 June 2014
8. Ridden, P.: The MetaWatch STRATA sportwatch wants to be friends with your smartphone (online). gizmag.com, 02/02/2012 (2012). http://www.gizmag.com/metawatch-strata-bluetooth-smartphone/23564/. Accessed 26 June 2014
9. Gallasch, E., Kenner, T.: Die Mikrovibration, eine Wechselwirkung zwischen kardiova-skulärem- und Neurosystem? Biomed. Tech. **57**(1), 131–133 (1992)

Preventing Health Emergencies in An Unobtrusive Way

Vittorio Miori[(✉)] and Dario Russo

Institute of Information Science and Technologies (ISTI),
National Research Council of Italy (CNR), Via Moruzzi 1, 56124 Pisa, Italy
{vittorio.miori,dario.russo}@isti.cnr.it

Abstract. The Ambient Intelligence (*AmI*) paradigm represents the vision of the next wave of computing. By relying on various computing and networking techniques, AmI systems have the potential to enhance our everyday lives in many different aspects. One area in which widespread application of this innovative paradigm promises particularly significant benefits is health care. The work presented here contributes to realizing such promise by proposing a functioning software application able to learn the behaviors and habits, and thereby anticipate the needs, of inhabitants living in a technological environment, such as a smart house or city. The result is a health care system that can actively contribute to anticipating, and thereby preventing, emergency situations to provide greater autonomy and safety to disabled or elderly occupants, especially in cases of critical illness.

Keywords: Ambient intelligent · Association rules · Data mining · DomoNet · Domotics · Home automation · Machine learning · Web services · XML

1 Introduction

Ubiquitous Computing and *Ambient Intelligence* (*AmI*) concepts refer to a vision of the future information society in which human living environments will be pervaded by intelligent devices that will be everywhere, embedded in everyday objects to provide the functionalities to integrate computing and telecommunications technologies.

According to the vision of Mark Weiser [1] (considered the father of ubiquitous computing), the most advanced technologies are those that "disappear": computer technology should become invisible, and the daily environment will enable innovative human-machine interactions in which autonomous and intelligent entities will act in full interoperability and will be able to adapt themselves to the user and even anticipate user needs [2]. Such innovative paradigms make *AmI* technology a suitable candidate for developing a wide variety solutions to real-life issues, including in the health care domain.

In this regard, one open issue regarding *AmI* is related to recognizing unusual or dangerous situations in order to anticipate health emergencies by monitoring users' habitual activities and capturing their normal behavior. Such functionalities can be implemented using systems based on machine learning techniques, which exploit artificial intelligence algorithms to learn users' habits by accumulating 'experience' on

© Institute for Computer Sciences, Social Informatics and Telecommunications Engineering 2015
R. Giaffreda et al. (Eds.): IoT360 2014, Part I, LNICST 150, pp. 242–247, 2015.
DOI: 10.1007/978-3-319-19656-5_35

their normal day-to-day activities in order to be able to recognize 'abnormal' situations. A system able to anticipate danger before life-threatening situations arise would certainly lead to faster and more effective intervention when used to predict health problems in time and can thus often save lives.

If we focus on the home, *AmI* services may be seen as a layer on top of the domotic system, per se. In order to make the advent of genuine *AmI* applications possible, there is a crucial need that the environment in which they act be fully interoperable [3]. However, the current immaturity of the field of domotics and, more specifically, the lack of definitions of application requirements, have led to the development of a large number of ad hoc proposals, which unfortunately are often limited and difficult to integrate.

2 Related Works

A large body of literature underscores the currently great research interest in *AmI* and methodologies for anticipating user needs. Chin [4] has classified three different categories of rules for programming an *AmI* system: pre-programmed rules, user-programmed rules, agent-programmed rules.

As regards the ability to identify user actions, Rashidi et al. [5] describe a system that identifies frequent behaviors using a powered *Hidden Markow Model* approach. Aztiria et al. [6] propose a similar system based on pattern recognition to understand users' behaviors and act accordingly to automate actions and devices. Chen et al. [7] present an interesting survey on user activity recognition.

Mileo et al. [8] uses logic programming techniques to reason about independent living. Another rule-based approach has been proposed by Aztiria et al. [9], while Puha et al. [10] provide a comparison between different methods for multiple people activity recognition.

3 Activity Recognition and Anticipating Needs

At the core of such *AmI* systems is activity recognition [11], whose goal is to identify user behaviors as they occur, based on data collected by sensors. In this regard, we define a '*scenario*' as a set of events occurring in the environment that are in some way related to each other and are recognized as such through the mediation of the domotic devices. Users must simply behave as usual within their living quarters, ignoring the technology surrounding them.

In order to recognize such scenarios and anticipate the needs of inhabitants we have built a system called *DomoPredict*, which is a software client component of the *DomoNet* project [12]. *DomoPredict* is able to act in place of users, basing its actions on the data collected while monitoring their behaviors.

DomoNet has the capacity to abstract the peculiarities of underlying, well-established heterogeneous domotic technologies (e.g. KNX, Lon, UPnP, etc.), enabling them to co-exist and interwork without eliminating their peculiar differences.

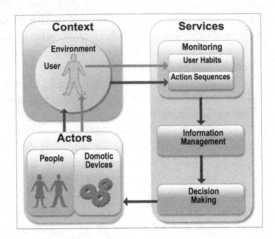

Fig. 1. Scheme of AmI based system

As shown in Fig. 2, *DomoPredict* is able to communicate with *DomoNet* and, through it, send commands to, and receive notifications of any state change in, any domotic device.

In particular, consistent with the *AmI* lifecycle (Fig. 1), *DomoPredict* functionalities can be divided into 4 steps:

- *Information Collection:* when a device changes state, an update message is sent from *DomoNet* to *DomoPredict*;
- *Collected Information Analysis:* identifying sets of actions that may lead to the recognition and creation of new scenarios;
- *Analysis:* recognizing if a new scenario is to be learned, or an existing one modified or removed;
- *Rules Execution:* the system applies a learned rule by invoking *DomoNet* to execute the corresponding commands to the appropriate domotic devices.

With the aim of learning as much information as possible, the system employs a hybrid method that exploits the advantages of two machine learning paradigms: data-mining and statistical approaches. Thus, the software is made up of two complementary, interoperating modules: the *association* and the *statistical rules managers*.

3.1 Association Rules Manager

The *association rules manager* is responsible for learning scenarios made up of a set of events or actions, called *itemsets*, habitually carried out by the user. These events are related to each other in the sense that they occur together within a specified short time interval, though they may be unrelated to any specific time of execution.

The manager applies a specific method for mining frequent sequences [13], in particular, associative rules. This enables the generation of opportune rules using binary partitions of the events determining the scenario being learned. An *unsupervised* learning technique has been adopted due to its ability to discover recurring sequences of sensor activities and in order to allow the creation of relationships and groupings between similar data [14].

By way of example, the system can learn a scenario that includes the two events: "switch on the light in the living room" and "switch on the TV". Once the user has switched on the light, it must be determined whether (s)he wants to turn on the TV as well. To do this, it is necessary to calculate the probability that the performance of one event (or group of events) implies execution of the other(s) in that same scenario.

The constraints of the *Apriori* data mining algorithm are used to define frequent scenarios. The algorithm finds *itemsets* commonly performed by the user and generates candidate action sequences via the standard method defined as *Fk-1 X Fk-1* [13].

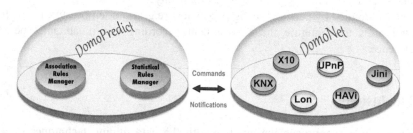

Fig. 2. *DomoPredict* is a *DomoNet* client

Such procedure requires a stage of data preprocessing, so as to determine the minimum set of events that enables recognizing the correct scenario.

Data mining algorithms are known to work well using large datasets. From this prospective, the usual techniques would seem unsuitable for our purposes, because our dataset is empty at startup and is populated in real time via the update broadcast messages sent by *DomoNet*. The solution adopted to overcome this obstacle is to act on the *support* parameter of the *Apriori* algorithm, bearing in mind that the few data available initially could lead to the acquisition of erroneous habits. In order to limit such inconvenience, the dataset is enriched with a new entry only when the *Apriori minimum support* parameter is greater than a prefixed threshold. So, simply increasing its value will make it more difficult for a given scenario to be learned, thereby preventing infrequent events from being considered.

When a change in learned habits or external factors occurs, the no longer valid scenario is modified or removed by the system using the *Apriori reinforcement* process, according to the newly acquired experience.

Lastly, decisions are translated into commands and sent to recipient domotic devices, which together with any reactions on the part of the human occupants, modify the initial settings.

3.2   Statistical Rules Manager

While recognizing and characterizing common normal activities, which account for the majority of the scenarios generated, is clearly crucial to the system's functioning, health applications require the ability to identify personal preferences as well as other events.

Thus a *statistical rules manager* has been designed to learn scenarios that are not captured by the *association rules manager*.

The data collected are recorded in tables, which indicate either the percentage time a device is in a particular state, or the percentage time that certain events occur [15].

The scenarios captured by the statistical rules manager are:

1. Scenarios made up of one or more events usually occurring at the same time of day or for a long period of time. If an action is performed every day at a certain time, we can assume that a relation exists between the action taken and the time of the day in question and we can thus perform it automatically.
2. Scenarios defined by personal living parameters (e.g. room temperature), which the system uses to configure the environment according the inhabitant's personal preferences.

4   Conclusions

Following a hybrid approach that applies both the data mining techniques of associative rule learning and statistical learning methods mitigates their respective limitations and leads to a more versatile and reliable domotic system.

The methods applied enable the system to anticipate user needs quite well, and system performance improved over time, as new experience was accumulated. The proposed method resulted also satisfactory in recognizing critical situations in advance.

To achieve more realistic results the prototype requires a dataset that is both more extensive and more detailed. The data acquired through the environmental sensors are simply not enough to achieve sufficiently reliability deductions. Such data must be integrated with the information that can be captured via wearable or implantable devices.

In the future it will be possible to design and develop smart environments able to instantly recognize not only different individuals interacting with the system, but also emotions subtly expressed by such individuals and respond to these emotions in an adaptive, personalized way. Consequently, such systems will aid in improving human health care by providing timely support and therapy.

References

1. Weiser, M.: The computer for the twenty-first century. Sci. Am. **265**(3), 94–104 (1991)
2. Aarts, E., De Ruyter, B.: New research perspectives on ambient intelligence. J. Ambient Intell. Smart Environ. **1**(1), 5–14 (2009)

3. Mudiam, S.V., Gannod, G.C., Lindquist, T.E.: Synthesizing and integrating legacy components as services using adapters. Sci. Comput. Program. **60**(2), 134–148 (2006)
4. Chin, J., Callaghan, V., Clarke, G.: A programming by example approach to customizing digital homes. In: IET-International Conference on Intelligent Environments, Seattle, pp. 21–22 (2008)
5. Rashidi, P., Cook, D.J., Holder, L.B., Schmitter-Edgecombe, M.: Discovering activities to recognize and track in a smart environment. IEEE Trans. Knowl. Data Eng. **23**(4), 527–539 (2011)
6. Aztirua, A., Augusto, J.C., Basagoiti, R., Izaguirre, A., Cook, D.J.: Discovering frequent user-environment interactions in intelligent environments. Pers. Ubiquit. Comput. **16**, 91–103 (2012)
7. Chen, L., Hoey, J., Nugent, C., Cook, D., Hu, Z.: Sensor-based activity recognition. IEEE Trans. Syst. Man Cybern. C Appl. Rev. **42**(6), 790–808 (2012)
8. Mileo, A., Merico, D., Bisiani, R.: Support for context-aware monitoring in home healthcare. J. Ambient Intell. Smart Environ. **2**(1), 49–66 (2010)
9. Aztiria, A., et al.: Discovering frequent user-environment interactions in intelligent environments. Pers. Ubiquit. Comput. **16**(1), 91–103 (2012)
10. Phua, C., Sim, K., Biswas, J.: Multiple people activity recognition using simple sensors. In: Proceedings of the International Conference on Pervasive and Embedded Computing and Communication Systems, pp. 313–318 (2011)
11. Singla, G., Cook, D., Schmitter-Edgecombe, M.: Recognizing independent and joint activities among multiple residents in smart environments. J. Ambient Intell. Humanized Comput. **1**(1), 57–63 (2010)
12. Miori, V., Russo, D., Aliberti, M.: Domotic technologies incompatibility becomes user transparent. Commun. ACM **53**(1), 153–157 (2010)
13. Tan, P.N., Steinbach, M., Kumar, V.: Introduction to Data Mining, 1st edn. Addison-Wesley Longman Publishing Co., Inc., MA (2005)
14. Dougherty, J., Kohavi, R., Sahami, M.: Supervised and unsupervised discretization of continuous features. In: Proceedings of the 12th International Conference on Machine Learning, Lake Tahoe, CA, pp. 194–202. Morgan Kaufmann, Los Altos (1995)
15. Hastie, T., Tibshirani, R., Friedman, J.: The Elements of Statistical Learning. Springer, New York (2009)

Web-Enabled Intelligent Gateways for eHealth Internet-of-Things

Jose Granados[1], Amir-Mohammad Rahmani[1(✉)], Pekka Nikander[2],
Pasi Liljeberg[1], and Hannu Tenhunen[1]

[1] Department of Information Technology, University of Turku, Turku, Finland
{josgra, amirah, pakrli, hatenhu}@utu.fi
[2] Department of Computer Science and Engineering,
Aalto University, Helsinki, Finland
pekka.nikander@aalto.fi

Abstract. The currently unfolding Internet of Things (IoT) technologies will enable health services that have higher quality and lower cost than those available today. However, the large majority of the current IoT research and development expects that the IoT "things" communicate wirelessly, leaving the question of their energy supply and communication reliability more-or-less open. The obvious alternative, wire line, has gained much less attention, perhaps since it is too well known. In this paper, we present an energy-efficient IoT architecture for healthcare applications that leverages clinical and home care scenarios, given their typically fixed, stationary nature, as the mobility of patients is in many cases confined to a room or a building. The architecture is based on intelligent, wired gateways that are power-efficient and low-cost. The gateways link wired/wireless medical sensors and hospital appliances to web services, enabling hospital automation and widespread data collection and aggregation of vital signs in a convenient, and cost-effective approach.

Keywords: Internet of Things · Web of things · WebSocket · Gateway · HTML5 · Healthcare · Smart Hospital · Home care

1 Introduction

The Internet of Things (IoT) refers to the extension of the current Internet services where the mundane everyday things are connected to the Internet, in addition to the already connected computers and smart phones [1]. This paradigm enables Electronic Health (eHealth), Mobile Health (mHealth) and Ambient Assisted Living (AAL) technologies that allow remote monitoring and tracking of patients living alone at home or treated in hospitals. These technologies provide health workers with the ability to check vital signs of patients from anywhere at any time [2].

In wireline, wireless, and hybrid situations, an IoT gateway could play an important role in health-related IoT applications. Initially, such a gateway may securely and reliably bridge legacy sensors and other medical equipment to traditional Internet Protocol (IP) based networks, such as a hospital intranet. In the longer run, such gateways may connect the devices to a (private) cloud-based service, allowing data

© Institute for Computer Sciences, Social Informatics and Telecommunications Engineering 2015
R. Giaffreda et al. (Eds.): IoT360 2014, Part I, LNICST 150, pp. 248–254, 2015.
DOI: 10.1007/978-3-319-19656-5_36

aggregation and sensor fusion across multiple sensors and all patients, both in hospitals and home care environments.

The IoT gateway may also be made responsible for intelligent processing and partial data aggregation of the vital signs signals, along with protocol conversion from the proprietary or primitive sensor data formats to those used IP based networks. When real-time asynchronous communication capabilities are desired, the WebSocket protocol [3] proves being useful by providing socket like capabilities for the Web.

Another potential benefit of the proposed approach is that sensors and actuators for both building automation and clinical appliances may be powered and networked by PoE (Power over Ethernet) [4] enabled technology. This allows building a Smart Hospital system where the medical devices and building automation, including safety and security, may become integrated. Furthermore, in the future even patients' own devices, such as cell phones, may be integrated to the system, increasing their awareness and self-responsibility of their situation.

In this paper, we propose an IoT architecture for healthcare applications based on energy-efficient web-enabled gateway design customized for health related data processing and transmission. The proposed architecture focuses on enabling wide-spread data collection from both wireless and wireline sensors, not only from the medical world but also from e.g. the building safety and security systems, in a unified way. The combination of this two realms of healthcare services and smart hospital realizations by taking advantage of PoE and web of things technologies represent a convenient, and cost-effective approach to healthcare services.

2   Related Work

In [5], a WebSocket based monitoring system for sensor activity over a 6loWPAN (IPv6 over Low power Wireless Personal Area Networks) network is proposed for feedback on building energy consumption, the WebSocket client is implemented in the sensor gateway and a web user interface based on HTML5 is used. The gateway however, does not serve as an energy source for the sensor nodes, leaving them to depend on batteries or third party power sources to work. In [6], authors present design and optimizations of a low power wireless gateway node that bridges data from wireless sensor networks to Wi-Fi networks on an on-demand basis. These works do not consider the use of intelligent processing of health related data on gateways. Ultimately the gateways in these works are used as connection points to external web servers instead of embedding the web connectivity on the gateway itself as proposed in this paper.

3   Motivation

IoT applications are based on the extension of Internet to resource-constrained network nodes that cannot take advantage of existing web services due to their high overhead and intricacy. Resources are accessed through RESTful interfaces in synchronous request/response fashion using methods such as GET, PUT, POST and DELETE and are identified by Universal Resource Identifiers (URIs) which allow for short lived transmissions only [7]. However, monitoring bio-signals required to estimate the overall user's health condition necessitates a constant connection for the non-stop transmission of live data from continuous and pulsed signals such as Electrocardiography (ECG), Electromyography (EMG), Electroencephalography (EEG), respiratory and heart rate. Each signal has a different bandwidth as shown in Table 1. Electrical activity often requires band-pass and notch filtering to remove baseline wandering, electric hum noise and motion artifacts. Depending on the need, the signal could be processed for feature extraction. In addition, classification of normal, deviant, risk and high risk conditions are performed in order to send notification to caregivers in order to take appropriate actions before a catastrophic event occurs. Many of these functions could be performed on the gateway in order to alleviate the burden that the sensor can carry.

A typical building automation system for hospitals is usually designed without taking into account the health data generated by biomedical sensors. Yet, a trend in modern healthcare is to go beyond the scope of traditional building management and integrate all kinds of data sources into a big data cloud repository for performing advanced analytics, improve forecasting and prioritize actions for increasing the bottom line while improving health services quality. As an example, room sensors sense the needs and preferences of staff and patients and allow to move from a traditional nurse call system based on buttons fixed to a wall to intelligent context aware nurse call system based on detecting hazardous situations (e.g. when a patient's temperature rise into fever or an abnormal heart condition is detected).

Table 1. Types of bio-signals and bandwidths.

Type of biosignal	Bandwidth	Signal nature
ECG	0.5–40 Hz	Continuous waveform
EMG	20–400 Hz	Continuous waveform
Continuous blood pressure	0–100 Hz	Continuous waveform
Systolic and diastolic blood pressure	–	Discrete measurements
Respiration rate	0.5–10 Hz	Continuous waveform
Heart rate	20–200 BPM	Pulses per minute
Blood glucose	–	Discrete measurements

4   Architecture

The intelligent gateway proposed features processing and web software components customized for the handling and transmission of healthcare related signals such as vital signs. On the sensor side, the gateway takes care of translation layers to accommodate vendor agnostic sensors using different communication protocols.

The system architecture is shown in Fig. 1. The biomedical sensors used for assessing physiological status serve as one of the data inputs to the system. These are wired or wireless sensors for biometrics such as ECG, EMG, EEG, temperature, pressure, heart rate, position, respiration rate, glucose levels, complete blood count, etc.

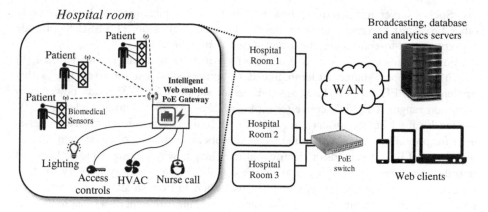

Fig. 1. Energy efficient IoT architecture for healthcare applications.

These sensors are connected to the gateway which receives the data, executes signal processing and/or feature extraction and forwards relevant information to a server, database or a directly to a web client.

In addition to remote patient monitoring, a smart building system is integrated consisting of IoT nodes used for building automation. These include traditional lighting, public address, access control and HVAC as well as hospital centric appliances namely next-to-bed controls and context aware applications such as intelligent nurse calling. The envisioned system is energy efficient by harnessing the PoE capabilities of the gateway, which allows for powering actuators and sensors directly without recurring to a different power grid or AC outlets. The back-end of the system consists of the two remaining components, the PoE enabled switch and a cloud computing platform that includes broadcasting, data warehouse and Big Data analytics servers, and finally Web clients as a graphical user interface for final visualization.

4.1 Medical Sensors

Medical sensors capture signals from the body used for treatment and diagnosing of a medical state. Examples are ECG, EMG and EEG signals for analyzing heart, muscles and brain conditions. The sensor contains transducers and electrodes for acquiring electrical signals that are converted to digital form using an analog front-end. The signal is then transmitted to the gateway via wireless or wired communication protocols such as Serial, SPI, Bluetooth, Wi-Fi or IEEE 802.15.4. The transmitted data contains information about the number of channels used and other status data such as lead-off detection.

4.2 Gateway

The gateway receives data from sensors and performs in-network processing e.g. data aggregation, filtering and dimensionality reduction. The gateway also contains a

WebSocket server for streaming data directly to web applications, or to interface to other broadcast servers. The WebSocket connection relies on TLS/SSL to provide encrypted, end-to-end secure client and server communications.

For the gateway role, we have designed a hardware platform known as *Ell-i* [8] which is an open source Arduino like development platform for fixed things that implements IEEE 802.3 at Power-over-Ethernet standard for 1–35 watts power consumption range. A DC/DC converter on board converts 48 V into 5 V and/or 3.3 V needed by the Microcontroller Unit (MCU), and an extra power supply converter is used for providing bulk power to the wired sensors and actuators of the system such as high-power LEDs, solenoids or electric motors. The gateway is designed to be low-cost in order to be massively deployed along a hospital (e.g. one gateway in every room or for every bed) so that low power wireless sensors benefit from small coverage area. The gateway receives commands over Internet to execute different tasks such as start streaming of sensor data which include processing and transmission over the WebSocket interface.

4.3   Smart Hospital Framework

The networking capabilities of the gateway can serve multiple roles in addition to monitoring patients. The same protocols used for connecting medical sensors are used in a similar way for managing building automation systems such as lighting, access control, indoor PA systems and HVAC controls and other more clinical centric as in the case of ambient-intelligent nurse calling systems. This setup enables the centralization of data acquisition not only for patient health data but also for hospital building management of an integrated Smart Hospital framework. The gateway serves not only as a managing node for the smart hospital controls but also as a smart power source by harnessing the power coming from the PoE cable. This makes the system more energy-efficient and practical compared to other architectures that use embedded solutions such as Raspberry Pi [9] as web servers.

5   Experimental Results

A test have been designed to assess the performance and practicality of the setup. We use the Ell-i platform with an e-health daughter board that includes signal conditioning circuitry to acquire ECG data from electrodes attached to a test patient (Fig. 2a). The data is digitally filtered in the gateway to remove power line noise and is streamed over Internet using the embedded WebSocket server via Ethernet. A JavaScript client plots the near real-time chart (1 s delay) of the signal (Fig. 2b). A set of commands is implemented to control transmission start-stop. Future work includes the expansion of the command set into a complete API for gateway management. The energy source comes from the PoE enabled Ethernet cable connected to the gateway which also powers the sensors.

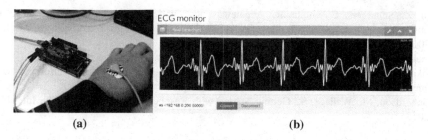

(a)   **(b)**

Fig. 2. PoE powered gateway with e-health daughter board and electrodes attached to a test patient for ECG monitoring (a). JavaScript client interface (b).

The signal is sampled at 500 SPS with 12-bit resolution. Samples are packetized into WebSocket messages of size 800 bytes and sent at an average rate of 1 KB/s. The cost of the system is estimated in $200 USD per patient.

6 Conclusions

We believe that focus on the IoT gateway design for healthcare applications represent an opportunity to solve IoT architecture challenges such as web connectivity, power efficiency and Smart Hospital integration. In this paper, an IoT architecture have been proposed that uses PoE powered gateways to serve as a bridge for medical sensors and hospital building automation appliances to IP based networks and cloud computing platforms. The proposed design of the gateway does processing and data aggregation of vital signs and includes streaming web server. In addition, the gateway harness the energy provided by the PoE enabled Ethernet cable to power sensors and actuators. The gateway is designed to be low-cost and allows massive deployment along the hospital facilities that together with PoE enabled network infrastructure result in an energy-efficient architecture for healthcare in hospitals and homes.

References

1. Singh, D., Tripathi, G., Jara, A.J.: A survey of Internet-of-Things: future vision, architecture, challenges and services. IEEE World Forum on in Internet of Things (2014)
2. Lopez, P et al.: Survey of Internet of Things technologies for clinical environments. In: International Conference on Advanced Information Networking and Applications Workshops (2013)
3. Fette, I., Google, Inc., Melnikov, A.: Isode Ltd.: The WebSocket Protocol. IETF RFC 6455
4. IEEE 802.3at standard for Ethernet. Amendment 3: Data terminal equipment (DTE) power via the media dependent interface (MDI) enhancements. IEEE Computer Society (2009)
5. Ma, K., Sun, R.: Introducing webSocket-based real-time monitoring system for remote intelligent buildings. Int. J. Distrib. Sens. Netw. **2013**, 1–10 (2014)

6. Jin, Z., Schurgers, C., Gupta, R.: A gateway node with duty-cycled radio and processing subsystems for wireless sensor networks. ACM Trans. Des. Autom. Electron. Syst. **14**, 1–17 (2009)
7. Shelby, Z.: Embedded web services. IEEE Wirel. Commun. **17**, 52–57 (2010)
8. Nikander, P., Vaddina, K.R., Liuha, P., Tenhunen, H.: Ell-i: an inexpensive platform for fixed things. SCPE J. **14**, 155–167 (2013)
9. Richardson, M., Wallace, S.: Getting Started with Raspberry Pi. O'Reilly Media, Inc., USA (2012)

Child Abuse Monitor System Model: A Health Care Critical Knowledge Monitor System

Tiago Pereira[✉] and Henrique Santos

ALGORITMI Centre, Information System Department,
University of Minho, Azurém Campus, 4804-533 Guimarães, Portugal
tiago.pereira@algoritmi.uminho.pt,
hsantos@dsi.uminho.pt

Abstract. The Childhood protection is a subject with high value for the society, but, the Child Abuse cases are difficult to identify. The process from suspicious to accusation is very difficult to achieve. It must configure very strong evidences. Typically, Health Care services deal with these cases from the beginning where there are evidences based on the diagnosis, but they aren't enough to promote the accusation. Besides that, this subject it's highly sensitive because there are legal aspects to deal with such as: the patient privacy, paternity issues, medical confidentiality, among others. We propose a Child Abuses critical knowledge monitor system model that addresses this problem. This decision support system is implemented with a multiple scientific domains: to capture of tokens from clinical documents from multiple sources; a topic model approach to identify the topics of the documents; knowledge management through the use of ontologies to support the critical knowledge sensibility concepts and relations such as: symptoms, behaviors, among other evidences in order to match with the topics inferred from the clinical documents and then alert and log when clinical evidences are present. Based on these alerts clinical personnel could analyze the situation and take the appropriate procedures.

Keywords: Health care knowledge sensitivity · Health care decision support system · Ontology · Health care knowledge security · Knowledge management · Topic models · Information retrieval · Text mining

1 Introduction

The health care information systems had evolved strongly and with the recent implementations of the electronic health record these information systems interoperate together and allow us to access patient information within of multiple healthcare organizations. This aspect brings new opportunities to develop new technologies to promote more patient or health care services benefits. Since health care information is highly sensible there are important aspects that cannot be neglected, such as: patients privacy, medical confidentiality, confidentiality of the clinical procedures and legal aspects. This context is prominent when we're dealing with child abuse matters. Child abuse cases are difficult to identify since they are more pervert and dissimulated [1]. When clinical personnel identify evidences by diagnosis in order to formulate the

© Institute for Computer Sciences, Social Informatics and Telecommunications Engineering 2015
R. Giaffreda et al. (Eds.): IoT360 2014, Part I, LNICST 150, pp. 255–261, 2015.
DOI: 10.1007/978-3-319-19656-5_37

accusation these evidences are not strong enough to do it. On the other hand, we assume that this difficulty could lead to a substantial number of cases that aren't identified. To address this problem we've developed a child abuse critical knowledge monitor system that based on medical expert knowledge alert and log when child abuses evidences are present in clinical documents. This is done automatically by the system using information retrieval and text mining techniques which allows to transform text in tokens, from tokens we infer topics, then we match them with an ontology that supports the child abuse evidences as concepts and finally, when there are present in documents clinical evidences of child abuse the system alerts and logs these evidences for further analysis by clinical personnel. In the Sect. 2 we explain what implicit considerations we should consider in patient privacy and health care information security, in Sect. 3 we defined the health care critical knowledge, in Sect. 4 we explain the research methodology that this research is based, Sect. 5 we describe the components of the child abuse critical knowledge monitor system model, in Sect. 6 we'll present the preliminary results of this research, finally, in Sect. 7 we'll describe the contribution to health care information systems.

2 Privacy and Health Care Information Security

2.1 Information Security and Privacy

Information is valuable for any kind of organization and when there are rights involved, such as: patient privacy, medical confidentiality, and information that could stigmatize persons in social context like health care, the needs of information preservation are even higher. Information security consists in the preservation of the security properties of information and based on many standards and work published in this field, we normally identify a set of three properties there are the core of information security: confidentiality, integrity and availability of information [2, 3]. In health care its easy to recognize these properties but we have to reinforce them with the right of privacy that cannot be affected by the promotion of the information security properties. In a concise form, we'll describe each of these aspects.

Confidentiality. It means that any information that is exchanged or stored by the systems is secret and only the authorized persons can access to it. In health care this property is fundamental because in all phases of the clinical process exists information exchange and can only be accessed by authorized personnel.

Integrity. Keep the integrity of information is keeping its accuracy, i.e., there should be guaranties that some modification of the information is intentional and made by authorized personnel. In this objective, we need three actions, not allow unauthorized modifications, keep updated the authorized personnel and keep the accuracy of the information.

Availability. It means that the information should be accessible permanently at all the time. In health care the access to the patient information could be vital to him, e.g. An anesthesiologist should have access to information of the patient about allergies and other diseases since that with anesthesia could lead the patient to a complicated situation.

Privacy. Privacy, more than an information security property, it's a right. In health care we should consider the privacy of the patient, medical and non-medical personnel. For this reason no mechanism implemented to support the information security properties could affect the privacy that consists in maintaining the secrecy of personal information which force to get it free from monitoring and unauthorized access. Typically, to access to the patient information a consent declaration is needed.

3 Health Care Critical Knowledge

The development of standards of health care software is a big step to the interoperability between information systems in this area. There are, at least, six entities that have developed standards in this field: The American Society for Testing and Materials with ASTM-E31, The American National Standards Institute with ANSI-HL7, The European Committe for Standardization with CEN-TC251, The International Organization for Standardization with ISO-TC215, The Association of Electrical Equipment and Medical Imaging Manufactures with NEMA-DICOM and IEEE with multiple standards [4]. With the evolution of the health care information systems the access to patient information using Electronic Health Record Systems (EHRS) is facilitated, e.g. Urgency treatment data, health monitoring data, among others. According to the health domain analysis report from the technical committee from HL7 about security and privacy of health care information, particularly, in exchange of information between information systems and according to HL7 Security and Privacy Ontology was possible for us to identify critical knowledge concepts in health care domain [5, 6]: Substances abuse, Sexual abuse and domestic violence, Genetic disease, Sexual transmitted disease, Sickle Cell, Sexuality and Reproductive, HIV/AIDS, Psychiatry and Taboo [6]. From this, we explore the subject General Abuses with the focus on the child abuse and based on regulations and legal documentation we have constructed an ontology that maps the concepts: symptoms, behaviour and other evidences of child abuse [7], see Fig. 1.

4 Research Methodology

For the different phases and objectives of this research we have used multiple research techniques: survey literature techniques, content analysis and proof of concept in Design Research context.

4.1 Design Science Research

"Design Science research is a research paradigm in which a designer answers questions relevant to human problems via the creation of innovative artefacts, thereby contributing new knowledge to the body of scientific evidence. The designed artifacts are both useful and fundamental in understanding that problem" [8].

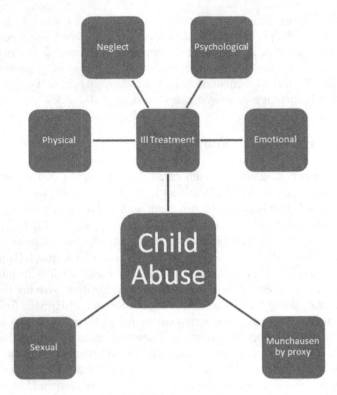

Fig. 1. Child abuse ontology

The design science research has its roots in the sciences of the artificial. Artificial as something that is created by humans that doesn't exists in Nature. Design Research is fundamentally a problem-solving paradigm. It consists in seeking innovation through ideas, practices, technical abilities and products obtained from a set of routines such as: analysis, design, implementation, and use of information systems concerning the effectiveness and efficiency achievement on organizations. The outputs forms of Design research could be: constructs (vocabulary and symbols), models (abstractions and representations), methods (algorithms and practices), and instantiations (implemented and prototype systems) [8].

5   Child Abuse Critical Knowledge Monitoring System

The model of the system is defined by four components: the knowledge capture component, the critical knowledge ontology component; the critical knowledge repository component; and the alert and log component. Each component is based on a variety of information systems fields [10, 11].

5.1 The Knowledge Capture Component (KC)

The knowledge capture component requisites are: extracting tokens from documents in a variety of formats, such as text and audio. Additionally, the implemented system supports other formats: video (extracting sound and text within the video), webpages, among others; and transform the tokens extracted in such format that could be searchable concerning the privacy and confidentiality, integrity and availability of documents. In order to do it, we have implemented a topic model approach using two methods, latent Dirichelet [12–14] and Pachinko allocation model (PAM) [15, 16]. The PAM has been chosen because it can establish relations between topics and topic descriptors. The use of the topic model approach is fundamental because allows to driven topics from documents and ignore (because of its lower occurrence within a document) personal data (names, contacts and addresses) complying with the privacy and information security properties. To use topic models from the extracted tokens from the documents we needed to filter [17] them, essentially, tokens less than four (configurable) characters and trivial discourse tokens such as "and", "or", punctuation, among others. As an output of this component we get a searchable set of descriptors clustered by topics that co-occur in the document.

5.2 The Critical Knowledge Ontology Component (CKO)

The critical knowledge ontology component requisites are: allowing the editing of the critical ontology; and matching the ontology with the output of the knowledge capture component. This component uses Portégé Editor and Portégé API, see acknowledgments, for the matching procedure with the topic descriptors.

5.3 The Critical Knowledge Repository Component

The critical knowledge repository component requisites are allowing the storage of the outputs from the KC and CKO. This component uses a document management tool with the control version capability. The control versions could be useful in future implementations and we could analyse multiple diagnosis of the same patient in an historical perspective.

5.4 The Alert and Log Component

The alert and log component requisites are: alerting the user by email of the probability of the document containing evidences about a child abuse; and register the evidences identified by the system of each document for further analysis. The system should select what cases should trigger an alert or register only. In order to do this we'll use artificial intelligence classification algorithms very well tested and implemented to assess the evidences and give value to the sensibility of the document in this context.

6 Preliminary Results

We have done tests in the laboratory only. The system is capable of identifying evidences within a document in many formats and in Portuguese and English languages, see Fig. 2. Documents with no relation to the subject of child abuse were tested, too, and they produce negative results, i.e., the system didn't identify evidences on these documents. The next step will be testing the system in real context. We'll test the system with documents from child abuse suspicion cases and confront the results with cases that was formulated an accusation. In order to evaluate the accuracy of the system by component we'll use the typical assessment models of knowledge management systems [18].

Topic 0		Topic 8	
child_young	0,14206	protection_child_young	0,02537
general_health	0,0566	health_bad	0,01202
situation_risc	0,00888	figure_algoritmo	0,01068
place_hospital	0,00666	framework_framework	0,00668
for_life_integrity	0,00555	integrity_physical_child	0,00668
physics_child_young	0,00555	nurse_medic	0,00668
parental_who	0,00555	abuse_neglect	0,00668
residence_child_young	0,00555	young_oposition	0,00534
court_family	0,00555	young_oposition_intervention	0,00534
model_report_for	0,00444	other_info	0,00534
procedure_intervention_for	0,00444	info_constant	0,00534
idea_suicidal	0,00444	intensive_when	0,00534
young_family_care	0,00444	for_fin	0,00534
health_primary	0,00333	health_for	0,00401
service_urgent_basic	0,00333	promote_health	0,00401
treatment_framework	0,00333	treat_intervention	0,00401
sindrome_munchausen	0,00333	inpatient_care_consult_external	0,00401
injuries_external_organs	0,00333	treat_care_health	0,00401
presence_sperm	0,00333	for_detection	0,00401
sperm_body	0,00333	uncomun	0,00401

Fig. 2. Topics captured from guide of detection of child abuse, the portuguese health general board document

7 Contributions of This Research

We propose a decision support system that addresses the problem of child abuse case identification. This subject is highly sensitive and valuable to the society and the community. This research has produced a child abuse ontology that could have many applications. In the information systems field, we bring to discuss the knowledge security: can we deal with knowledge security like we do with information security? The sensitivity of knowledge is fundamental when dealing with knowledge preservation?

Acknowledgement. This work is financed by FEDER funds through the Competitive Factors Operational Program – COMPETE and Portuguese national funds through FCT – Fundação para a ciência e tecnologia in project FCOMP-01-0124-FEDER-022674.

This work was conducted using the Protégé resource, which is supported by grant GM10331601 from the National Institute of General Medical Sciences of the United States National Institutes of Health.

References

1. JN: Maus tratos a crianças cada vez mais perversos e difíceis de identificar. Jornal De Notícias. Controlinveste (2013). www.jn.pt
2. ISO: ISO/IEC 27001:2013 Information technology - Security techniques - Information security management systems – Requirements. ISO (2013)
3. Oladimeji, E.A., Chung, L., Jung, H.T., Kim, J.: Managing security and privacy in ubiquitous eHealth information interchange, vol. 10, pp. 26:1–26 (2011)
4. IRMA: User-Driven Healthcare: Concepts, Methodologies, Tools, and Applications: IGI Global (2013)
5. H. S. O. WG: HL7 Version 3 Standard: Security and Privacy Ontology, Release 1, Version 3 ed: HL7 (2013)
6. S.W.g.o. HL7: Composite Security and Privacy - Domain analysis Model Report, Ballot, HL7, May 2010
7. P. M. o. Health: Despacho n.º 31292/2008, in 236, ed. Diário da república: INCM (2008)
8. Hevner, A., Chatterjee, S.: Design Science Research in Information Systems. Design Research in Information Systems, pp. 9–22. Springer, Heidelberg (2010)
9. March, S.T., Hevner, A.R., Park, J., Ram, S.: Design science in information systems research. Manage. Inf. Syst. Q. **28**, 75–105 (2004)
10. Pereira, T.R., Santos, H.: Critical knowledge monitor system model: healthcare context. In: European Conference on Knowledge Management, Cartagena, Spain (2012)
11. Pereira, T., Santos, H.: Health care critical knowledge monitor system model: health care critical knowledge ontology component. In: SHEWC2013 - XIII Safety, Health and Environment World Congress, Porto, Portugal, p. 002 (2013)
12. Blei, D.M., Ng, A.Y., Jordan, M.I.: Latent dirichlet allocation. J. Mach. Learn. Res. **3**, 993–1022 (2003)
13. Hofmann, T.: Unsupervised learning by probabilistic latent semantic analysis. Mach. Learn. **42**, 177–196 (2001)
14. Steyvers, M., Griffiths, T.: Probabilistic topic models. In: Landauer, T., McNamara, D.S., Dennis, S., Kintsch, W. (eds.) Handbook of Latent Semantic Analysis, vol. 427, pp. 424–440. Erlbaum, Hillsdale (2007)
15. Mimno, D., Li, W., McCallum, A.: Mixtures of hierarchical topics with pachinko allocation. In: Proceedings of ICML, pp. 633–640 (2007)
16. Li, W., McCallum, A.: Pachinko allocation: DAG-structured mixture models of topic correlations. In: Proceedings of the 23rd International Conference on Machine Learning, Pittsburgh, Pennsylvania (2006)
17. Sharda, R., Delen, D., Turban, E.: Decision Support and Business Intelligence Systems, 9th edn. Prentice Hall Press, Upper Saddle River (2010)
18. Pereira, T.R., Santos, H.: The matrix of quality dimensions of knowledge management: knowledge management assessment models review. Knowl. Manage. Int. J **12**, 33–41 (2013)

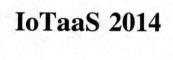

COLT Collaborative Delivery of Lightweight IoT Applications

Michael Vögler$^{(\boxtimes)}$, Fei Li, Markus Claeßens, Johannes M. Schleicher,
Sanjin Sehic, Stefan Nastic, and Schahram Dustdar

Distributed Systems Group, Vienna University of Technology,
Argentinierstraße 8/184-1, 1040 Vienna, Austria
{voegler,li,claessens,schleicher,sehic,nastic,dustdar}@dsg.tuwien.ac.at
http://dsg.tuwien.ac.at/

Abstract. Todays IoT solutions are typically delivered by domain-specific solution providers. In these solutions, components are highly customized for specific project requirements, limiting their users to the offerings of their providers. To overcome these limitations, we propose a novel mechanism that opens the market for OEMs and third-party developers. This paper introduces the IoT Application Market, where a range of stakeholders can distribute, sell, share and contribute features for lightweight device-specific IoT applications. Based on the offerings in the IoT Application Market, users can buy applications and deploy them in their environment through self-service.

Keywords: Internet of things · IoT applications · IoT market · IoT PaaS

1 Introduction

The overall process of delivering an IoT solution is typically orchestrated by solution providers for specific projects [1,8]. Since this delivery process is mostly vendor-specific, a big challenge in the Internet of Things domain, is to establish an environment that allows various stakeholders to share, contribute and distribute applications collaboratively. The scale of IoT solutions can range from a simple application that monitors and reacts to a temperature sensor, to a full-blown enterprise application that manages and controls a set of buildings. In this paper we focus on lightweight applications that can be executed on gateways [9–11], which are used to connect heterogenous devices and handle resources efficiently. These lightweight applications are software services that carry out various tasks autonomously by executing application code directly on the embedded runtime environment of the device, resulting in a small footprint in terms of resource and memory consumption. The drawback of this approach is that the actual development of these gateway-dependent applications requires deep knowledge of the runtime environment, which significantly increases the efforts for development, and limits the involvement of more developers. As a result providers are

© Institute for Computer Sciences, Social Informatics and Telecommunications Engineering 2015
R. Giaffreda et al. (Eds.): IoT360 2014, Part I, LNICST 150, pp. 265–272, 2015.
DOI: 10.1007/978-3-319-19656-5_38

interested in distributing and selling their applications to a broad audience to cover their efforts. To save time and costs as well as expand their market coverage, providers are eager to collaborate with other stakeholders to reuse their solutions, which will only work in an ecosystem that allows not only distribution but also a model to collaborate.

In this paper we present a novel ecosystem, where application providers can share, contribute to and distribute IoT applications. The core idea is to realize an IoT Application Market, that opens the application delivery process to OEMs and third-party developers. To facilitate and integrate the offerings of the mentioned stakeholders, the market supports application providers to form collaborations with other stakeholders to create and distribute applications. Furthermore the market allows users to search for suitable applications, purchase and deploy them in their local environment through self-service.

The paper is structured as follows: Sect. 2 presents a motivating industrial use case, Sect. 3 illustrates the overall approach, Sect. 4 describes the implementation details, in Sect. 5 the related work is compared, and finally the paper concludes in Sect. 6.

2   Motivation

This work is motivated by a real-world scenario in Building Management Systems (BMS). The scenario is based on a case study we conducted in our lab in collaboration with an industrial partner. In the case study we have identified the following: generally a BMS provides efficient management of building facilities to save energy and reduce operational costs. A BMS consists of a vast number of sensors, other smart devices and a platform that connects and handles these resources and is developed by an *Application Provider* for a specific *Customer*. During the process of delivering a BMS, the provider gathers information about the target building, installs and integrates suitable hardware into an infrastructure and finally connects it to a platform that provides specific control and management applications. This approach has the following limitations: (i) the customer is limited to the applications and services offered by his provider, and (ii) providers have to develop tailored applications based on customer demands and their respective installed solution, which is both time- and cost-ineffective. To address these limitations we want to open the process of developing customer specific applications to the following contributing stakeholders. *Third-party developers* develop and offer lightweight applications that run on specific IoT devices. Based on the installed device-set, a customer can choose suitable applications. This gives the customer more flexibility and the provider the opportunity to outsource some of the application development. *OEMs* provide complete applications or just contribute features that are tailored for specific hardware devices. These offerings can be reused by both third-party developers and providers for new requirements or different physical environments. Based on this scenario we identified the following requirements: (i) a market-based collaboration and distribution environment, and (ii) a solution to manage the deployment and execution of lightweight IoT Applications.

3   IoT Application Market

In order to address the previously mentioned requirements we propose an app-roach that consists of the following key components: *IoT Application, IoT Application Market* and *IoT PaaS*.

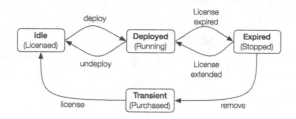

Fig. 1. IoT Application lifecycle

In this paper we focus on lightweight IoT Applications, which are used to automatically tune building facilities, acquire data from different sensors, monitor devices, and automatically report a certain device status. In our approach, an IoT Application is represented as a self-contained archive with corresponding metadata, containing the following information: (i) a *Name* that uniquely identifies the application, (ii) a natural language *Description* that can be read by humans and a structural one that can be understood by software (i.e. the market) in order to provide a reliable search, (iii) *Provider* name and id, who created and uploaded the application, (iv) a list of *Suitable Devices* the application can be deployed and executed on. This list can always be updated by the provider, to react on new emerging compatible devices, and (v) a *Version* number that uniquely identifies the current release of the application.

The lifecycle of an application is depicted in Fig. 1 and has the following states: *Transient, Idle, Deployed* and *Expired*. An application that is purchased is in state *Transient*. Once the application is licensed by the market it is in state *Idle*. As soon as the user deploys the licensed application on the gateway device, the gateway checks if the license is valid, initializes the startup process and sets the state to *Deployed*. If the gateway detects that the license is expired, it interrupts the execution and sets the application to *Expired*.

3.1   IoT Application Market

The IoT Application Market represents an ecosystem, where *Application Providers* offer and users browse and retrieve applications. The overall process, involved components and stakeholders are depicted in Fig. 2. The market stores the uploaded applications in the *IoT Application Repository*, which is an open service repository that hosts applications as self-contained archives with corresponding metadata. The market provides the following core components.

The *Stakeholder Management* is responsible for handling the management of users, their authentication and authorization within the market. We identified

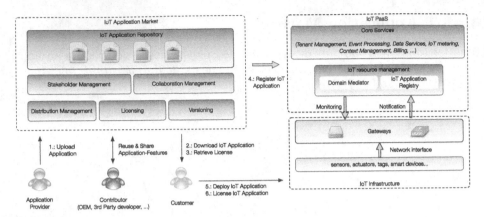

Fig. 2. IoT Application Market and IoT PaaS

the following groups of users based on [3]: *Application providers* develop applications and upload them to the market. Additionally the provider can decide to share features with other users of the market and form a collaboration. Users invited to collaborations are called contributors. *Contributors* can reuse shared features for other or new applications and provide new or improved code for the collaboration. Based on this collaboration, involved parties can decide if and how they want to distribute the outcome and decide on an appropriate revenue sharing model. Users of the market, which are not involved in the development process are called customers. *Customers* browse the market and search for interesting and suitable applications e.g. if the release of an application can be deployed and executed on the owned IoT devices. The *Collaboration Management* supports and manages the collaboration among the application provider and contributors. For each group of users that formed a collaboration, the market provides a specific private repository, where the group can store their application code and other required artifacts. This repository can only be accessed by the members of the collaboration and provides the basic features of a conventional source code management (SCM) and revision control system. Additionally it supports different plugable metrics to track the contribution of each member of the collaboration, e.g. one of the easiest models, calculates the contribution based on the number of committed code-lines. The Collaboration Management uses the data provided by the respective metric to calculate the revenue share. The *Distribution Management* monitors and controls the distribution of applications. A monitoring component keeps track of all downloads and a control component regulates if a user is allowed to download a specific application, based on historic data e.g. punctual payment of bills. The *Licensing* component governs the use or redistribution of an application. A typical license in our model grants the user permission to use an application on a defined set of field devices.

After downloading the application from the market and deploying it on the gateway, the user needs the corresponding license file that triggers the actual instantiation and startup process of the application.

Based on the user's inputs (e.g. used device group, subscription schema) the market generates a license file that can now be deployed on the gateway. The gateway detects the deployed license and triggers the startup process of the corresponding application. During the execution of the application the gateway may detect that the license is expired and passivates the execution. The user can now decide if he wants to extend the license or undeploy the application from the device. In case the user wants to prolong the license he can retrieve an extended license in the market. To keep track of multiple releases of the same application the market uses a *Versioning* component. Since in the market we need to handle a vast amount of applications, we need an efficient mechanism to deal with different releases of the same application. Therefore, whenever a provider uploads a new release to the market, he has to decide if it is either a major (significant improvement) or minor (bug fixes) release. This approach has the following advantages: (i) developers can decide for which release they want to provide updates and which are no longer supported, (ii) users can easily decide which release is the most suitable for their environment, and (iii) the market can notify the user about updates or known issues for a certain release.

3.2 IoT PaaS

IoT PaaS [7] is a domain-independet Platform as a Service framework. In general, IoT solutions are highly domain-specific, so the IoT PaaS framework is build to be generic and extendable enough to be used in different IoT domains. The framework provides essential platform services on cloud that can be used and extended by IoT solution providers. Additionally IoT PaaS offers a registration point for devices, gateways and control applications, to handle the vast number of IoT resources. This registration point is the *IoT resource management* and uses *Domain Mediators* to mediate between different gateway interfaces. To handle events and notifications that can be pushed by IoT applications, we extended the resource management of IoT PaaS and added the *IoT Application Registry*. The registry is a constantly evolving catalog of information about the available and deployed applications, which guarantees that the platform always knows what kind of application and how many of them are deployed. The necessary information about the current status of an application is published by two components: the IoT Application Market and connected gateways, respectively the deployed application.

4   Implementation

The prototype of the presented approach is implemented in Java. We utilize several open-source products from WSO2[1]. We used the Application Server for hosting the service-based components. To provide a flexible and scalable solution the prototype uses the ESB to connect and integrate the components. For the

---

[1] http://wso2.com.

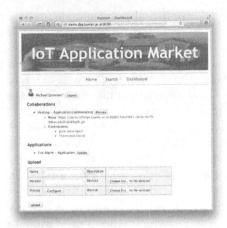
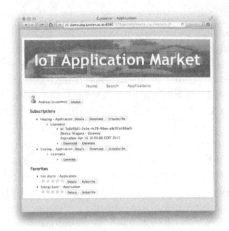

(a) Provider Perspective   (b) Customer Perspective

Fig. 3. IoT Application Market

IoT Application Repository we implemented a custom repository, based on the Governance Registry and Repository. The *Stakeholder Management* is based on an Identity Server that handles users and their respective roles and additionally provides sophisticated security management of services and APIs. For the *Collaboration management* we utilized Gitorious[2] and integrated the statistical analysis tool gitinspector[3]. The communication of IoT Applications with IoT PaaS is based on push notifications implemented by JMS Queues, Publishers and Subscribers supported by Apache ActiveMQ[4]. As our Gateway environment we used the Niagara Framework[5]. The implementation of the IoT Application Lifecycle facilitates Niagara's Component Lifecycle[6] mechanism. Furthermore we facilitated the Niagara Licensing[7] methodology for custom applications, for our *Licensing* implementation.

To demonstrate our prototype we will discuss two stakeholder perspectives of the market. The Application Providers' perspective is depicted in Fig. 3a and displays the provider's collaborations and for each collaboration the repository provided by the market and the contributors with their respective role are shown. Additionally the screen displays applications that got uploaded by the provider and a form to add new offerings to the market. Figure 3b depicts the customers' perspective. The screen displays subscriptions, which the customer received for purchasing an application. For each subscription the customer can generate a

---

[2] https://gitorious.org.

[3] https://code.google.com/p/gitinspector/.

[4] http://activemq.apache.org.

[5] http://www.niagaraax.com/cs/products/niagara_framework.

[6] https://community.niagara-central.com/ord?portal:/blog/BlogEntry/254.

[7] https://community.niagara-central.com/ord?portal:/blog/BlogEntry/269.

new or download a license file that is required for deploying the application. Applications that are currently not purchased can be searched and added as favorites.

5   Related Work

The key concept, the overall terminology and used components of the Internet of Things is well-defined in the literature. In comparison the definition of applications in IoT is not that clear. Recent approaches [4,6] define IoT applications, as applications that are developed on top of a resource abstraction layer. Zhu et al. [11] define two different types of IoT applications. An application that is embedded in and an enterprise application that is build on the Gateway. In contrast to the aforementioned approaches, this paper proposes lightweight IoT applications that are directly deployed and executed on IoT devices (gateways), which brings advantages in terms of scaling and resource consumption.

Bohli et al. [2] describes a market that offers a platform to collect and trade all kinds of sensor information in a WSN. They identified several entities that play an important role in the market and discuss possible pricing schemes and strategies. As the current development of IoT solutions is mostly driven by big industrial players, [5] proposes a set of connected marketplaces where users and developers can create and share innovative IoT artifacts. Although, they share similarities with our approach regarding opening the IoT service delivery process the authors solely concentrate on including users to enable innovation. Contrary to them, our market provides an ecosystem that empowers providers to collaborate with various stakeholders to reduce the costs of the delivery process. Furthermore [5] is mainly focused on providing concepts for the overall approach, whereas we implemented a prototype to demonstrate our market's capabilities.

6   Conclusion and Future Work

This paper proposes the IoT Application Market – a novel open market model for managing the distribution of IoT applications. In the IoT Application Market stakeholders can share, contribute and distribute their lightweight and device-specific IoT Applications. Based on the offerings users can browse the market for interesting and suitable applications. Then they can buy, deploy and execute them in their own local environment through self-service. To efficiently handle the deployment and execution of the vast amount of applications this paper utilizes the IoT PaaS framework. This domain-independent framework provides a set of essential platform services and eases the overall management of IoT Applications. As future work we plan to extend our approach beyond the domain of building management systems. We will also try to identify further participants in the overall market and distribution model. Furthermore, we intend to integrate pricing and revenue sharing models that allow more stakeholders that are involved in the development process, to collaborate.

Acknowledgment. This work is sponsored by Pacific Controls Cloud Computing Lab (PC^{3}L), a joint lab between Pacific Controls L.L.C., Scheikh Zayed Road, Dubai, United Arab Emirates and the Distributed Systems Group of the Vienna University of Technology. (http://pc3l.infosys.tuwien.ac.at/)

References

1. Atzori, L., Iera, A., Morabito, G,: The Internet of Things: a survey. Comput. Netw. **54**(15), 2787–2805 (2010)
2. Bohli, J.M., Sorge, C., Westhoff, D.: Initial observations on economics, pricing, and penetration of the Internet of Things market. SIGCOMM Comput. Commun. Rev. **39**(2), 50–55 (2009)
3. Dustdar, S., Li, F., Truong, H.L., Sehic, S., Nastic, S., Qanbari, S., Vögler, M., Claeßens, M.: Green software services: from requirements to business models. In: 2013 2nd International Workshop on Green and Sustainable Software (GREENS), pp. 1–7. IEEE (2013)
4. Guinard, D., Ion, I., Mayer, S.: In search of an Internet of Things service architecture: REST or WS-*? A developers' perspective. In: Puiatti, A., Gu, T. (eds.) MobiQuitous 2011. LNICST, vol. 104, pp. 326–337. Springer, Heidelberg (2012)
5. Kortuem, G., Kawsar, F.: Market-based user innovation in the Internet of Things. In: 2010 Internet of Things (IoT), pp. 1–8 (2010)
6. Kovatsch, M.: Firm firmware and apps for the Internet of Things. In: Proceedings of the 2nd Workshop on Software Engineering for Sensor Network Applications, SESENA 2011, pp. 61–62. ACM, New York (2011)
7. Li, F., Vögler, M., Claeßens, M., Dustdar, S.: Efficient and scalable IoT service delivery on cloud. In: 2013 IEEE 6th International Conference on Cloud Computing (CLOUD) (2013)
8. Miorandi, D., Sicari, S., De Pellegrini, F., Chlamtac, I.: Internet of Things: vision, applications and research challenges. Ad Hoc Netw. **10**(7), 1497–1516 (2012)
9. ThereCorporation: ThereGate. http://therecorporation.com/en/platform
10. Tridium: JACE Controller. http://www.tridium.com/cs/products_/_services/jace
11. Zhu, Q., Wang, R., Chen, Q., Liu, Y., Qin, W.: IoT gateway: bridging wireless sensor networks into Internet of Things. In: 2010 IEEE/IFIP 8th International Conference on Embedded and Ubiquitous Computing (EUC), pp. 347–352 (2010)

An Approach Towards a Service Co-evolution in the Internet of Things

Huu Tam Tran[✉], Harun Baraki, and Kurt Geihs

Distributed Systems Group, University of Kassel, Kassel, Germany
{tran,baraki}@vs.uni-kassel.de, geihs@uni-kassel.de
http://www.vs.uni-kassel.de

Abstract. In the envisioned Internet of Things (IoT), we expect to see the emergence of complex service-based applications that integrate cloud services, connected objects and a wide variety of mobile devices. These applications will be smarter, easier to communicate with and more valuable for enriching our environment. They interact via interfaces and services. However, the interfaces and services can be modified due to updates and amendments. Such modifications require adaptations in all participating parties. Therefore, the aim of this research is to present a vision of service co-evolution in IoT. Moreover, we propose a novel agent architecture which supports the evolution by controlling service versions, updating local service instances and enabling the collaboration of agents. In this way, the service co-evolution can make systems more adaptive, efficient and reduce costs to manage maintenance.

Keywords: Service co-evolution · IoT services · Web services

1 Introduction

In this paper, we address the challenge of coordinated services in the scope of IoT by employing an agent-based approach. Service providers may depend on third party services to deliver quality products to customers and to other service providers as well. To prevent outages and failures by individual service modifications and updates coordinated evolution (hereafter co-evolution) is required in such complex systems, i.e. they need a co-evolution for services in order to ensure that no interruptions occur. A centralized solution would not be realizable due to administrative and technical reasons. It would not be scalable, in particular, in the area of IoT, and security issues would complicate the whole approach. Consequently, service providers have to be responsible for the evolution of their own services. The required actions have to be coordinated with other providers in the IoT environment. The objective is to automate the coordinated evolution as much as possible.

Recently, agent-based models have been suggested for IoT as they can capture autonomy, and proactive and reactive features. Beside that, they can include ontologies for cooperation and different contexts [1,2]. Within the scope of IoT,

© Institute for Computer Sciences, Social Informatics and Telecommunications Engineering 2015
R. Giaffreda et al. (Eds.): IoT360 2014, Part I, LNICST 150, pp. 273–280, 2015.
DOI: 10.1007/978-3-319-19656-5_39

agent approaches address application levels and can use services provided by smart objects in order to achieve co-evolution.

Service co-evolution in IoT has received barely attention so far. Thus, there are some needs for detailing the vision of service co-evolution and solutions to provide benefits for IoT users. However, there are many challenges and requirements to tackle to meet an overall tradeoff between aspects like the satisfaction of clients, the resource consumption of provided interface versions and the efforts to update them. Consequently, this paper will analyze the roles of this evolution regarding potential results, challenges and its requirements as well as the solution.

It is not the intention of this paper to present details of Web service evolution as that has been done elsewhere [4,5]. This paper aims at promoting the idea of co-evolution of web services in IoT by (i) illustrating how a service co-evolution is carried out, what should be involved, why it is essential, and what should be prepared in order to meet the co-evolution requirements, (ii) highlighting a novel agent architecture for service providers in the IoT environment and explaining how this agent can be used in service co-evolution environments, (iii) discussing some potential research challenges of service co-evolution. Thus, the main contribution of this paper is to make software engineers aware of the power of service co-evolution and make systems more adaptive, efficient and reliable.

The rest of the paper is structured as follows. Section 2 illustrates an overview of our solution and its key components. Section 3 analyzes the coordination of services and discusses research challenges in service co-evolution. Section 4 introduces a number of existing researches and compares them with our approach, and finally Sect. 5 draws conclusions on our current results and provides an outlook for future work.

2   Solution Overview

Services running on heterogeneous systems and offered by different providers have de-coupled lifecycles, in particular, in IoT. Single services will be updated due to amendments or refinements or to provide further functionalities. Other providers may cut back the functionalities without taking notice of remaining clients that try to apply the removed functions. Business processes and applications that depend on services require appropriate coordination and adaptation by the participating parties. The solution we worked out equips every service with an agent, called EVA (EVolution Agent), that is capable to undertake these tasks. The internal structure and the rough composition of an EVA is depicted in Fig. 1. The next sections introduce the main components of an EVA and their interactions.

2.1   Analysis

The information interaction flow within our model is as follows. When an EVA receives first an Evolution Request, it is analyzed by the Analysis module.

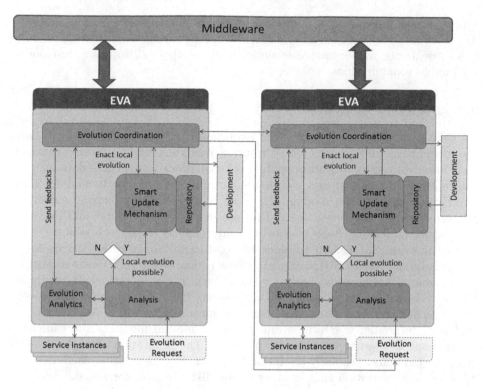

Fig. 1. Architecture of the EVA: global view

An Evolution Request demands for adaptation to be able to take part in future interactions. The Analysis module has to decide whether an evolution should take place and, if so, whether a local evolution is possible or whether the evolution has to be coordinated with other EVAs. For this reason, it assesses firstly the significance of the Evolution Request by evaluating the importance, the reputation and the number of partners who sent the request. The importance of a partner will increase, the more clients are affected by him. The significance will rise too, if the local service strongly depends on the other service and if there are no alternative services available. If either resources are becoming scarce or if it takes high efforts to satisfy the request, then lowly rated Evolution Requests may be rejected. Service instances not requested for a long time can be switched off to free resources for crucial service instances.

To estimate the efforts required for adaptation, the Analysis module considers initially local knowledge that includes information about locally available update mechanisms, the different service instances realizing different versions of the service, and the dependencies that the service versions might have towards other services. In case the Analysis module accepts the Evolution Request and a local update would satisfy the request, it will instruct the Smart Update Mechanism module, as presented below, to execute the local update and to provide eventually a new service instance. If a pure local update is not available or not sufficient due to an interplay between several services, the Evolution Coordination module has to deal with a coordinated evolution and possibly ask software developers for further configurations.

2.2 Evolution Analytics

As time passes, the Analysis and the Evolution Coordination module can take more sophisticated decisions. The Evolution Analytics module collects runtime data about successful and unsuccessful evolution procedures. These data include information about local and coordinated evolutions since both modules feed the Evolution Analytics module. The goal is to discover promising evolution patterns by fostering successful and proven evolution procedures and preventing unsuccessful ones. Success does not only depend on smooth running in a technical sense, but has to consider the cost-performance ratio, the revenue, the reputation and QoS (Quality of Service) parameters too. Costs comprise, for instance, hardware and human resources which can be estimated hardly in the very beginning. If a new configuration has been implemented, the developer specifies the total man-hours spent. By means of Evolution Analytics EVA will learn to predict worthwile evolutions while minimizing costs and time and maximizing the own revenue and reputation. The reputation of an EVA may decrease if it denies regularly Evolution Requests. Here, Evolution Analytics has to weigh the reputation against other factors like the costs for updates and the future revenue. To estimate reputation, costs and QoS, we will make use of our two prediction algorithms presented in [7].

For reasons of bootstrapping, EVAs are allowed to share parts of their knowledge with other EVAs. Special know how that affects only the service supervised by the EVA, has to be left out.

2.3 Evolution Coordination

In the event that a pure local evolution is not applicable, the Evolution Coordination module will co-operate with other EVAs and possibly interact with software developers. For example, the service is providing a method that depends on data delivered by a third party. To customize the interface for the client sending the Evolution Request, the Evolution Coordination will determine first the involved third parties and send them an Evolution Request. A continuous feedback between the EVAs is required to keep all parties up-to-date and to recognize future developments early. If a third party rejects the Evolution Request or if it is not available anymore, the Evolution Coordination can start a search for suitable services. To this end, we will adopt our service selection algorithms proposed in [8]. If the latter fails due to a lack of matching services, the Evolution Coordination will instruct the service provider or a responsible software developer to adapt the service. For this purpose, the developer may implement a configuration that is subsequently executed by the Smart Update Mechanism.

2.4 Smart Update Mechanism

The Smart Update Mechanism encompasses mainly two types of evolution capabilities. Firstly, it is aware of the different versions of the services running as service instances on the local machine and the versions used in the past. If one of them is fulfilling the conditions required, then it will be assigned to the requesting party. The second approach is a specification of the evolution rules and constraints that represent the possible service re-configurations and adaptations. In MUSIC [6] application developers specified the possible variants of an application and their dependencies on the runtime context; this was exploited by the adaptation manager in the middleware to achieve optimized application adaptation in different situations.

An EVA maintains up-to-date evolution models of its services. The models expose the possible configuration and adaptation paths. The EVA may govern multiple instances and versions of the same service at the same time, in order to accommodate different applications that may have different needs with respect to the service. Eventually, out-dated alternatives will be slowly retired.

The Analysis and Evolution Coordination modules introduced in the previous sections decide which configuration or version will be used for a specific client. In this connection, they do not only consider the possibilities offered by the Smart Update Mechanism, but take also into account the Evolution Analytics to optimize criteria like revenue, reputation, response time and own operability.

2.5 Repository and Middleware

The Smart Update Mechanism makes use of a repository where several configurations were made available by developers. Developers can add new configurations to the repository during the lifetime of a service, for instance, if the Smart Update Mechanism did not find appropriate ones to update the service.

Since objects or mobile devices are free to enter or leave the system, the middleware enables EVAs to communicate with each other in an asynchronous and loosely coupled manner. Beside that, the EVA itself can be divided into its modules such that each module may run on another device. This allows to make use of powerful runtime environments while energy constrained IoT devices that deliver the data offered by the service are spared.

3 Challenges of Service Co-evolution

Service co-evolution needs to be managed in a decentralized fashion since a centralized approach constitutes a bottleneck and would not be scalable. The services have to be responsible for their own evolution and should coordinate their actions with other services according to the knowledge they have of their own capabilities and that of the other services.

Coordinating the evolution of services is a major challenge since it is a complex process that requires multiple interactions, as well as continuous feedback to understand whether the distributed evolution is proceeding as desired. To prevent never-ending negotiations between service providers about which service has to adapt first or to change at all, we introduce an algorithm that gives a clear path for the evolution. Therefore, we include the number of clients of each concerned service and their overall reputation.

The EVA that is managing an affected service is either interested in an adaptation or rejects it. For this reason, an EVA can vote for (vote = +1) or against (vote = -1) the evolution of a used service. The higher the reputation of a service and the higher its number of clients, the higher the vote of the EVA that is managing the service is weighted. Thus, the overall feedback is comprised of the multiplication of the vote and the weight that consists of the reputation and the number of clients. This means that services that satisfy and affect more clients have a higher impact. A step-wise structure of the proposed algorithm is given in the following:

STEP 1: *An EVA x receives an evolution request from another EVA y.*

STEP 2: *x is asking the EVAs $c \in C$ of its clients whether they would accept or reject the required adaptation.*

STEP 3: *x is summing up the feedbacks of $c \in C$ by considering their vote and their reputation and number of clients that are both scaled into the range $[0, 1]$.*

STEP 4: *x is dividing the summed up feedbacks by the number of clients to obtain f_{agg} and compares f_{agg} with a predefined threshold value ϵ.*

STEP 5: *x is striven for the co-evolution if $f_{agg} \geq \epsilon$. In this case, the aforementioned steps of Sect. 2 will be executed. Otherwise, the evolution requests will be rejected.*

Mostly, evolution cannot be fully automated. In general, it is a multi-step process that a service must go through to transition from a problematic configuration, to a more acceptable new one. This transition may involve adaptation mechanisms that are already in-place, as well as offline activities, such as requirements gathering and software development. Although software evolution mechanisms have been deeply studied in the last decades, service co-evolution offers further research challenges:

- Heterogeneous services in IoT have de-coupled lifecycles, meaning that single services may be updated, or newly developed, while others are still in operation. Any evolution that we perform on a service requires that this action be coordinated with other actions paramount if we want to preserve the applications overall functionality and quality of service.

- The evolution of such complex systems will require that we harness and understand the horizontal and vertical relationships that exist between services, so that we can have them evolve in a coordinated fashion. This can be achieved through modeling and analytics, and through detailed runtime analysis, e.g., runtime testing and formal verification. Given the decentralized nature of the application environment, all these tools need to rely on local knowledge of the service itself and of its surroundings.

4   Related Work

Joo Pimentel et al. [11] outlined the reasoning required in order to support forward and backward co-evolution of service-oriented systems. But this paper only analyzed how to assess the mutual impact of requirements and architecture changes on other service oriented systems and how to react to these changes in order to prevent misalignment between them.

The paper in [12] also provides a theoretical framework and language-independent mechanisms for controlling the evolution of services that deal with structural, behavioral, and QoS level-introduced service changes in a type-safe manner. In particular, the authors distinguished between shallow changes (small-scale, localized) and deep changes (large-scale, cascading). However, the authors only focused to deal with shallow changes. In contrast, our paper tries to deal with vital aspects of deep changes with an adaptive agent approach.

Authors in [10] introduced a change-oriented service life-cycle methodology and described its phases. They discussed when a change in a service is triggered, how to analyze its impact, and the possible implications of the implementation of the change for the service providers and consumers. Nevertheless, a formal model for deep changes based on the one for shallow changes is missing. Additionally, their approach did not mention about the IoT environment which differs from our approach.

The Chain of Adapters technique [13] is an alternative approach for deploying multiple versions of a Web service in the face of independently developed unsupervised clients. The basic idea is to resolve the mismatches between the expected by the consumers and the supported by the implementation interface [12]. It can prove useful in self-configurations. However, it is not clear whether the approach would scale to a high number of Web services.

In fact, there are many agent-based approaches available to support interoperable IoT devices and their services nowadays [1–3,9]. Nonetheless, the adaptation mechanisms and the collaboration characteristics in these agents are not sufficient in order to achieve coordinated service evolution. Furthermore, it needs a global vision which can predict potential effects, challenges and requirements for participating service providers.

5   Conclusion and Future Work

The main goal of this paper is to introduce a new vision of service co-evolution and to provide a common evolution management model and reference architecture for developers. It represents a focused effort to provide a foundation for realizing the full potential of the Internet of Services and other service-based architectures. For this reason, the challenges in the co-evolution of services that cover the wide spectrum from IoT to Cloud Computing, are analyzed too.

This paper also adopts a novel conceptual agent as a solution for service co-evolution. Evolution tasks like the assessment and coordination of evolution requests, updating and versioning the interfaces and selecting matching services can be performed automatically or semi-automatically by EVAs, inter alia, by exploiting already existing self-adaptation techniques.

In future, first research prototypes and scenarios on the coordination of EVAs shall be delivered to evaluate the prospect of this approach. A further path for future work is to develop an evolution description language for service co-evolution. In this way, systems can be made more adaptive, efficient and reduce costs to manage maintenance.

References

1. Atzori, L., Iera, A., Morabito, G.: The internet of things: a survey. Comput. Netw. **54**(15), 2787–2805 (2010)
2. Ayala, I., Amor, M., Fuentes, L.: An agent platform for self-configuring agents in the internet of things. In: Infrastructures and Tools for Multiagent Systems, pp. 65–78 (2012)
3. Roalter, L., Kranz, M., Möller, A.: A middleware for intelligent environments and the internet of things. In: Yu, Z., Liscano, R., Chen, G., Zhang, D., Zhou, X. (eds.) UIC 2010. LNCS, vol. 6406, pp. 267–281. Springer, Heidelberg (2010)
4. Leitner, P., Michlmayr, A., Rosenberg, F., Dustdar, S.: End-to-end versioning support for web services. In: IEEE International Conference on Services Computing, SCC 2008, vol. 1, pp. 59–66. IEEE (2008)
5. Fokaefs, M., Mikhaiel, R., Tsantalis, N., Stroulia, E., Lau, A.: An empirical study on web service evolution. In: 2011 IEEE International Conference on Web Services (ICWS), pp. 49–56. IEEE (2011)
6. Floch, J., Frà, C., Fricke, R., Geihs, K., Wagner, M., Gallardo, J.L., Cantero, E.S., Mehlhase, S., Paspallis, N., Rahnama, H., Ruiz, P.A., Scholz, U.: Playing music - building context-aware and self-adaptive mobile applications. Softw. Pract. Exper. **43**(3), 359–388 (2013)
7. Baraki, H., Comes, D., Geihs, K.: Context-aware prediction of qos and qoe properties for web services. In: 2013 Conference on Networked Systems (NetSys), pp. 102–109. IEEE (2013)
8. Comes, D., Baraki, H., Reichle, R., Zapf, M., Geihs, K.: Heuristic approaches for QoS-based service selection. In: Maglio, P.P., Weske, M., Yang, J., Fantinato, M. (eds.) ICSOC 2010. LNCS, vol. 6470, pp. 441–455. Springer, Heidelberg (2010)
9. Yu, H., Shen, Z., Leung, C.: From internet of things to internet of agents. In: Green Computing and Communications(GreenCom), 2013 IEEE and Internet of Things, IEEE International Conference on and IEEE Cyber, Physical and Social Computing, (iThings/CPSCom), pp. 1054–1057. IEEE (2013)
10. Papazoglou, M.P., Andrikopoulos, V., Benbernou, S.: Managing evolving services. IEEE **28**(3), 49–55 (2011)
11. Pimentel, J., Castro, J., Santos, E., Finkelstein, A.: Towards requirements and architecture co-evolution. In: Bajec, M., Eder, J. (eds.) CAiSE Workshops 2012. LNBIP, vol. 112, pp. 159–170. Springer, Heidelberg (2012)
12. Andrikopoulos, V., Benbernou, S., Papazoglou, M.: On the evolution of services. IEEE Trans. Softw. Eng. **38**(3), 609–628 (2012)
13. Kaminsi, P., Müller, H., Litoiu, M.: A design for adaptive web service evolution. In: Proceeding of the 2006 International Workshop on Self-Adaptation and Self-Managing Systems, May 21–22, 2006, Shang Hai, China (2006)

Identity Management in Platforms Offering IoT as a Service

Juan D. Parra Rodriguez[✉], Daniel Schreckling, and Joachim Posegga

Institute of IT-Security and Security Law, University of Passau,
Innstraße 43, Passau, Germany
{dp,ds,jp}@sec.uni-passau.de

Abstract. We describe a generic attribute-based identity management system. It aims to support the large variety of security requirements induced by applications for the IoT. Hence, we discuss various management options for system entities. We show how attribute assurance can be used to reliably define attributes within groups of identities. Apart from enabling personalized identity and policy enforcement schemes, this provides a feasible trade-off between the flexibility and scalability needs and the policy definition and enforcement requirements in the IoT. We provide a proof-of-concept implementation of our framework.

Keywords: Identity management · Internet of Things · Platform as a service · Attribute based access control · Federated identity management

1 Introduction

There is a growing need for an Internet of Things (IoT) runtime ecosystem in which services using actuators and data from sensors can coexist. Such an ecosystem would not only expose functionalities as reusable services. It could also provide usage control; ensuring that data processing is compliant with the security requirements of individual device owners. These inherently diverse requirements, ask for fine-grained and expressive security policy frameworks. Such security frameworks, in turn, require a flexible identity management (IDM) system for *things*, services processing IoT-data, owner or users of *things*, and other related entities. Thus, we propose an infrastructure to identify, authenticate, and manage the security principals in an IoT platform. The three main contributions of this paper can be summarized as follows:

- Identification of challenges faced when users define their own IDM scheme in a platform offering IoT as a service.
- Analysis of possible approaches to enable users to share identity information with each other, while comparing the computational complexity induced in the policy decision process.
- Providing mechanisms designed to ensure the reliability of identity information and enabling users to share such information, without a significant increase of computational complexity in the policy evaluation process.

© Institute for Computer Sciences, Social Informatics and Telecommunications Engineering 2015
R. Giaffreda et al. (Eds.): IoT360 2014, Part I, LNICST 150, pp. 281–288, 2015.
DOI: 10.1007/978-3-319-19656-5_40

2   Challenges

2.1   Support for Access and Usage Control

IoT platforms have to manage and process data of myriads of devices used for different applications. Controlling access to such devices using mandatory access control (MAC) is infeasible. In contrast, discretionary access control (DAC) needs to offer the flexibility required for different application for independent users. While role based access control (RBAC) may efficiently combine both worlds, it strictly requires a unified hierarchy of roles.

Fortunately, attribute based access control (ABAC) [1–3] is able to merge the abilities of MAC, DAC, and RBAC [4] without imperatively enforcing a centralized role management. It enables technologies which grant access based on attributes assigned to subjects, objects, or the environment. Flexible and domain specific security policies can be defined easily. With an IDM supporting attributes it is also possible to implement sophisticated systems which support fine-grained policy decisions such as $UCON_{ABC}$ model [5]. This is beneficial for the processing of security sensitive data in IoT platforms as coarse grained policies based on system principals or resource levels are insufficient and inflexible. Instead, attributes enable domain and application specific control mechanisms. Policies and their enforcement can be adapted to specific needs by considering individually defined and trusted attributes.

As a consequence, the IDM presented in this contribution addresses the specific needs and security enforcement technologies feasible for IoT systems. Thus, a reliable attribute-based principal management that enforces the correct and authorized declaration and definition of attributes becomes inevitable.

2.2   Attribute Assurance

Once users can define their own identity schemes in the platform, they start to resemble small identity 'silos' with their own self-defined attributes. As a result, enabling users to interact and exchange identity information becomes critical. To exemplify the challenges to be tackled, we consider the following scenario.

Two companies provide sensor data through an IoT platform: *SensIoT*, and *fakeIoT*. Further, assume each company creates an attribute called "produced by" containing the name of the company. Most likely, sensor containing the attribute "produced by" with value *SensIoT* will be used more. However, unless there is a mechanism enforcing that only devices belonging to *SensIoT* can assign the value *SensIoT* to the attribute "produced by", *fakeIoT* could start faking attribute values to fool customers. Even though this example could be solved by including a simple customized verification, the question is, how to enable companies, or groups of users, to define attributes which require approval before those attributes are considered reliable. We call this process *attribute assurance*, given its affinity to a more process driven aspect of Federated Identity Management (FIDM), called identity assurance [6,7].

2.3   Sharing Attributes with Other Users

Users should be able to decide whether they consider attribute values approved by other users, or groups of users, to be sufficiently reliable for supporting policy decisions. This is a parallel challenge to managing trust in FIDM [6] with an additional pitfall: the inclusion of users' preferences should not increase the complexity of policy decisions. We discuss two possibilities to manage trusted attributes and analyse their computational complexity. For this purpose, let n be the number of attribute values for a device, service, or user that require approval according to a policy[1] and let the cost of verifying the approval status for a given attribute be in $O(1)$.

The first possibility is to use a **global and centralized repository of attribute values** and to authorize selected users to globally approve attributes. In this case policy evaluation could be in $O(n)$. Only the verification of an approval flag would be required for each attribute value. Policy evaluation becomes trivial as an approved attribute is automatically trusted system-wide. However, authorized users won't be elected freely, declining the possibility to benefit from approval mechanisms to most of the users in the IoT platform; also, the attribute approvals become unmanageable for a limited number of authorized users.

A completely opposite approach is to allow users to set and approve attribute values. In such an **ad-hoc sharing scheme for attributes** the most important question is whether an attribute value has been approved by a trusted user. This notion can be implemented by adding credibility to attributes [8]. Users specify a list of trusted users for each attribute used in a policy. Let k be the number of users in the system. K is both, the upper bound of attribute approvals for a given attribute value, as well as the upper bound of trusted users chosen for each one of the n attributes. In this case, the computational complexity of the policy evaluation is in $O(n \cdot k^2)$. For each approval, it must be verified whether a trusted user approved the value. Although flexible, this approach induces high computational complexity during evaluation. Hence, we propose a trade-off between flexibility required for IoT environments and the complexity imposed on policy evaluation.

3   Identity Management Scheme

Identities are simply a computer's representation of an *entity* [9]. They are required when their corresponding entity is either providing some functionality or involved in some access/usage control decision. Thus, in our IoT platform, we consider users, device representation (sensors, actuators), and services. Including these entities beyond users allows us to control access/usage on data generated by devices, services or the devices, and services themselves.

---

[1] Filtering which attribute values from the user, service or device correspond to the attributes referenced by the policy is disregarded (same algorithm for every case).

3.1   Entity Management

Users can create their own groups (e.g., organizations, family, friends). To have significance for security, groups must implement access control mechanisms. This is achieved trough mutual agreement on group memberships.

A group membership is defined as a tuple *(u,r,g)* where user u has role r in group g. Further, before memberships are considered effective by the IDM system, it has to be approved by two parties: the administrator of g, and u. In this way users cannot be misplaced in a group, and groups only contain approved users. Due to this property, groups are the cornerstone for attribute assurance and for the sharing of attribute values among users (Sects. 3.3 and 3.4).

3.2   System Structure

The IDM system contains eight modules shown in Fig. 1. Every API call to the prototype comes from the bottom of the picture; consequently, it must go through the authentication and authorization module before it reaches any other module. Afterwards, if the request is related to the creation or deletion of a user, group, or an entity, it will go directly to the appropriate registry. Note that users are both in the user and entity registry for readability reasons, and also because they could be handled by a third party, such as an user authentication server.

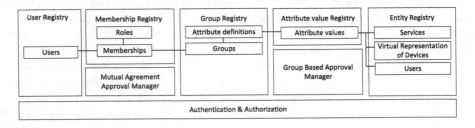

Fig. 1. Internal identity management architecture

If there is a request for the creation, deletion or approval of a user membership, it must go through the *Mutual Agreement Membership Manager*, which will take care that memberships are updated only by the right users. Similarly, if the request concerns the approval of an attribute, it will go through the *Group Based Approval Manager*, which judges whether the user trying to approve an attribute value has the right permissions in the correct group.

3.3   Attribute Definition and Assurance

Figure 2 shows how attribute definitions, attribute values, and groups are related to each other. Attributes are defined in a per-group basis. For attribute assurance purposes, attribute values are only valid after they have been approved

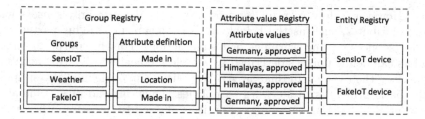

Fig. 2. Attribute definition

by administrators of the group where the attribute definition is registered in. Figure 2 shows two groups (SensIoT and FakeIoT) that have an attribute called "Made in", and also two devices with approved attribute values for the "Made in" attribute definitions in each group. Also, both devices have values pointing to the same attribute definition (approved by the same authority) for the "Location" attribute, previously defined inside the weather group. This implies an approval from an administrator of Weather group for "Himalayas" (both devices).

3.4 Sharing Attributes with Other Users

Given the properties described in the previous section, groups are employed as a mechanism to let users express which users (in a group) are considered trusted. Here is the advantage in terms of policy evaluation: when users refer to the attribute definition directly in their policies (e.g. "Made in" attribute definition inside SensIoT), the complexity[2] of the policy evaluation algorithm is $O(n)$ since for every attribute value, only the approval state of the attribute value needs verification. Most interestingly, attribute assurance is not lost since only administrators from the group can approve the attribute value. Further, the proposed schema is still flexible enough to support an ad-hoc approval where users provide just the name of the attribute, the expected value, and the trusted groups for approval in their policies; nevertheless, this is not encouraged due to computational complexity (see Sect. 2.3).

3.5 Access Control Integration

We briefly illustrate the power of our IDM for policy enforcement. Assume a variety of sensors deployed in an alpine area. They have a virtual representation in our platform and can be used by different services. Further, suppose independent service providers use these sensors to report on slope conditions, generate warnings for mountaineers, or shutdown cable cars. A slope condition service simply uses attributes to determine whether a sensor is on a specific slope. Such attributes may change over time and confuse users but they are not

---

[2] n is number of attribute values for the entity, such as the SensIoT device.

critical. However, safety relevant services need to make sure only sensors with assured attributes, such as the height or location, are used. This particularly holds for services casting warnings or taking actions. For this purpose, service providers can define policies described by simple predicates validating attribute and checking their values. In this way ABAC policies can be defined also supporting the basic principles of $UCON_{ABC}$ policies. Thus, instead of accumulating the potentially changing set of IDs of entities allowed to access another entity and assigning them some property, our IDM supports direct filtering based on attributes. This simplifies the task to implement domain specific access control, avoids administrative overhead, and prevents burdensome reimplementaitons.

As we offer IoT services hosted in one platform we also support decentralized evaluation of policies at the entity level. During entity deployment local PDPs extract required information from the registries tagged to the respective entities. In this way, access control decision on services, for example, boil down to simple and localized value comparisons.

4   Related Work

Contributions using attributes in IDM systems are manifold and were inspired by the first designs of ABAC [10]. Based on these models implementations for ABAC have been proposed. The prominent contribution by Bonatti and Samarati [11] introduced a framework to logically specify and reason about service access and disclosure constraints in open environments. While this contribution recognizes the relevance of ABAC for $UCON$ and the flexibility to describe entities of a system with attributes, it neither focuses on their management nor does it consider their ad-hoc definitions. Similar holds for the modelling of ABAC in a logic-based framework [1] where policies defined on attributes are logic programs with recursion allowing for powerful and efficient evaluation.

Yuan and Tong apply ABAC to the web service domain [2]. An authorization and policy definition architecture is described but it remains unclear how attributes could be defined in a flexible manner. ABMAC [12], an extension of the ABAC model, faces the same problem. Comparable to our IDM, ABMAC also aims towards the support of multiple heterogeneous policies. Yet, it does not consider attribute assurance as presented in this contribution.

Another popular approach is the use of attribute certificiates [13–17]. They bind entity attributes and their values to a domain. Apart from the propblem to setup up a commonly accepted PKI, these solutions induce impractical overheads in terms of management, during policy evaluation and challenge scalability.

In contrast, Cabarcos et al. introduce a dynamic scheme for federations among IDM systems [18]. They define a P2P reputation system with dynamic trust lists. If entities out of this list provide attribute values, reputation values can be queried to decide on the reliability of the information. Reputation is defined by domain administrators. Although this system enables dynamic and gradual trust, users cannot individually administer their policy domain.

A similar approach is taken in the Liberty framework, a federated IDM system. It uses the Identity Web Service Framework (ID-WSF) [19] to store principal attributes which can also be used for policy decisions. However, the attribute declaration is strongly centralized and only security providers can define new attributes and does not allow to select specifically trusted attributes or authorities.

5   Conclusion

We have designed and implemented a prototype[3] for a generic attribute-based IDM for a platform offering IoT as a service. In such system, every user can define his own attribute scheme, and use mechanisms to ensure reliability of attribute values to other users in the platform. Furthermore, users of the platform can choose trusted groups to approve attribute values before they are used by the PDP. Additionally, the proposed solution offers a good trade-off between flexibility and complexity increase for the policy evaluation process.

Acknowledgements. The research leading to these results has received funding from the European Union's FP7 project COMPOSE, under grant agreement 317862.

References

1. Wang, L., Wijesekera, D., Jajodia, S.: A logic-based framework for attribute based access control. In: Proceedings of the ACM Workshop on Formal Methods in Security Engineering, FMSE 2004, pp. 45–55. ACM, New York (2004)
2. Yuan, E., Tong, J.: Attributed based access control (ABAC) for web services. In: Proceedings of the IEEE International Conference on Web Services, pp. 561–569, July 2005. doi:10.1109/ICWS.2005.25
3. Hu, V.C., Scarfone, K., Kuhn, R., Sandlin, K.: Guide to attribute based access control (ABAC) definition and considerations. Technical report, Nation Institute for Standards and Technologies, January 2014
4. Jin, X., Krishnan, R., Sandhu, R.: A unified attribute-based access control model covering DAC, MAC and RBAC. In: Cuppens-Boulahia, N., Cuppens, F., Garcia-Alfaro, J. (eds.) DBSec 2012. LNCS, vol. 7371, pp. 41–55. Springer, Heidelberg (2012)
5. Park, J., Sandhu, R.: The $UCON_{ABC}$ usage control model. ACM Trans. Inf. Syst. Secur. **7**(1), 128–174 (2004)
6. Jensen, J.: Federated identity management challenges. In: Seventh International Conference on Availability, Reliability and Security, pp. 230–235. IEEE, August 2012
7. Beres, Y., Baldwin, A., Mont, M.C., Shiu, S.: On identity assurance in the presence of federated identity management systems. In: Proceedings of the ACM Workshop on Digital Identity Management, DIM 2007, pp. 27–35. ACM, New York (2007)
8. Thomas, I., Meinel, C.: Enhancing claim-based identity management by adding a credibility level to the notion of claims. In: 2013 IEEE International Conference on Services Computing, pp. 243–250 (2009)

---

[3] https://github.com/nopbyte/compose-idm.

9. Bishop, M.A.: The Art and Science of Computer Security. Addison-Wesley Longman Publishing Co., Inc., Boston (2002)

10. Johnston, W., Mudumbai, S., Thompson, M.: Authorization and attribute certificates for widely distributed access control. In: Proceedings of the 7th Workshop on Enabling Technologies, pp. 340–345. IEEE Computer Society, Washington, D.C. (1998)

11. Bonatti, P.A., Samarati, P.: A uniform framework for regulating service access and information release on the web. J. Comput. Secur. **10**(3), 241–271 (2002)

12. Lang, B., Foster, I., Siebenlist, F., Ananthakrishnan, R., Freeman, T.: A flexible attribute based access control method for grid computing. J. Grid Comput. **7**(2), 169–180 (2009)

13. Thompson, M.R., Essiari, A., Mudumbai, S.: Certificate-based authorization policy in a PKI environment. ACM Trans. Inf. Syst. Secur. **6**(4), 566–588 (2003)

14. Chadwick, D.W., Otenko, A.: The PERMIS X.509 role based privilege management infrastructure. In: Proceedings of the Seventh ACM Symposium on Access Control Models and Technologies, SACMAT 2002, pp. 135–140. ACM, New York (2002)

15. Alfieri, R., Cecchini, R., Ciaschini, V., dell'Agnello, L., Frohner, A., Gianoli, A., Lõrentey, K., Spataro, F.: VOMS, an authorization system for virtual organizations. In: Fernández Rivera, F., Bubak, M., Gómez Tato, A., Doallo, R. (eds.) Across Grids 2003. LNCS, vol. 2970, pp. 33–40. Springer, Heidelberg (2004)

16. Guo, S., Lai, X.: An access control approach of multi security domain for web service. Procedia Eng. **15**, 3376–3382 (2011)

17. Cha, B.R., Seo, J.H., Kim, J.W.: Design of attribute-based access control in cloud computing environment. In: Kim, K.J., Ahn, S.J. (eds.) Proceedings of the International Conference on IT Convergence and Security. Lecture Notes in Electrical Engineering, vol. 120, pp. 41–50. Springer, Netherlands (2012)

18. Arias Cabarcos, P., Almenárez, F., Gómez Mármol, F., Marín, A.: To federate or not to federate: a reputation-based mechanism to dynamize cooperation in identity management. Wireless Pers. Commun. **75**(3), 1769–1786 (2014)

19. Tourzan, J., Koga, Y. (eds.): Liberty ID-WSF web services framework overview (Version 2.0). Technical report, Liberty Alliance Project (2006)

Network and IT Infrastructure Services
for the IoT Store

Gaël Fromentoux and Nathalie Omnès[✉]

Orange Labs, 2 avenue Pierre Marzin, 22 300 Lannion, France
{gael.fromentoux, nathalie.omnes}@orange.com

Abstract. IoT, Internet of Things, is a major revolution dragging along new requirements that impact the network & IT infrastructure under development. Actually, the network infrastructure is evolving to embed virtualization techniques to gain in flexibility. For this purpose, new architectures are drawn-up such as the one proposed by the ETSI NFV. In this article, we first highlight a new business model: the IoT store. We then show how it benefits from the network & IT infrastructure services. After presenting the main actors of this business model, we actually provide the overview of an NFV-based architecture that fulfills new IoT requirements. We thus show that the move towards a network & IT infrastructure benefiting of Cloud and virtualization solutions can highly serve the IoT deployment.

Keywords: Infrastructure · Network · IT · IoT · Cloud · NFV · Business model · Store

1 Introduction

While the availability of mature IT virtualization techniques has led the IT infrastructure to successfully evolve to the Cloud, the network infrastructure still has to find its way to virtualization. This trend is on its way, in particular thanks to NFV (Network Function Virtualization), currently under standardization by the ETSI, but also with solutions put forward by vendors. Hence the evolution towards a new digital network & IT infrastructure is a revolution that has begun.

IoT, Internet of Things, is another major revolution. Billions of connected objects are upcoming, covering numerous areas ranging from health to entertainment, for example with pointless objects [1]. As a matter of fact, IoT encompasses a large variety of connected "things", including IoO (Internet of Objects) and its passive objects, M2M (Machine to Machine) and smart communicating devices / connected objects. These billions of objects drag along new requirements impacting the network & IT infrastructure under definition [2].

In this paper, we investigate how the network & IT infrastructure can fulfill some requirements issued from IoT.

The paper is organized as follow: the IoT store's business model is depicted in the Sect. 2. In the Sect. 3, we present how to move forward to offer an infrastructure service on line with IoT needs. The Sect. 4 then presents the actors and general architecture, while the Sect. 5 presents the architecture into more details. We finally conclude in the Sect. 6.

© Institute for Computer Sciences, Social Informatics and Telecommunications Engineering 2015
R. Giaffreda et al. (Eds.): IoT360 2014, Part I, LNICST 150, pp. 289–296, 2015.
DOI: 10.1007/978-3-319-19656-5_41

2   IoT Store Business Model

The application store business model, which relies on a multitude of web designers and developers, emerged thanks to the application of DIY (Do It Yourself) to web technologies. With the open hardware revolution, DIY now applies to the electronic field. By bringing a disruption into hardware conception, open hardware does not only lead to inventiveness, it also paves the way to the creation of many connected objects and start-ups. Hence the IoT store business model may emerge as a double-sided business, benefiting on one side of the multitude of connected objects' inventors, and on the other side of the relationship with the customers [3, 6].

The IoT store also benefits to connected objects' inventors by offering them a window display and by simplifying the distribution of their products. The IoT store manager should further provide inventors with a large customer basis so that their invention has a real opportunity to be widely exposed and adopted.

The IoT store benefits to consumers, by helping them into finding a way through the boiling universe of connected objects. In particular, connected objects shall get through a test phase so that only the reliable ones are published on the store. Billing, research and recommendation functions must also be implemented within the store to allow the consumers to buy objects and to let them be guided to new experiences or usages.

Thanks to all these elements, the IoT store business model becomes as safe as the application store business model, and multiple actors are enticed to grasp this opportunity. Please note that the main elements of this business are depicted within white rectangles in the following Fig. 1.

3   Towards Network and IT Infrastructure Services for IoT

Unlike web applications, connected objects have numerous and specific needs, while the related standards or technical trends are not clear yet. In particular, there are many possible access technologies, including 6LowPan, ZigBee and BLE (Bluetooth Low Energy), and none of them clearly appears currently as the sole possible answer. Furthermore, strong access control and authentication on the one hand and privacy and safety on the other hand are key issues, as stated by Vint Cerf [5], that must be addressed for the general public to gain confidence in connected objects and the associated data processing. Consider for example a connected lock letting authorized users to get into your home even when you are away. The corresponding requirements are very stringent and require a rigorous technical answer!

These stringent requirements will turn into the advantage of the actor that will combine the IoT store business model with the appropriate network service in terms of cost, QoS, connectivity and security. For instance, the IoT store itself cannot prevent customers from pervasive monitoring of the data received and emitted by their objects. However, that is the job of the network & IT infrastructure. The services developed over the network & IT infrastructure may encompass for example secured network links for exchanging information with connected objects, data storage within a cloud, gateways to link the IoT objects to the web or the secured access to the connected objects.

The main lines of this new business model are depicted on the following Fig. 1. The white rectangles correspond to the IoT store business model, while the grey ones are specific to the IoT store enriched with infrastructure services. Thanks to this business model, the store manager can win new business partners.

As depicted in the Figure, the key partners are a crowd of inventors, object designers and start-ups. The first need to fulfill is to provide a large customer basis to the IoT inventors. This is capital but however far from enough. Actually, it is necessary to provide inventors and consumers a common framework encompassing all the required functions and interfaces needed over the network & IT infrastructure (e.g. IP gateways, signaling gateways, authentication schemes, cloud resources). It is indeed the abilities to connect objects, but also to authenticate and associate with all involved actors the right bunch of objects, to bill, to provide secured network connections and advanced services which are keys for the success of the IoT store.

The value propositions are firstly to ease connected objects' distribution and advertizing for inventors and secondly to help consumers to step into the IoT through a trusted store. The customer relationship is indeed achieved through stores, online or not. The customer segments are very wide, as connected objects are likely to concern all mankind, from youth to elderly, at work, at home and on leisure time. The source of income for the IoT store actor is a percentage on all sales. Note there is also an indirect income linked to the actor's brand. Finally, the cost revenue must be kept very low, for the ARPO (Average Revenue Per Object) will be very low, if not nonexistent. This can be achieved with the dynamic sharing of network & IT resources thanks to virtualization. Furthermore, for this business model to be fully effective, API (Application Programmable Interface) must be designed and carefully opened.

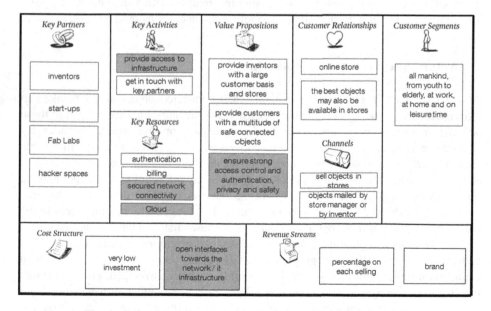

Fig. 1. Infrastructure service IoT store: a new business model

If we keep in mind that there will soon be billions of connected objects offered by multiple actors of different kind and for multiple different applications, there are a lot of challenges ahead!

The connected lock example highlights for example the need to make the distinction between different types of actors: the **owner** will have the right to deliver permanent or temporary access to a list of beneficiaries, a **user** will only have the right to unlock the door, while the **store manager** may have the right to remove all rights for unlocking the door. The related digital rights will have to be stored securely in a referential. Yet this digital rights inventory implies referencing connected objects thanks to metadata. This raises in particular the issue of identifying connected objects, issue that is not solved yet to our knowledge.

Therefore one or several IoT referential will have to be created, allowing the IoT store actor to identify, localize, characterize and group connected objects according to different points of view and types of actors. These referentials must in particular map objects, actors and rights related to each object. Managing and delivering access rights to a huge range of objects of various types is challenging, and so is managing access rights to billions of objects. The data stored in the IoT referentials also allows the objects' owners and users to have an overview of all the objects they are related to on a single web page, through a single interface. By providing the objects' location and state, it can further be used for managing the objects' end of life.

Another distinctive feature of connected objects is their huge diversity. They rely on different sources of energy, including none. They are connected to different types of access networks, including very low range connections. Some of them are connected by intermittence, either to preserve their battery or because they are intended to connect to an intermediate device that will provide them with the access to the service. This is for example the case of a NFC tag exchanging information with a smartphone. Hence a lot of basic connected objects will need to rely on a gateway to send and receive data.

4 Actors and General Architecture

As we have seen in the previous section, each connected object may be linked to different actors, including in particular its owner, its user and its manager. Each of these actors is interested by different kinds of information on the object. Consider for example an anemometer placed close to a kite surf spot and fed by a windmill. This anemometer thus provides wind information when the windmill can provide enough energy. Yet, when an anemometer does not provide any information, the owner may be interested by knowing whether it is because there is no wind or because the anemometer has broken down, while the users are only concerned by having access to the wind information. Furthermore, providing an overview of all available anemometers on a given geographical area and keeping an up-to-date inventory of them is an issue to address. More generally, managing any fleet of objects and providing its owner with exploitation information is a service that should be widely developed. For performing this, the store manager needs to build an IoT referential, including all metadata related to the object and in particular: an identification of each object, of each actor linked to the object and all access rights to each of these objects.

The main actors are depicted in the following figure. They include on the one side the object **user** that actually uses the object and the object **owner** that buys and maintains the object, both depicted on the left-hand lower corner of the figure. On the other side, the **inventor** specifies, designs and possibly markets connected objects. As an intermediate between these two actors lies the **store manager**, responsible for delivering, advertising and marketing applications and services related to IoT. To achieve these actions, the store manager relies on a convergent and virtualized network & IT infrastructure. IoTaaS services are provided on top of this virtualized infrastructure, providing on the fly resources such as applicative gateways and including also an IoT referential, matching objects, actors and access rights (Fig. 2).

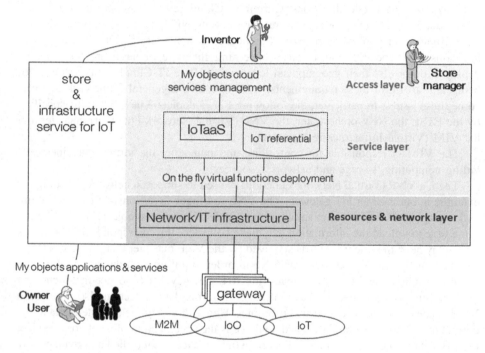

Fig. 2. Actors and general architecture

Thanks to this infrastructure, the store manager can identify and authenticate objects and objects' users and owners. Correlating this authentication to the IoT referential is indeed crucial for respecting strong access control and authentication, privacy and safety, required for the general public to gain confidence in connected objects. Furthermore, the store manager must provide interfaces to the inventors on the one side and to the objects' users and owners on the other side for them to manage the pool of connected objects they are related to, as we are going to depict into more details in the following Sect. 5.

5 Overview of the Network and IT Infrastructure Architecture

In this section, we give an overview of the network & IT architecture for addressing IoT requirements. More precisely, we show how the ETSI NFV architecture framework [4] can be used to support the IoT store.

Having access to a gateway between IoT on one side and service platforms on the other side is a recurrent issue. We have seen we will soon be surrounded by billions of connected objects. We therefore need to build these gateways on a scalable framework, in which one will pay only for what he actually uses. These are part of the founding principles of Cloud services, and hence we believe the answer shall be found in virtualization and Cloud directions. Currently, Cloud services are mature for the IT infrastructure, but not yet for network resources. With NFV, the ETSI currently defines the virtualization applied to network functions. As a matter of fact, some network functions have specific requirements concerning the type of hardware they can be deployed on or else their geographical localization. Pure IT Cloud infrastructures not being able to fulfill these requirements, NFV specifies a general framework to overcome these issues. In particular, the following Fig. 3 depicts 3 new functions specified by the ETSI: the NFV orchestrator, the VNF (Virtual Network Function) manager and the VIM (Virtual Infrastructure Manager).

The **VIM** is responsible for controlling and managing the virtual machines providing computing, storage and network resources.

Then, a **VNF** (Virtual Network Function) is used to support a network function, for example in our case an IoT gateway. The **VNF manager** is responsible for controlling and managing all VNFs. For example, if thousands of connected objects wake up at the same time to upload the information they have collected, the correspond IoT gateway's VNF may need to scale up. This is achieved by the VNF manager that asks the VIM to allocate a new virtual machine to the VNF in order to put up with the new traffic load.

When uploading its collected data, the IoT gateway needs to get in touch with another network function: the data collection. But this data collection also relies on a VNF, made of one or several virtual machines. Hence directing the collected data to the correct location is not straightforward, and needs the specification of a network service: the IoT data collection in our case. This **network service** is controlled and managed by the **NFV orchestrator**. In particular, the orchestrator has a complete knowledge of all deployed IoT gateways and data collectors together with the links between them. It can further create a new gateway when necessary, for example for scalability of localization issues.

Unlike IT resources, the geographical location of network functions is indeed crucial. In particular, the IoT gateway cannot be deployed anywhere in the network, but only in precise and defined locations. The ETSI NFV addresses this issue by allowing specific constraints to be added when requiring a virtual machine, including hardware and localization constraints. Thus NFV can bring an appropriate answer for deploying IoT gateways geographically distributed throughout a territory.

The following Fig. 3 depicts other elements, and in particular a portal to which the objects' owners and users are related. This IoT portal offers several services, within

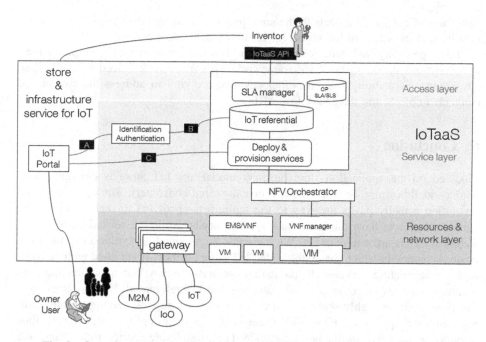

Fig. 3. Overview of the Network and IT Infrastructure Services Architecture

which the IoT dashboard. To build this dashboard, the IoT portal requires the access to the IoT referential. For security and safety issues, this access to the IoT referential must be protected thanks to an identification and authentication function. We thus highlight new interfaces, A and B, depicted in red in the Fig. 3.

The above Figure highlights another new interface, labeled C, between the IoT portal and another function named "deploy & provision services". This function is responsible for interacting with the NFV orchestrator to create new network services or update existing network services for instance in terms of features, topologies, resources. This new interface is restricted to the store manager and does thus not need other actors to authenticate.

The **IoT referential** is also implemented within a VNF, using one or several virtual machines. We have seen this referential must have knowledge concerning all objects, including the **identification,** the **type** of connected object and type of object's authentication. The object's **location**, crucial when deploying IoT gateways, shall be referenced within this IoT referential function. The list of each object's users and owner shall also be stored within the referential. This list must be dynamically updated each time a digital right is either created or removed by the object's owner. This referential shall further be improved by the network & IT infrastructure, which provides in particular location and status information.

Smartphones as widely distributed and smart connected devices are likely to play a particular role, acting as gateways and digital rights repository. The IoT referential can be linked to a push notification server and provide relevant information concerning a collection of connected objects to the smartphone, including for example the owners' identity and the status of the object (alive, unreachable, low battery…).

More generally, IoT requirements can be fulfilled by dynamically implementing new functions thanks to the NFV framework. This framework indeed offers the key advantage of scalability and cost-efficiency that are vital to address the tsunami of connected objects and their very low ARPO.

6 Conclusion

Modeled on the application store business model, the IoT store is emerging as a double-sided business between the IoT inventors and consumers. The open hardware revolution actually paves the way to the multiplication of IoT inventors. However, connected objects have numerous and specific needs, while the related standards or technical trends are not clear yet. We have thus highlighted an evolution of the store business model, in which the double-sided IoT store business is enriched with network & IT infrastructure services. In particular, we have shown that new functions are required and must be combined: IoT gateways and IoT referential. Because these new functions must be highly scalable and cost-efficient, we suggest relying on the virtualization techniques – see ETSI NFV framework - for their deployment. We have thus provided an overview of this new network & IT infrastructure service architecture. We indeed believe that the IoT stringent requirements will turn into the advantage of the IoT store actor that will be able to offer the appropriate network & IT services in terms of cost, QoS, connectivity, flexibility and security.

References

1. Boujemaa, F., et al.: Internet of things, the newt Wave of Internet, Final synthesis, September 2012
2. Ropert, S.: Internet of Things, Outlook for the top 8 vertical markets, Idate, Septembre 2013
3. Berkers, F., Roelands, M.: Contructing a Multi-Sided Business Model for a Smart Horizontal IoT Service Platform. In: 17th International Conference on Intelligence in Next Generation Networks, October 2013
4. Chiosi, M., et al.: Network Functions Virtualisation – Introductory White Paper, at the "SDN and OpenFlow World Congress", Darmstadt-Germany, 22–24 October 2012
5. http://www.networkworld.com/community/blog/google%E2%80%99s-vint-cerf-defines-internet-things-challenges
6. http://phx.corporate-ir.net/phoenix.zhtml?c=176060&p=irol-newsArticle&ID=1923514 &highlight

Multipath Bandwidth Scavenging in the Internet of Things

Isabel Montes[1]([⊠]), Romel Parmis[1], Roel Ocampo[1], and Cedric Festin[2]

[1] Computer Networks Laboratory, Electrical and Electronics Engineering Institute,
University of the Philippines Diliman, Quezon City, Philippines
isabel.montes@upd.edu.ph
[2] Networks and Distributed Systems Group, Department of Computer Science,
University of the Philippines Diliman, Quezon City, Philippines

Abstract. In order to achieve the capacity and geographic scope required by IoT applications, service providers should explore mutually-beneficial modes of collaboration such as through cooperative packet forwarding by IoT nodes and cooperative gatewaying through fixed backhauls. To promote such resource pooling while minimizing negative impact on collaborating providers, we developed a transport-layer approach that combines multipath techniques with less-than-best effort (LBE) congestion control methods to enable IoT nodes to opportunistically scavenge for idle bandwidth across multiple paths. Initial tests using TCP-LP and LEDBAT congestion control algorithms on scavenging secondary flows show that this desired functionality can be achieved, while our use of standard TCP congestion control on primary flows ensures that IoT nodes are guaranteed at least one flow that can compete for fair share of the network capacity.

Keywords: Internet of things · Bandwidth scavenging · Less-than-best-effort · Congestion control · Multipath flows

1 Introduction

The Internet of Things (IoT) will place new demands on service providers for connectivity, including fixed infrastructure-based gateway services and backhaul to cloud services for further aggregation, processing, storage and distribution of data from devices and smart objects. Prudent design would dictate that such gateways and backhauls be engineered to appropriately handle peak aggregate traffic from potentially large numbers of data sources. In addition, sufficient coverage over large geographic areas would ensure continuous connectivity even in the face of mobility. Moreover, the strategic placement of access points and gateways would help minimize energy-consuming packet forwarding within the wireless network of objects.

All these technical requirements will result in design challenges and significant capital and operating costs to IoT service providers in the future. In order to avoid having to engineer for peak loads and maximum coverage, one possible

© Institute for Computer Sciences, Social Informatics and Telecommunications Engineering 2015
R. Giaffreda et al. (Eds.): IoT360 2014, Part I, LNICST 150, pp. 297–304, 2015.
DOI: 10.1007/978-3-319-19656-5_42

approach for IoT providers servicing overlapping areas would be to enter into mutually-beneficial bilateral commercial agreements enabling cooperative access and transit through their peers nodes and infrastructure. Such cooperation may further be enhanced if nodes are available to concurrently exploit the multiple forwarding paths through the additional resources made available by cooperating providers.

1.1   Multipath Bandwidth Scavenging

Although current routing techniques allow packets from a single origin to be forwarded via multiple routes and gateways, naively striping packets from a single flow into multiple paths may cause problems for transport layer protocols with reliable in-order delivery and congestion control functionality. Uneven path delays and loss characteristics may trigger timeouts and unnecessary retransmissions, requiring endpoints to heavily buffer out-of-order received packets [4,5,16]. A better alternative would be to intelligently partition application flows into subflows and enforce per-subflow reliability and congestion control mechanisms. This has been the general approach taken by the Internet community with Multipath TCP (MPTCP), which, along with coordinated congestion control between subflows, will provide TCP the capability to utilize multiple paths between source and destination for redundancy and better resource usage [15].

MPTCP can potentially provide the multipath capability we require. However, it is possible that a provider will not wish to fairly share bandwidth with a competitor that opportunistically uses bandwidth on top of what it can already obtain from its own network. In other words, an IoT service provider might only allow a competitor to scavenge whatever remaining unused bandwidth is available.

1.2   Less-Than-Best Effort Congestion Control
as a Scavenging Mechanism

If opportunistic scavenging subflows are too aggressive, these may negatively impact the ability of other nodes to use the network and thus defeat the purpose of allowing scavenging in the first place. Indeed, a paramount concern in scavenging scenarios is to minimize impact on entities volunteering the use of their idle resources [13]. This may be achieved through the use of a class of congestion control mechanisms called less-than-best-effort (LBE) mechanisms, that detect the onset of congestion more quickly than conventional packet loss-based ones [14]. A desirable side effect is that when LBE flows mix with TCP flows in a bottleneck link, the former yield bandwidth to the latter. In the absence of any competing flows, an LBE flow will also attempt to maximize the use of the available bandwidth. These characteristics make LBE congestion control techniques well suited to the task of opportunistic bandwidth scavenging.

Inspired by current work on LBE congestion control and MPTCP, we developed a hybrid transport-layer approach that would enable concurrent multipath bandwidth scavenging by combining MPTCPs multipath mechanisms with LBE congestion control. Our design and validation efforts are described in the rest of this paper.

2 MP-LBE Design

Similar to MPTCP, two communicating endpoints start by establishing a single primary subflow that uses standard TCP-like congestion control. Any additional paths that are discovered will carry secondary subflows, and use LBE congestion control mechanisms. These secondary subflows are essentially the ones that scavenge bandwidth from the rest of the network, opportunistically using resources from both its own and from cooperating providers.

2.1 Congestion Control in Secondary Subflows

Our work aims to explore the use of the LBE class of congestion control methods in secondary subflows in order to achieve low-impact multipath bandwidth scavenging. We start by evaluating TCP-LP and LEDBAT as candidate congestion control methods in our secondary subflows.

TCP-LP is a congestion control algorithm that manages the congestion window of the sender based on the delay experienced by the traffic on a bottleneck [9]. TCP-LP uses variations in one-way delay to infer congestion earlier than standard TCP through a simple threshold-based algorithm. TCP-LP calculates one-way delay (owd) upon receiving an ACK by computing the difference between the receiver's timestamp in the ACK and the timestamp taken when the sender sent the packet, which the receiver copies into the ACK and echoes back to the sender. A smoothing parameter γ is used to get a weighted average of the current owd measurement with the previous owd measurement. When the smoothed owd rises above a fraction δ of the difference between the maximum owd (d_{max}) and minimum owd (d_{min}), congestion is inferred. TCP-LP will then reduce the congestion window by half and enter an inference phase where it awaits further congestion indication. If congestion is detected during the inference phase, $cwnd$ is reduced to 1. Otherwise, TCP-LP proceeds with an additive increase of $cwnd$.

LEDBAT, like TCP-LP, measures owd using the timestamps in the ACKs received at the sender side [12]. In place of TCP-LPs threshold-based algorithm for inferring congestion, LEDBAT makes use of a target queuing delay value. When queuing delay becomes higher than the target, congestion is assumed and LEDBAT reduces its $cwnd$ to alleviate the potential congestion in the network. LEDBAT regulates the $cwnd$ size using a proportional-integral-derivative (PID) controller, which varies the $cwnd$ proportional to the difference of the queueing delay and the target value.

2.2 Congestion Control in Primary Subflows

Our primary subflows use TCP SACK, which is a loss-based congestion control algorithm. As such, it does not detect congestion as early as the delay-based algorithms of TCP-LP and LEDBAT.

3   Evaluation

We used an existing NS-2 MPTCP implementation [11] and disabled congestion control coupling between subflows. We further modified it by assigning its
first subflow to use standard TCP, and any succeeding subflow added to the
connection takes on an LBE congestion control algorithm. We implemented two
versions of MP-LBE: one that uses LEDBAT for its secondary flow and one that
uses TCP-LP. Our LEDBAT implementation uses a target queueing delay value
of 12 ms. We used $\gamma=1/8$ and $\delta=0.25$ for the TCP-LP implementation.

The topology used in all the simulations is shown in Fig. 1. An MP-LBE connection is configured with two subflows, one primary and one secondary subflow,
and each of these share a bottleneck link with a TCP connection. The bottleneck links each have a capacity of 5 Mbps and 5 ms delay. The link used by the
primary subflow will be referred to as the top link, while the link used by the
secondary subflow will be referred to as the bottom link.

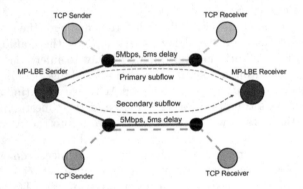

Fig. 1. The topology used for the simulations. Each access link is configured with a
capacity of 100 Mbps, with 5 ms delay.

3.1   Bandwidth Scavenging

In this simulation, both subflows compete with standard TCP traffic. MP-LBE's
primary subflow should share its evenly link with the competing traffic, while
the secondary subflow should back off. Halfway into the simulation, the TCP
connection on the bottom link ends, and the secondary subflow should react by
maximizing the available bandwidth once the link becomes idle. Both MP-LBE
(LEDBAT) and MP-LBE (TCP-LP) are able to achieve this behavior, as seen
in Fig. 2. When the secondary flow is using LEDBAT,it is able to maximize the
available bandwidth better than TCP-LP. We observed that LEDBAT achieves
a steadier throughput because its *cwnd* size does not change as drastically as
that of TCP-LP.

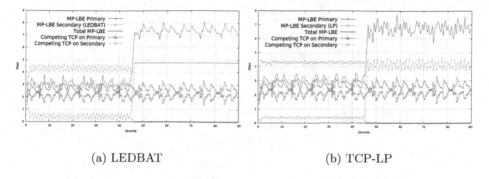

(a) LEDBAT   (b) TCP-LP

Fig. 2. Bandwidth scavenging behavior of MP-LBE.

3.2 LBE Behavior

In this experiment, we disabled the competing TCP connection on the bottom link at the start of the simulation. This allowed the secondary flow to maximize 5 Mbps capacity of the link. At 45 s, a TCP connection begins on the bottom link, which should cause the secondary subflow to back off. Figure 3 shows the simulation results. MP-LBE using TCP-LP on its secondary subflow was able to back off more rapidly than LEDBAT, but both demonstrated correct LBE behavior when the bottom link stopped being idle.

3.3 Goodput

In multipath connections, even if the aggregation of bandwidth effectively improves throughput, the goodput achieved is usually not as high due to the out-of-order arrival of packets. To evaluate the MP-LBEs goodput performance, we recorded the data-level sequence numbers (DSNs) received by the destination node and plotted this against time. For this experiment, we eliminated all competing TCP traffic. We ran the simulation using regular MPTCP, in addition to

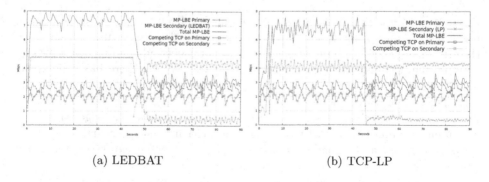

(a) LEDBAT   (b) TCP-LP

Fig. 3. LBE Behavior of MP-LBE.

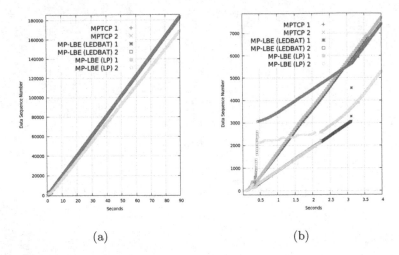

(a)   (b)

Fig. 4. DSNs received at the destination. The y-axis is scaled to 1:536, as DSNs are in increments of 536.

the simulation runs for MP-LBE (LEDBAT) and MP-LBE (TCP-LP). The simulation results (Fig. 4) show that the rate of DSN increase of both MPTCP and MP-LBE (LEDBAT) is the same, while MP-LBE (TCP-LP) achieves much lower DSN within the given time. For the first 4 s of the experiment (Fig. 4(b)), the MP-LBEs primary subflow (for both LEDBAT and TCP-LP) received DSNs at a slower rate than the secondary subflow, causing the goodput to suffer because only the DSNs on the secondary subflow are arriving, and all the DSNs sent through the primary subflow are delayed in arriving. In the case of MP-LBE (LEDBAT), when the delayed packets finally arrive a little after 3 s, the primary subflow has picked up its pace. After this point, the rate of DSN increase of MP-LBE (LEDBAT) matches that of MPTCP.

4   Related Work

Resource scavenging is not a new concept, having been previously used to harness idle computing resources to perform useful calculations for users other than the resource owner [13]. Our approach focuses on network bandwidth scavenging through a transport layer multipath approach. While there has been some recent similar work on the development of a multipath version of LEDBAT called LEDBAT-MP [1], we are interested in the more general class of LBEs and intend to comparatively evaluate several of the representative algorithms for our intended application. Furthermore, our approach makes a crucial distinction between primary and secondary flows, ensuring that nodes can rely on at least one flow, the primary one, to compete fairly within the network.

In order to achieve cooperative gatewaying among providers, we need mechanisms to enable concurrent access to their respective fixed wireless infrastructure.

BeWifi [2], a service rolled out by service provider Telefonica, allows users to use idle capacity through neighbors access points within range, while CableWiFi [3] employs a multi-provider model, allowing customers from five ISPs access to the consortiums infrastructure. One mechanism that can enable cooperative gatewaying is offered by BaPu (Bunching of Access Point Uplinks) [8], which employs packet overhearing to pool together WiFi uplinks that are in close proximity to one another. BaPu was designed primarily for uploading user-generated content over the Internet and cannot be used for downloads.

The ability to concurrently exploit multiple paths for bandwidth scavenging may also be viewed as a problem of bandwidth aggregation. Application layer solutions such as DBAS [7] typically do not require changes in the underlying protocols or infrastructure, but instead rely on an application-layer proxy residing within the endpoint to intercept traffic, and manage the scheduling, reordering, and transmission of that traffic over multiple network interfaces. We preferred to take an endpoint-based approach since it offers an end-to-end solution, covering both the fixed and wireless portions of the network.

5   Conclusion and Future Work

We proposed an approach for multipath bandwidth scavenging in the Internet of Things through the introduction of a transport-layer protocol that uses TCP-like congestion control for primary subflows and LBE congestion control for secondary subflows. Our simulations demonstrate that our MP-LBE design can effectively improve throughput when an idle link becomes available for a secondary subflow to utilize. Such an ability to scavenge additional bandwidth and paths may offer the ability for sensors and devices to transmit information at higher-than-minimum levels of spatial and temporal resolution, or to explore shortcut fast paths to accelerate local aggregation and processing of data by peer devices within the IoT. When no additional links are available, the primary subflow is able to maintain the throughput of a standard single-flow TCP, and secondary flows are able to rapidly utilize the links once they become idle.

Smart objects and devices in the Internet of Things will undoubtedly have to dedicate most of their resources to their primary tasks of sensing and aggregating data, and to execute any local processing and cognitive functionality required. It is a challenge therefore to minimize the resource footprint of any new functionality being introduced, including multipath bandwidth scavenging. The management of concurrent multipath TCP flows is known to introduce additional buffering resource requirements in endpoints [6], with approaches ranging from smart packet transmission scheduling [4,5] and network coding [10] having been proposed as mitigating solutions. We intend to investigate these approaches further, with the view of achieving low-overhead implementations.

References

1. Adhari, H., Werner, S., Dreibholz, T., Rathgeb, E.P: LEDBAT-MP on the application of lower-than-best-effort for concurrent multipath transfer. In: Proceedings of

the 4th International Workshop on Protocols and Applications with Multi-Homing Support (PAMS), Victoria, British Columbia/Canada, May 2014. ISBN 978-1-4799-2652-7

2. BeWifi, Accessed on 30 June 2014. http://www.bewifi.es
3. Cable WiFi : Internet access brought to consumers through a collaboration among U.S. Internet Service Providers, Accessed on 30 June 2014. http://www.cablewifi. com
4. Chebrolu, K., Raman, B., Rao, R.R.: A network layer approach to enable TCP over multiple interfaces. Wirel. Netw. **11**(5), 637–650 (2005)
5. Evensen, K., Kaspar, D., Engelstad, P., Hansen, A.F., Griwodz, C., Halvorsen, P: A network-layer proxy for bandwidth aggregation and reduction of ip packet reordering. In: IEEE 34th Conference on Local Computer Networks. LCN 2009, pp. 585–592. IEEE (2009)
6. Ford, A., Raiciu, C., Handley, M., Barre, S., Inyegar, J.: Architectural Guidelines for Multipath TCP Development. RFC 6182, RFC Editor, March 2011
7. Habak, K., Youssef, M., Harras, K.A.: DBAS: a deployable bandwidth aggregation system. In: 2012 5th International Conference on New Technologies, Mobility and Security (NTMS), pp. 1–6, May 2012
8. Jin,T., Huu, T.V., Blass, E.-O., Noubir, G.: BaPu: efficient and practical bunching of access point uplinks. CoRR, abs/1301.5928, 2013
9. Kuzmanovic, A., Knightly, E.W.: TCP-LP: low-priority service via end-point congestion control. IEEE/ACM Trans. Netw. **14**(4), 739–752 (2006)
10. Li, M., Lukyanenko, A., Tarkoma, S., Cui, Y., Yl-Jski, A.: Tolerating path heterogeneity in multipath TCP with bounded receive buffers. Comput. Netw. **64**, 1–14 (2014)
11. Google Code Project. Multipath-TCP: Implement Multipath TCP on NS-2, Accessed on 30 June 2014. http://code.google.com/p/multipath-tcp
12. Shalunov, S., Hazel, G., Iyengar, J., Kuehlewind, M.: Low Extra Delay Background Transport (LEDBAT). RFC 6817, RFC Editor, December 2012
13. Strickland, J.W., Freeh, V.W., Ma, X., Vazhkudai, S.S.: Governor: autonomic throttling for aggressive idle resource scavenging. In: Second International Conference on Autonomic Computing, ICAC 2005. Proceedings, pp. 64–75. IEEE (2005)
14. Welzl, M., Ros, D.: A Survey of Lower-than-Best-Effort Transport Protocol. RFC 6297, RFC Editor, June 2011
15. Wischik, D., Raiciu, C., Greenhalgh, A., Handley, M.: Design, implementation and evaluation of congestion control for multipath TCP. NSDI **11**, 8–8 (2011)
16. Zinner, T., Tutschku, K., Nakao, A., Tran-Gia, P.: Using concurrent multipath transmission for transport virtualization: analyzing path selection. In: 2010 22nd International, Teletraffic Congress (ITC), pp. 1–7, Sept 2010

BETaaS Platform – A Things as a Service Environment for Future M2M Marketplaces

Sofoklis Kyriazakos[1]([✉]), Bayu Anggorojati[1], Neeli Prasad[1],
Carlo Vallati[2], Enzo Mingozzi[2], Giacomo Tanganelli[2],
Novella Buonaccorsi[3], Nicola Valdambrini[3], Nikolaos Zonidis[4],
George Labropoulous[4], Belen Martinez Rodriguez[5],
Alessandro Mamelli[6], and Davide Sommacampagna[6]

[1] Center for TeleInfrastructure, Aalborg University, Aalborg, Denmark
{sk, ba, np}@es.aau.dk
[2] Department of Information Engineering, University of Pisa, Pisa, Italy
{c.vallati, e.mingozzi, g.tanganelli}@iet.unipi.it
[3] Intecs S.p.A., Roma, Italy
{novella.buonaccorsi, nicola.valdambrini}@intecs.it
[4] Converge ICT Solutions and Services S.A., Athens, Greece
{nzonidis, glabropoulos}@converge.gr
[5] Tecnalia Research & Innovation, San Sebastian, Spain
belen.martinez@tecnalia.com
[6] Hewlett-Packard Italiana S.r.l., Roma, Italy
{alessandro.mamelli, davide.sommacampagna}@hp.com

Abstract. Building the Environment for Things as a Service (BETaaS) is a novel platform for the deployment and execution of content-centric M2M applications, which relies on a local cloud of gateways. BETaaS platform provides a uniform interface and services to map content with things in a context-aware manner. Deployment of services for the execution of applications is dynamic and takes into account the computational resources of the low-end physical devices used. To this aim, BETaaS platform is based on a suitable defined IoT model, allowing the integration of the BETaaS components within the future Internet environment. In this paper we present the BETaaS concept, the high level platform architecture and application scenarios that extend the state-of-the-art in M2M communications and open the horizon for future M2M marketplaces.

Keywords: IoT · M2M communications · TaaS

1 Introduction

Marketplaces of applications became a trend over the past years within this decade and this trend is a game-changer by providing a different business model. Usually the app marketplaces are linked with smart phones, but are not limited to that. Recently operating systems make use of such models and even TV manufactures is using this 'channel' to differentiate from the competitors in the smart TVs world. M2M communications, which imply the elimination of the human in the loop, are not only a

© Institute for Computer Sciences, Social Informatics and Telecommunications Engineering 2015
R. Giaffreda et al. (Eds.): IoT360 2014, Part I, LNICST 150, pp. 305–313, 2015.
DOI: 10.1007/978-3-319-19656-5_43

trend, but is the natural evolution of the marketplaces. The IoT that integrate objects into the Internet, has opened new horizons in the M2M communications and we consider this as a unique opportunity to come up with a Things as a Service Environment that will increase the spectrum of M2M applications.

This paper is organized around 5 sections. After the first section, which is this introduction, we present in Sect. 2 the current approaches, the limitations and the constraints of M2M applications and IoT. The section finishes with the challenges that are addressed from BETaaS platform, that are described in more detail under Sect. 3, BETaaS platform. In this section the concept, the high level architecture and the Things as a Service model are described, which are the basis of the BETaaS project and the major innovation of this approach. In Sect. 4 we focus on M2M applications that can be available in future marketplaces, requiring the flexibility offered by BETaaS approach. Finally, in the conclusions section we focus on the next step and the vision of BETaaS in the IoT and M2M world.

2   M2M Applications and IoT

2.1   Current Approaches, Limitations and Ways to Address These Challenges

The main limitations coming from the world of M2M applications and IoT is certainly related to fragmentation of standards and technologies. A lot of them are available on the market and platforms are often designed to work with specific subsets, depending on the applications. BETaaS architecture includes a specific layer in charge of adapting to specific technologies and protocols. Furthermore the platform is based on a software framework that allows plug-ins to be dynamically added, making it easy to cope with the fragmentation of the M2M market referred above. Besides that, BETaaS focuses on the ETSI M2M standard that is going to be a promising solution to next M2M systems. The platform then opens to this class of sensor networks that is likely to soon become the most widespread M2M standard, partially representing a solution to fragmentation. Another class of limitations is related to the heterogeneity of ontologies that have to be harmonized and integrated when several applications and devices need to talk each other. BETaaS faces this issue through the construction of an ontologies network. Concerning the implementation patterns of M2M systems, a strong limitation often comes from their vertical and closed architecture. It commonly happens that each infrastructure serves a single M2M application, excluding any interoperability pattern between other systems, applications or things. Thus, when new M2M applications are needed, providers have to re-create M2M communication platforms and data representation formats. BETaaS differentiates itself from this kind of model, implementing a horizontal approach and defining a single common reference model that can be used by different applications and devices to build M2M services.

2.2 Challenges

BETaaS is providing a new vision about the way to expose and manage things in the Internet of Everything environment. The BETaaS platform is using semantic technologies and stays close to the M2M nodes, through the creation of local clouds among nodes in concrete contexts. That ease the development and execution of content centric user applications, thus allowing the definition of new M2M applications whose scope spans across different domains. Evaluating the advances of BETaaS compared to existing approaches, there are significant improvement in aspects like QoS, interoperability aspects, discovery, security and trust, and the integration of Big Data analytics capabilities. At QoS level, the BETaaS improvements include QoS negotiation support, support to real-time applications, energy-efficient selection of things and QoS assurances in a distributed environment. BETaaS defines a comprehensive QoS management framework that comprises a general QoS model in order to differentiate IoT/M2M services based on appropriate QoS measures, and optimized resource reservation and allocation to services. BETaaS extends the current state-of-art of SLA creation and negotiation for enabling the BETaaS QoS model in the relevant M2M application scenarios. Regarding interoperability, BETaaS integrates different IoT/M2M systems and exploits different capabilities of different IoT/M2M systems. As far as discovery is concerned, BETaaS supports distributed discovery of thing services and look-up of thing services based on context and with regards to security and trust, BETaaS focuses on the secure access to thing services and trust establishment in the overall system. BETaaS also enables virtualization in ARM-based devices, so it is possible to perform more complex tasks in the local environment. In addition, BETaaS leverages innovative Big Data capabilities to build a highly scalable and efficient architecture that is capable of handling the large amount of highly distributed information generated by things, and then enabling to query data with low complexity.

3 BETaaS Platform

3.1 BETaaS Approach

BETaaS platform provides a runtime environment relying on a local cloud of gateways to support the deployment and execution of content-centric M2M applications. BETaaS platform seamlessly integrates existing heterogeneous M2M systems by means of a network of gateways. Each gateway runs the BETaaS run-time environment that forms a logical overlay. The logical federation of networks forms a local cloud in which each gateway shares the functionalities offered by the smart objects of its M2M systems with the rest of the network. The run-time platform running on each gateway provides M2M applications connected to any of the BETaaS gateways a common interface to access their respective things, regardless of location and technology. In order to account for heterogeneity, the BETaaS platform builds upon a baseline reference model and architecture, Things-as-a-Service (TaaS), providing an abstract and uniform description of the underlying M2M systems. The TaaS paradigm defines for each thing connected to the platform, a *thing service* is created to represent the *basic service*(s) that can be provided to each application. The BETaaS platform is content-centric in the sense that it provides services that depend on the type of data that they provide and on the context in which that data is used. The circumstances that have not been considered in BETaaS as part of the context of a thing are its battery level, its available computing capacity, the communication protocol used and its location. BETaaS uses semantic technologies and natural language processing to unify the information that comes from heterogeneous things and to deal with the dynamic nature of their context. Following this purpose, we have built the BETaaS ontology, a network of ontologies created reusing ontologies that are relevant in their domains and that model the BETaaS scenarios. In particular, we have used the following ontologies: SSN [1], Time [2], CF [3], Phenonet [4], MUO [5], FIPA [6] and GeoNames [7]. To promote standardization, the contextual information related to things (type of thing, location, etc.) is translated to WordNet [8] synsets whenever possible, and stored in the ontology. Wordnet is a lexical database that groups English words into sets of synonyms (synsets), and whose organization is based on the semantic relationships between synsets (hypernymy, hyponymy, holonymy and meronymy). All synsets inserted in the BETaaS ontology are stored following these relationships, through SKOS, [9] which offers a common data model to organize classifications in a hierarchical way. The relationships between the terms are used as a mechanism of knowledge inference. Inference can be applied at the time of the execution of applications: e.g. if an application demands the temperature at home, a temperature sensor installed in the kitchen is valid (*kitchen* is meronym of *home*). Inference can also be applied when registering things in the BETaaS ontology: e.g. a new thing described as moistness sensor, would be added to a family in the ontology described as humidity sensors (*moistness* and *humidity* belong to the same WordNet family). The contextual information associated to each of the things connected to a gateway allows the platform to create a thing service for each of those things, following the nomenclature *setLocationType/getLocationType* (e.g. *getKitchenTemperature*).

3.2   BETaaS High Level Architecture

BETaaS high level architecture is depicted in Fig. 1. A layered structure is adopted to guarantee at the top the proper level of abstraction to applications and at the bottom the flexibility necessary to integrate different system characterized by different technologies.

The core component of the BETaaS architecture is the Thing as a Service layer (TaaS) that is implemented in a distributed fashion this layer exposes a service oriented interface to access the things connected to the platform, regardless of their technology and physical location. Build on top of the TaaS layer BETaaS platform exposes the service layer to applications. A basic service that exposes directly one or more thing services, or can be an extended service installed on the platform to provide to custom services.

Transparent integration of existing systems is achieved through the definition of adaptation layers. An adaptation layer implements a common interface towards TaaS layer to access the functionalities of the physical system in a uniform manner regardless of its technology. The definition of an adaptation layer allows the integration without requiring any modifications to the original system which is BETaaS-unaware, though at

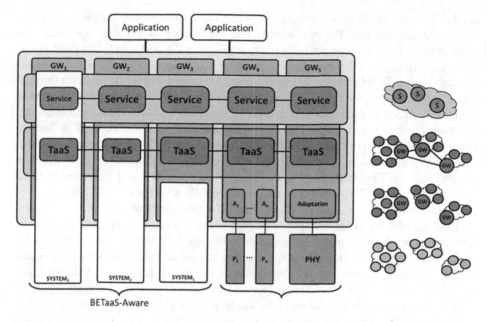

Fig. 1. BETaaS architecture.

the cost of possible replication of some functionalities. When modifications to the original systems are allowed, a more efficient integration can be achieved introducing a set of modifications which make the original system BETaaS-aware, through the implementation of some of the BETaaS layers. Some or all of the BETaaS function-alities are implemented by the integrated system in a fully interoperable manner, i.e. compliant with BETaaS internal interfaces.

3.3   Things as a Service

The major impediment of the current IoT galaxy is its fragmentation. Current IoT is made of vertical isolated systems characterized by different technologies and com-munication protocols, often proprietary and not interoperable. In this context the BETaaS goal is to build the environment for the integration of these systems into a horizontal architecture on which the next generation of applications will leaverage. At this aim, one of most important feature of the platform is providing a unified interface to applications in order to enable seamless access to smart objects abstracting their technology and location. At this aim, the BETaaS platform defines at its core a Service Oriented interface, the Things as a Service model, *TaaS* for short. Goal of the TaaS is to abstract all the details behind each thing, e.g. location, technology, communication protocol, through a common representation, the *Thing Service*. Defined in [11], the Thing Service is the logical representation of a basic functionality that can be offered by a physical smart object. The role of the TaaS model within the BETaaS platform is illustrated in Fig. 2. As can be seen the TaaS model is implemented in the platform by the TaaS layer, which is at the core of the BETaaS architecture, between the lower layers (Adaptation and Physical layers) and the higher layers (Service layer and applications). TaaS main responsibility is to implement the bridge between the "*service providers*" (things) and the "*service consumers*" (services and applications). Smart devices from different physical IoT systems are integrated within the platform through the Adaptation layer: for each IoT system a different Adaptation instance is installed to implement a common interface that is used by the TaaS to discover and access things. For each device, one or more Thing Services are created to be exposed to Service Layer. TaaS layer represents also the foundation for the BETaaS distributed architecture. Implemented in a distributed manner over the local cloud of gateways that characterizes BETaaS deployments, the TaaS allows services, and indirectly applications, to access the Thing Services not only regardless of their specific interface or communication protocol, but also independently of their physical location. Retrival and exploitation of context information is of paramount importance for TaaS operations. Semantic capabilities, in particular, are included in the TaaS implementation to process the context associated with each thing to derive the set of Thing Services. At this aim the TaaS Context information are also exploited to provide Look-up functionalities to services which can request a Thing Service through its contextual requirements. In order to support deployment of real-time applications the TaaS layer includes Quality of Service (QoS) funcitonalities that can be used by the Service Layer to request a certain QoS for invoking a Thing Service. In order to support heterogeneous requirements that characterize IoT deployments, the QoS is negotiated to stipulate a SLA. For this reason, a negotiation procedure is implemented in the TaaS to allow services to negotiated the QoS level necessary to fulfill application needs. QoS is enforced through an efficient managing of resources, which is performed exploiting the

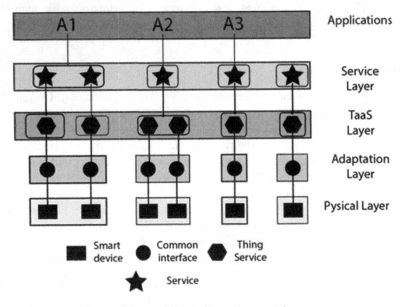

Fig. 2. Thing as a service model.

concept of Equivalent Thing Services, Thing Services that can provide the same functionality equivalently.

4 Application scenarios

4.1 Smart City

The Smart City scenario is mainly focused on the integration of Smart Things belonging to different systems. This scenario shows how BETaaS can adapt to different data sources, how it can be used to build a complete system and how it can provide an added value to existing ones.

4.2 Building Blocks

The scenario is built upon:

- A smart lighting system that controls public lamp posts in a parking lot
- A system to manage cars access to a restricted area of the city based on the car's positions
- A traffic system that receives data from traffic sensors installed along a network of roads.

The smart lighting system is completely implemented through a single BETaaS gateway connected to ETSI-enabled devices: light intensity tunable lamp posts and infrared presence sensors. A second BETaaS gateway is in charge of receiving users' position, matching them to the city map. It is intended to implement a service to check the access to Low Emission Zones (LEZ), making users to pay a fee as they enter. In this case Things are represented by on-board cars' GPS receivers. The traffic system is then a completely independent system called SIMIS (Sustainable and Intelligent Mobility Integrated System). It allows to check the current status of roads and parking lots, also providing traffic data to external applications. In this scenario it is shown how BETaaS can be easily extended to receive data from it.

4.3 Integration through BETaaS

In this smart city scenario the two BETaaS gateways described above are then used to make up a single BETaaS instance. Once they are configured to join each other, they start sharing their resources. Gateways resources are mainly represented by the Thing Services they created on top of the Things: lamp posts, presence sensors, traffic sensors and cars' GPS receivers. BETaaS allows to add an application logic inside the instance through extended services. In this scenario two extended services are included:

- The smart lighting extended service on the first gateway. It not only exploits the presence sensors directly connected to the gateway itself but it also considers the traffic data provided by the other gateway. Lamp light is then intensified or dimmed also based on the current traffic density.

- The LEZ extended service not only uses the cars' position to make users pay a fee once they enter the restricted zone. It also exploits traffic data coming from SIMIS to compute dynamic fees based on the current roads congestion.

Extended services may also be accessed by BETaaS users from their external applications. So in this case users access the platform through mobile applications from their cars, being notified about the current fee that is currently applied, depending on their position and traffic intensity.

4.4 Home domain

The Home Domain scenario is focusing on a typical need of Smart Homes and Building Management Systems, which is the exploitation of existing infrastructures. BETaaS concept aims to prove through this scenario, that it can extend proprietary systems in order to result in integrated solutions with multiple services and capabilities. The first sub-scenario of the Home Domain presents the steps that a user would do in order to cover a need, which is the deployment of an application that is managing the garden watering. In this scenario, the main actor downloads the app from a marketplace and is exploiting a number of proprietary systems that can be upgraded into BETaaS enabled gateways. Therefore devices such as thermometer, humidity sensor, etc. can be exploited from the home BMS. Additional devices that are required, e.g. electronic watering valve, has to be installed and controlled by another BETaaS gateway. The second sub-scenario of the Home Domain is focusing on the case of a user who already has an alarm system installed for his home, but still he would be interested for an extension of the alarm to cover the entry points of the building, i.e. front door of the building and garage automatic door. In this scenario, again he downloads (or writes) an application that exploits the capabilities of the home alarm, which is upgraded to become BETaaS enabled, and extends its services by managing some additional devices (Things) that are required to extend the coverage of the alarm.

5 Conclusions

The paper presents the Things as a Service environment for future M2M applications, proposed by BETaaS. The challenges and the implementation of BETaaS are described, as well as the indicative scenarios and applications. Unlike many IoT and M2M approaches, BETaaS is a tangible platform that aims become an open-source community to further develop the source code and achieve the highest impact. We strongly believe the clear advances of BETaaS and in the future work we are considering to prepare the community and all stakeholders for the evolution of M2M applications.

Acknowledgment. This work has been carried out within the activities of the project "Building the Environment for the Things as a Service (BETaaS)", which is co-funded by the European Commission under the Seventh Framework Programme (grant no. 317674).

References

1. SSN. http://www.w3.org/2005/Incubator/ssn/XGR-ssn-20110628
2. Time. http://www.w3.org/2006/time
3. CF. http://www.w3.org/2005/Incubator/ssn/ssnx/cf/cf-property
4. Phenonet. http://www.w3.org/2005/Incubator/ssn/ssnx/meteo/phenonet
5. MUO. http://purl.oclc.org/NET/muo/muo
6. FIPA. http://www.fipa.org/specs/fipa00091/PC00091A.html
7. GeoNames. http://www.geonames.org/ontology/ontology_v3.1.rdf
8. WordNet. http://wordnetweb.princeton.edu
9. SKOS. http://www.w3.org/2004/02/skos/intro
10. Teixeira, T., Hachem, S., Issarny, V., Georgantas, N.: Service oriented middleware for the internet of things: a perspective. In: Abramowicz, W., Llorente, I.M., Surridge, M., Zisman, A., Vayssière, J. (eds.) ServiceWave 2011. LNCS, vol. 6994, pp. 220–229. Springer, Heidelberg (2011)
11. Thoma, M., et al.: On iot-services: survey, classification and enterprise integration. In: 2012 IEEE International Conference on Green Computing and Communications (GreenCom). IEEE (2012)

Context Sensitive Smart Device Command Recognition and Negotiation

Frank Bauerle, Grant Miller[⊠], Nader Nassar, Tamer Nassar,
and Irene Penney

IBM Corp., Somers, NY, USA
{fbauerle,millerg,nnassar,tamer,sprouts}@us.ibm.com

Abstract. The Internet of Things (IoT) represents a dramatic shift in how computing and communication interrelate. Devices can potentially connect to anything at any time in any place. While many researchers focus on how to make the IoT seamless, faster, and add more devices into the mesh, our approach is to introduce a new approach whereby devices not only communicate, but also have a level of context awareness that results in optimal intelligence among the mesh of connected devices.

Keywords: Iot · Negotiation · Context-sensitve · Mobile

1 Introduction

The numbers of smart devices are increasing almost exponentially. The capabilities of these devices are increasing daily. The ability for these devices to interact is increasing exponentially as mobile and telecom networks continue to expand. In the past, smart devices and their associated network were built for purpose. A network of medical devices knows which other devices are or may be available and understand how to interact.

It is when an unknown number or type of devices exist on the same network that the specifics of how these devices interact and respond to commands becomes a problem. An algorithm and approach for determining which device is best suited to respond to a command must be implemented.

1.1 Background

Imagine walking into a room full of smart devices. There are tablets and phones. An Xbox360 is sitting next to the SmartTV. A DVR sits next to the television. Smart remotes sit on the coffee table. A laptop sits on the coffee table (Fig. 1).

When a command[1] is made to turn the television on, which device should respond? When a command is issued to watch a movie, which device should respond?

---

[1] Throughout this paper, unless the situation is specific to voice commands, we use the term "command" to refer to directives that are given by any input method (voice, keyboard, or other).

© Institute for Computer Sciences, Social Informatics and Telecommunications Engineering 2015
R. Giaffreda et al. (Eds.): IoT360 2014, Part I, LNICST 150, pp. 314–330, 2015.
DOI: 10.1007/978-3-319-19656-5_44

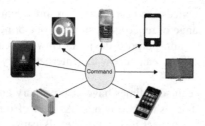

Fig. 1. Command to smart devices

Today, it seems simple. We know which device the movie is on or which remote we need to use to turn on the television.

In the future, this will not always be the case. There will be multiple smart devices that can respond to a command whether it is a smart phone or tablet that have embedded television remote applications or the Xbox360® that can respond to a command to play a movie that may also be available on the television or DVR.

As smart devices become smarter, the ability for these different devices to recognize and respond to different commands will only increase. If multiple smart devices attempt to respond to a command, the result could be chaos. A movie could begin playing on the Xbox, the television, and even the Netflix™ application on a tablet.

To help bring order to this potential chaos of having a multitude of devices respond to a command, a method of having these smart devices negotiate amongst themselves to determine which device should respond is needed.

In order to support this capability, it is clear that smart devices will need to evolve. Given the rate at which these devices are currently evolving, it is not a stretch to assume that in the near future smart devices will become smarter and have the ability determine through the context of the device, its location, and the type of command issued, which is the best device to respond.

In this paper, we lay out the case for a context-aware negotiation-based command determination method.

1.2   The Evolution of Smart Devices

There are many types of devices becoming connected. There are many examples of "smart things" that exist, such as wireless sensor and actuator networks, and embedded devices [1]. Smart devices began as single purpose devices. They were purpose-built to satisfy a single use, or command, or set of commands that they were built to satisfy. A thermostat is a great example of a built-for-purpose smart device. An individual can interact with the device to set the temperature in the house. The same individual can create a program to raise and lower the thermostat during the course of a day. But, other than potentially providing some history on the thermostat settings that is all the thermostat can do.

These built-for-purpose smart devices are typically hardware based and have limited ability to learn.

Today, multipurpose devices are becoming more prevalent. These are devices that are capable of fulfilling a range of requests. A smart phone or next-generation television are excellent examples of multi-purpose devices. They are capable of responding to multiple types of requests. They can access the Internet. They can play movies. They can make phone calls.

Multi-purpose devices can sometimes have also primary and secondary purposes – the primary purpose of a television is obvious. As part of our interconnected world, televisions are now able to connect to the Internet. Because of these secondary capabilities, devices such as smart televisions may be able to fulfill multiple types of request – but may not be the most appropriate device in the network to respond to a request.

1.3   Problems with Current Networks of Interconnected Devices

When the network of devices is known and the purpose and function of each device is clearly defined, it is relatively straight forward and simple to define which device should respond to which command.

It is when there are several, or many independent devices available for a similar task that challenges rise. Part of the challenge is to achieve interoperability between connected devices while maintaining their "smartness" and allowing for adaptive and autonomous behavior [2]. This implies that the devices need to remain true to their purpose, but also capable of negotiating with other devices trying to fulfill similar tasks.

There are precursors to the connectivity of autonomous devices to build from. Sensor networks are collections of connected devices that are autonomous, but coordinate and communicate for a single purpose. Each device in the network has the same task and is responsible for collecting and transmitting data. The design of these networks focused on coordination to transmit data (see Fig. 2).

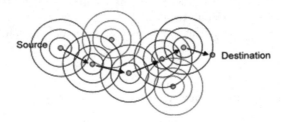

Fig. 2. Source-destination

Early challenges with sensor networks, such as network discovery, control and routing, collaborative information processing, tasking and querying, and security all set a foundation for connecting smart devices and the basis for this proposal [3]. Pervasive computing also set a foundation for communication between devices and coordination around responding to requests [4].

Networks of smart devices have advanced to become ecosystems of devices all collectively providing a function for a "user". Examples of hospitals with many monitoring devices or automated homes such as shown in Fig. 3 with devices provided an array of functions.

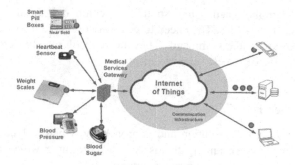

Fig. 3. Internet of Things

Even in these advanced ecosystems, the coordination and negotiation between devices is not for who can fulfill a request, but connecting, authorizing, and transferring collected data.

When several devices can fulfil a request and only one is required to do so, a whole new type of negotiation is needed. The next figure represents the high level steps required for this next evolution of negotiation (Fig. 4).

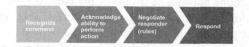

Fig. 4. Negotiation as a service process overview

The first step is discovery and identification: what the request being made, who is requesting it, and why it is needed. This request might be sent to multiple devices all capable of responding to a request. Once discovered and identified, the devices need to collaborate on a proper response. Previous work has been done providing a coordinated layer response [5].

The proposal for this paper is to go beyond the existing work. Many proposals focus on a centralized coordinator for devices, which may be possible in dedicated networks of known systems [1]. In an IoT environment, each device is autonomous and may not exist in a known or dedicated environment. To do that, the context of a request needs to be taken into account. A coordinated response among entities using services, nodes, equipment, and the infrastructure must use a specific context [6].

2   Proposed Solution

When the network and paths are not predefined, the ability of this dynamic network of smart devices to interact with each other becomes much more difficult. Our goal is to establish negotiation between a set of existing intelligent devices, all of which are capable of performing the same or similar task, to determine which device should perform a task.

In order to determine whether to respond to a command, the devices need to be aware of a number of variables. They need to be aware of where they are. They need to be aware of who issued the command. They need to ultimately determine through negotiation which device is best suited to respond.

2.1 Solution Overview

In this paper, we describe a solution and approach by which a dynamic network of smart devices can negotiate among themselves to determine which device is algorithmically better to respond to a given command.

Our focus is on two aspects of this solution.

1. The devices themselves – what must they be capable of supporting and doing to support the contextual response required. The devices must be capable of responding to a given command in order to be viable.
2. The interactions between the devices - how must the interactions be identified, the context understood, and the negotiations between the devices be done to determine best fit and most appropriate response

It must be clearly stated that being context aware is key to this solution. The devices and the device interactions must all be aware of the context of the command.

Within this solution, a command is given – spoken, sent, etc. – over standard protocols – and the appropriate devices respond to the request.

The response must be given in context – meaning that the responding device must understand:

(1) Is it capable of responding – can it fulfill the command being given?
(2) Where is the device now – understanding the context of location and network
(3) Who gave the command – understanding the context of the command giver
(4) Is the device authorized to respond to the command?
(5) Is it the appropriate device to respond? Is there another device in the network that can fulfill the response more effectively?

In this context sensitive device interaction, when a command is spoken, there may be multiple devices that are capable of responding. The following diagram shows a command being issued to a potential set of devices (Fig. 5).

These devices must understand that there are other devices in the area that may be capable of responding. When a command is given, the devices must collaborate, and based on the available contexts (who gave the command, where was the command given, etc.), determine how to respond. As the following diagram shows, as the number of enabled smart devices grows, the networks of devices can become increasingly complex. Having a standard way of determining which device should respond will become increasingly important (Fig. 6).

The first decision is both the simplest and potentially the most complex to address. For single-purpose devices, the decision is simple – am I equipped to fulfill the request or am I not. A toaster is not capable of responding to a request to turn on the television – or to find directions to the nearest sushi restaurant.

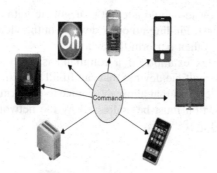

Fig. 5. Command issued

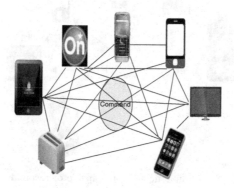

Fig. 6. Devices interact

The simplest case is when there is a single device in the area that can fulfill a request. For example, if a request is made to toast some bread, the only device that has the capability to perform that action is the toaster (Fig. 7).

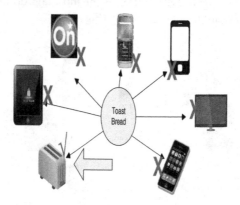

Fig. 7. Device wins simple negotiation

In this instance, the toaster would attempt to negotiate with any devices that might be able to fulfill the request. Finding no other devices in the vicinity that can fulfill the request, the toaster would then perform the action.

Using a more complex example, if a command is given, such as 'turn on the television', there may be multiple devices that can fulfill the request. Smart phones and tablets now can run applications that allow the device to perform as a television remote control. The second question must be addressed by the network of devices – which device should respond (Fig. 8)?

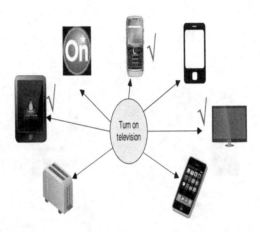

Fig. 8. Multiple devices are capable of responding

In this example, when the command is given, the devices must first answer the question "can I fulfill the request?" For the purpose of simplicity, only 2 of the smart phones, the tablet, and the smart television are all capable of turning on the television. The question that must be answered is – which device (of those four) is the most appropriate to respond to the request.

In the example above, the television itself is the most appropriate device to respond and so, responds by turning on the television (Fig. 9).

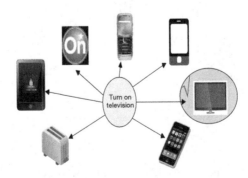

Fig. 9. Devices wins complex negotiation

Another factor is understanding and determining which devices are authorized to respond. A device may be capable of responding – but it may not be authorized to respond.

In defining this, we look at both implicit and explicit authorization, as well as rule sets. Implicit authorization may be leveraged for simple commands – which device should turn on the television. When the devices negotiate, there may be multiple devices that are capable of responding. The devices may have no explicit rules set up for responding (or not responding). Instead, the device that best satisfies the rules will win the handshake between the devices.

In the example of a command being given to 'turn on the television', the network of devices must determine which devices can respond. During negotiations, those devices that are capable of responding should determine which device is implicitly the best device to respond – in this instance, the television is capable of turning on directly without going through a remote. In this instance, the television will turn on directly.

Explicit authorization exists in this model to satisfy multiple situations. First, the owner of the device may elect to change the rules so that the remote takes precedence over the smart television. In this situation, when the command is given, the rule establishing the order of precedence and which device should respond has been set to authorize the smart remote instead of the smart television directly.

In other situations, explicit authorization is important to prevent accidental or intentional misuse. If a command to 'phone home' is given, the devices must be intelligent enough to understand the nature of the request and who is typically associated with that request. In a network of devices, each device must understand that based on the context of the request that it and it alone are qualified to make the request.

Before responding to the request, the device should know who gave the request. It may not be sufficient for the device to simply respond to the request based on whether it was capable of responding or was the best device based on feature/function. It must also be authorized to respond. In this case, commands to dial the phone is restricted to the phones owner (Fig. 10).

If the person who spoke the command is not the phones owner, the request will be ignored. Another smart device in the network may be set up to respond to that request – but the smart device that we are referring to is explicitly set up to only respond to the owners voice for this particular command.

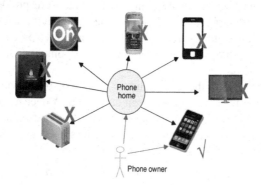

Fig. 10. Context sensitive – device owner

Finally, the device must be aware of where it is located. Many devices today have this capability in some limited fashion. For example, smart phones and tablets are aware of surrounding wi-fi networks – and automatically connect to the appropriate SSID when the opportunity presents itself – as well as being aware of their physical location via GPS coordinates.

This solution carries the analogy a bit further. The smart device must know where it is located in order to know whether it should respond to a particular request (Fig. 11).

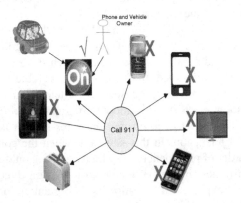

Fig. 11. Context sensitive – device location

In the case when a call to 911 is made in a vehicle, the enabled smart devices must recognize where they are. As the devices begin negotiating to determine which device should respond, the Onstar device should assert that it is the most appropriate device to respond because it is part of the vehicle – as such, it should take responsibility for making the call. Based on the negotiation rules, all other enabled smart devices should submit to this assertion.

2.2   The Solution Stack

Logically, the solution adds a 'negotiation layer' to smart devices that helps the devices negotiate and determine which device is the best device to respond (Fig. 12).

The solution stack diagram above describes the basic device stack. It begins once a command is given – either to a software-enabled smart device or a hardware-enabled smart device. These commands are received and responses provided on a defined transport layer.

Within the device, once the command is received, the device must determine whether it is capable of responding to a given command. A decision not to respond can be made because the device is not capable of responding or because according to the rules associated with the command on the device, it is not authorized to respond.

Starting from the top of the stack and moving down,

1. The transport and protocol for communicating between devices should not matter to this solution. Because Bluetooth® technology is prevalent today, we assume that it

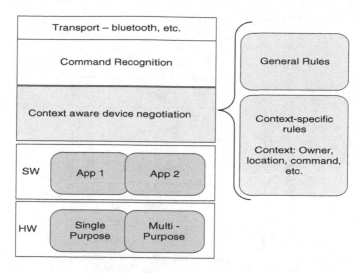

Fig. 12. Smart device solution stack

is the transport for the inter-device communications today, but it is not a requirement for our proposal. As technologies evolve, other transport technologies may take precedence and become the standard.

2. All devices must have the capability of recognizing the command - and be able to respond based on some set of rules. This context-aware negotiation module is used to determine whether a device should respond to a given command and to negotiate with other devices on which device in the network is most appropriate to respond.

3. Assuming more complex smart devices, there are special purpose software modules that may exist on the device and that may be able to respond to a request.

4. All devices will have some level of hardware involved - this layer is shown to capture the fact that both simple and complex devices are part of this ecosystem.

Responding to a Command. Assuming a device is capable and authorized to respond, when a command is recognized, the context aware device negotiation module is invoked and needs to determine how to respond.

When a command is issued, the sequence for determining which device responds should be as shown in Fig. 13 - Command Processing.

Defining the Rules for Responding to a Command. When the command is received by a device, the device should determine whether it is capable of fulfilling the request. Each of the devices that validate, authenticate, and authorize the command, will then negotiate with the other devices in the network to determine which device is best suited to respond.

There will be times when the negotiation is simple – in the case of a smart toaster in a network of smart devices, only the toaster is capable of responding to a command to 'toast bread'.

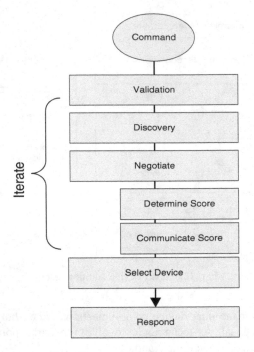

Fig. 13. command processing

In other instances, multiple devices may be capable of responding to a command. In this instance, a set of rules to sort and prioritize devices must be established. Rules should be established to understand

- Who spoke the command? Is the owner of the device the person who spoke the command?
- Where was the command spoken?
  - Was it spoken in a car?
  - What network is the device on currently? Wi-fi? 4G? etc.
- What is the social weighting of the application?
- How did the owner of the device rate or prioritize the applications on their device?

Weights or scores will be assigned to the different contexts and rules to help the devices respond with their ability to respond and their worthiness of responding. Weight may be given to the owner of the device in many cases to allow device affinity. In other cases, the network or connectivity of a device to a network – whether the device is LTE or 4G capable and can respond on a higher speed network - may skew the command toward a particular device.

Using the iteration or recursive model, the devices will broadcast their scores to the other devices. The device with the highest score will be confirmed – that device will then respond to the command.

Table 1. Proposed rules

Rule	Description
First in, first out	First device to respond to the command takes precedence
Owner of device	if voice is recognized as owner, takes priority. If the command is given using the owners voice, that device should take precedence.
Device purpose	If the device has a specialized purpose, it should (or could) take precedence.
Command location	Where was the command issued? Was it on a local network? Was it on a wi-fi network? Was it on the devices 'home network'?
Device connectivity or utilization	A rule could be set up to determine if connectivity or responding to a command would cost the owner. example - wireless vs. wifi, exceeding monthly limits
Quality of signal	For some commands, quality of signal may be critical. A device that has a higher quality of signal might need to take precedence.
Timestamp comparison	earliest timestamp takes precedence examine correlated packets - use packet timestamp to concede to packet with earliest timestamp
Deadlock break	Multiple devices may receive and indicate their ability to respond almost simultaneously. A method of breaking deadlocks must exist
<other rules>	...

If it is determined that the message is a new command, a set of rules will be evaluated - the attached table provides an example set of potential rules that could be embedded within each device (Table 1).

For some devices, the rules will be rigid - especially for single purpose devices. The rules for those devices that are multi-purpose may be customizable - through the device settings - or through a special application.

Where the time to respond to a command is critical, rules may be established to immediately execute the command without iteratively negotiating with other devices. In the case of a call to emergency services, it is more critical to reach emergency services than to determine the best device to execute the call. To prevent mis-use of this feature, rules may be embedded to only allow commands to be completed if initiated by the device owner.

Rules can be stored locally or centrally – depending on how the solution is ultimately implemented, there can be multiple layers of rules – general and context specific.

- Static rules will exist when a device only has one purpose (in the case of a toaster who can only toast bread) or soft rules
- Context sensitive rules will exist when the context of a command needs to be evaluated before responding to a request.

Whether stored centrally or distributed on each device, the rules must all be uniquely identified and associated with a given command. When the device recognizes the

Table 2. Define rules

Attribute	Definition
Command	Command that rule applies to
Rule ID	Rule identifier
Rule	Rule definition
Priority	User or system defined priority of the command
Weight	Weight of rule
Time window	Time window in which rule applies

command, it would retrieve or consult the rules for that command and determine whether the device should respond and if so, how it should respond (Table 2).

Negotiating Iterating to Determine Which Device Should Respond. Once a device receives a command and responds with its intent to respond, it should evaluate the rules for the given command and respond to the network of other devices that have indicated they can satisfy the command.

The device will evaluate the rules and respond with a message that indicates the command that was given, the timestamp that the device responded, the device-specific command ID, and the other information (Table 3).

Table 3. Response message format

Attribute	Definition
Command	Command given
Timestamp	Timestamp the device responded to command
Command ID	Unique identifier for the command on the device
Score	Score from evaluating the rules for the context-aware device

After evaluating the rules, each receiving device will respond with a status - it could indicate that it is a viable device - it could also concede because it doesn't fit the rules.

There may be instances when the weights or scores reported by the devices in a network will be the same – in that case, a set of rules to break the deadlock condition should be established – in many cases, the first device to react to the negotiation request will be given priority to respond to the command.

In the example of a command to 'find a sushi restaurant', each of the devices capable of providing a response to that command should consult their rules database and determine the weight or score of their response.

The score may be influenced by the default application on a particular device, who spoke the command, or the location of the device. In the example of a device owner asking, the device may assign a higher score because of device ownership – or even the fact that the device is OnStar capable device and the command was spoken in a car.

The device will communicate their score to the other devices in the network. Those that are still vying to fulfill the request will evaluate the scores against their score.

The devices will broadcast a response indicating whether they want to assume control or will submit to one of the other devices in the network.

Using the context sensitive device negotiation solution, the devices would interact with each other and based on a set of general or context-specific rules determine how to respond.

The devices will iterate in the context sensitive negotiation phase until only a single device responds. With our solution, devices can understand – based on the network of other devices and the rules governing the device – which device should respond to a request. With the ever increasing proliferation of smart devices in our world, being able to issue a command and have the appropriate device respond is becoming increasingly important. In this solution, based on a command, the enabled devices in the network can determine which devices are capable of responding and then negotiate which device should respond to the request.

2.3 Negotiating as a Service

The negotiation described thus far is peer-to-peer between devices to determine the best device between a set of acknowledged devices. In some situations, this may not be enough.

There are cases where 2 or more devices may be capable of handling a request just as well as any other. In these cases, an arbitrator could help decide which device to select.

Additionally, in a known location, you may want to control which device responds to a command even if you don't "own" the devices in the network. Examples of this include a hospital device ecosystem where you only want certain devices responding and you want to control which devices respond in a given situation. Even though a device may be authorized to be on the network, you may not want it to perform some actions.

Another example can be found in the workplace where smart phones are often allowed to access the corporate network. You may want to authorize the phone to respond to some commands but not others – for example, "download file" may not be a command that you want to allow your phone to fulfill.

Negotiation as a service is centered by the existence of an arbitrator. The arbitrator would understand which devices, commands, and rules it may arbitrate. The arbitrator would also recognize all commands and receive all responses from available devices. The arbitrator would then arbitrate and evaluate all responses – and determine which device should respond to a given command. The next figure shows a high level view of this (Fig. 14).

The negotiation starts with each device that has similar capabilities contacting the arbitrator and sending its identification. The arbitrator uses the identity of the devices and their capabilities to determine the appropriate device to respond.

The next 2 figures illustrate this interaction (Fig. 15).

The processing done by the arbitrator includes a similar set of rules that were described in the peer-to-peer model. After the arbitrator selects a device, the user may

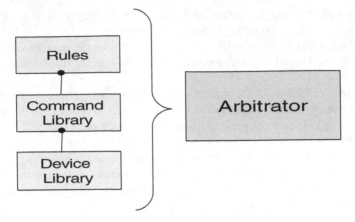

Fig. 14. Rules arbitration

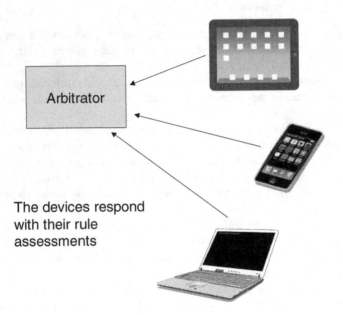

Fig. 15. Arbitrator asssess response

override that selection for another device. That override is collected and saved as a rule adjustment by the arbitrator. In this way, a social aspect of arbitration is introduced as people build up the rule engine for which devices work in certain conditions for certain sets of devices (Fig. 16).

Arbitrators can exist in multiple configurations. They can be distributed, centralized, or tiered. Tiered arbitrators can first department, then division, then corporate-wide.

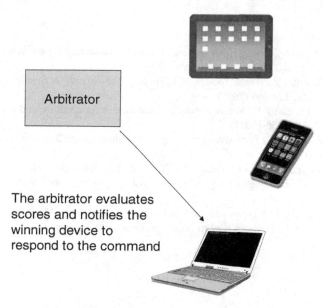

Fig. 16. Arbitrator selects device

3   Conclusion

In conclusion, we introduced a new approach focusing on context awareness that could be implemented in the Internet of Things. Commands are responded to based on many factors that theIoT could negotiate to determine the best device to respond. This approach would add an additional layer of intelligence into the IoT landscape. This approach paves the way for IoTaaS where IoT are integrated through a layer of context awareness that enables the whole paradigm as a service.

We also introduced how negotiation could be done as a service to give and addition layer of "intelligence" to the IoT device ecosystem.

4   Future Work

There are several areas we have identified that warrant further investigation. One of these areas is around security. If you, or someone else, gives a verbal command that a set of IoT devices are capable of responding to, but not owned by the requestor, how is that handled? Can I request that my neighbors' oven turn on? A level of authentication and authorization needs to be introduced into the system.

We are planning to build a prototype to illustrate the context awareness aspect and command negotiation in IoT. In addition, we are looking at the concept of device training where the IoT is updated or reduced by one or more devices. How the device introduce itself to the mesh of things, and how the network will be updated to included new contexts that been monitored by the new devices.

References

1. Guinard, D., Trifa, V., Wilde, E.: A resource oriented architecture for the Web of Things. In: Internet of Things (IOT), pp 1–8, December 2010
2. Heuser, L., Nochta, Z., Trunk, N.-C.: ICT Shaping the World: A Scientific View. Wiley Publication, ETSI, London (2008)
3. Chong, C.-Y., Kumar, S.P.: Sensor networks: evolution, opportunities, and challenges. Proc. IEEE **91**(8), 1247–1256 (2003)
4. Saha, D., Mukherjee, A.: Pervasive computing: a paradigm for the 21st century. Computer **36** (3), 25–31 (2003)
5. Future internet: The Internet of Things. In: 2010 3rd International Conference on Advanced Computer Theory and Engineering (ICACTE), vol. 5, pp. V5-376–V5-380, 20–22 Augest 2010
6. Sarma, A.C., Girão, J.: Identities in the Future Internet of Things. Wirel. Pers. Commun. **49** (3), 353–363 (2009). Find out how to access preview-only content

DIMCloud: A Distributed Framework for District Energy Simulation and Management

Francesco G. Brundu[1]([✉]), Edoardo Patti[1], Matteo Del Giudice[2],
Anna Osello[2], Enrico Macii[1], and Andrea Aquaviva[1]

[1] Department of Control and Computer Engineering, Turin, Italy
{francesco.brundu,edoardo.patti,enrico.macii,andrea.acquaviva}@polito.it
[2] Department of Structural, Construction and Geotechnical Engineering,
Politecnico di Torino, Turin, Italy
{matteo.delgiudice,anna.osello}@polito.it

Abstract. To optimize energy consumption, it is needed to monitor real-time data and simulate all energy flows. In a city district context, energy consumption data usually come from many sources and encoded in different formats. However, few models have been proposed to trace the energy behavior of city districts and handle related data. In this article, we introduce DIMCloud, a model for heterogeneous data management and integration at district level, in a pervasive computing context. Our model, by means of an ontology, is able to register the relationships between different data sources of the district and to disclose the sources locations using a publish-subscribe design pattern. Furthermore, data sources are published as Web Services, abstracting the underlying hardware from the user's point-of-view.

Keywords: Smart city · Middleware · Ubiquitous computing · Pervasive computing · Internet of things · District

1 Introduction

A single district and urban model is necessary for many purposes, including: (i) design or refurbishment of buildings; (ii) maintenance and monitoring of energy consumption; (iii) data visualization for increasing user awareness. Unfortunately, the design of such model is more difficult than collecting and analyzing data. For example, the different technologies used to collect such data produce heterogeneous information, which is difficult to integrate. Moreover, data coming from different platforms are encoded with a specific data format, and therefore not portable. Furthermore, data is usually stored in different locations and accessed using different protocols.

A common scenario involves different technologies. For instance, Building Information Model Systems (BIMs) [7] build a 3D parametric model of buildings, enriched with semantic information, such as measures, materials and costs [11].

© Institute for Computer Sciences, Social Informatics and Telecommunications Engineering 2015
R. Giaffreda et al. (Eds.): IoT360 2014, Part I, LNICST 150, pp. 331–338, 2015.
DOI: 10.1007/978-3-319-19656-5_45

On the other hand, Geographic Information Systems (GISs) [15] map the geographical location of buildings, energy distribution networks or other elements (such as smart meters). GISs are used for data automation and compilation, management, analysis and modeling of advanced cartography [5]. Finally, it is possible to have System Information Models (SIM) databases, to outline the structure of energy distribution networks with a 3D parametric model, and measurements databases, to store data collected by sensors.

In addition, a district model must satisfy the following constraints: (i) the use of underlying hardware (e.g. sensors) must be transparent from the user's point-of-view; (ii) each data source must be able to be registered into the system without needing to restart the whole infrastructure; (iii) the system must communicate by means of shared open protocols; (iv) the system must handle the data integration; (v) the data format must be open and independent from data source.

Currently, we believe there is a lack of interoperability, regarding information exchange, in district information management. Hereby we propose a distributed infrastructure for district management, which integrates and interconnects different models [6] and data sources, and delivers information by means of Web Services. This article is organized as follows: Sect. 2 presents the state-of-art in the fields of heterogeneous devices integration and BIM/GIS integration. Section 3 introduces the DIMCloud concept, outlining the different aspects of the system. Finally, Sect. 4 reports conclusions and future directions.

The research is funded by EU, FP7 SMARTCITIES 2013 District Information Modelling and Management for Energy Reduction (http://dimmer.polito.it).

2   Background

Nowadays, one of the major challenges in Ubiquitous Computing and Internet of things concerns the interoperability between heterogeneous devices. Considering a district context, this problem is even more challenging. However, middleware technologies and Services Oriented Architectures (SOA) [10] can be considered as the key issue to provide low-cost integration for enabling the communication between such heterogeneous devices. In the context of big environments, such as buildings and public spaces, middleware technologies should implement the abstraction software layer, which is the key issue to achieve a true interoperability between heterogeneous devices. In addition, they should also integrate the already existing and deployed Building Management Systems. The authors of [2] developed a modular open infrastructure, which is a complete SOA ecosystem designed to provide the capabilities of the integrated embedded devices. Finally, Stavropoulos et al. [14] introduces the aWESoME middleware, which provides uniform access to the heterogeneous Wireless Sensor and Actuator Networks (WSAN), enabling fast and direct discovery, invocation and execution of services.

Several concepts have been proposed to integrate heterogeneous data and to promote information exchange. For instance, [8] integrated BIM and GIS data to provide a Supply Chain Management framework for Construction. In this case, the BIM model traced cost and materials, while the GIS model minimized the logistics costs. Microsoft Access was used for information exchange. The authors of [4] proposed the USIM concept, an Indoor GIS Building Information Model for context-aware [3] applications. The compatibility was achieved following the IFC standard. In [8] the integration of GIS and BIM models optimized the installation of tower cranes. The GIS model located tower cranes to minimize conflicts between them. On the other hand, the BIM model represented each tower crane area to check the spatial coverage of the system, and was used to estimate the operator point-of-view. The BIM model was exported using a database (e.g. with Microsoft Access). In [9] the authors used Schema-Level Model Views, i.e. partial sub-models taken from the BIM (IFC) model and translated to the geo-spatial context into a ESRI Geodatabase (geo-spatial[1] database) or a ESRI Shapefile (a file format used to represent the geo-relational model[2]).

On the other hand, from the district energy consumption point-of-view, [16] introduced the CDIM (City District Information model) concept, which aim at integrating and managing data, to support the conception and the simulation of district energy consumption. CDIM integrates data by means of object-relational databases.

In our work, we propose a framework for simulation and visualization of energy consumption in a district context, by means of middleware and SOA concepts. To achieve it, the framework enriches BIM and SIM with real-time data collected by devices deployed in buildings and energy distribution networks.

3   Distributed Framework for District Energy Simulation and Management

In a Smart Cities context, we designed our concept DIMCloud (District Information Model Cloud) to ease the visualization and simulation of energy consumption in a city district. DIMCloud (depicted in Fig. 1(a)) links the district energy consumption data with semantic and geographic information, such as the building in which the data has been collected. In this way, it is possible to monitor in real-time the district as a whole or with a more fine-grained perspective, e.g. each single house, abstracting the pervasive distributed infrastructure of sensors. DIMCloud abstracts data sources by means of a set of specific proxies, contained in the data layer. Each proxy responds to data requests retrieving the correspondent data, adapting them to a district context (for instance, labeling them as belonging to a specific building) and converting them to a shared unique format. There are two types of proxy: Device-proxy, if data comes from a device (see Sect. 3.1), Database-proxy, if data comes from a database (see Sect. 3.2). The requests enter the integration layer and are dispatched to the correct proxy by

---

[1] http://support.esri.com/en/knowledgebase/GISDictionary/term/geospatial+technology.

[2] http://support.esri.com/en/knowledgebase/GISDictionary/term/georelational+data+model.

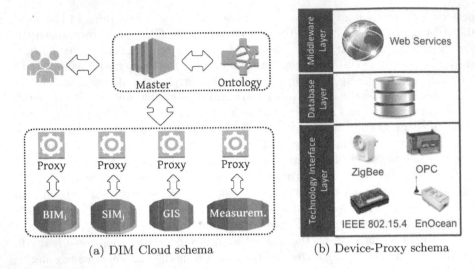

(a) DIM Cloud schema   (b) Device-Proxy schema

Fig. 1. Framework for energy simulation and management in the district.

the cloud's master node, as shown in Fig. 1(a). The references between different databases are modeled by means of an ontology and are exploited by the master node during the integration of different data (for instance, to integrate the data of a building with its geographical location and sensors measurements).

DIMCloud exploits the SEEMPubS service-oriented middleware [12]. It provides components, called managers, to develop distributed software based on both user-centric and event-based approaches. SEEMPubS, thanks to the *Network Manager*, is in charge to establish a peer-to-peer communication across the different entities in the middleware network. The SEEMPubS event-based approach is given by the *Event Manager*, which implements a publish/subscribe model. Hence, the middleware allows the development of loosely-coupled event-based systems removing all the explicit dependencies between the interacting entities. Finally, the concept of SEEMPubS *Proxy* [13] has been extended to enable the interoperability between heterogeneous devices and also to integrate the different databases, as described respectively in Sects. 3.1 and 3.2. It abstracts and eases the integration of a specific technology, device or service into a SEEMPubS application providing Web Services and registering it at a Network Manager.

3.1   Enabling Interoperability Across Heterogeneous Devices

Figure 1(b) summarizes the schema designed to implement the Proxy, which integrates heterogeneous devices into the DIMCloud and enables the interoperability between them. The Device-Proxy is a service layer for abstracting the underlying heterogeneous wireless and wired technologies. Different Device-Proxies, one for each considered technology, were developed to provide the following main features:

- enabling the integration of heterogeneous devices and interfacing them to the whole proposed infrastructure by means of Web Services, through which access sensor data;
- collecting environmental data coming from sensor nodes into a local database, which can be accessed in an asynchronous way and protected against network failures;
- pushing environmental information into the infrastructure via an event-based approach, thanks to the Event Manager;
- allowing the remote control of actuator devices.

Therefore, the Device-Proxy, as shown in Fig. 1(b), is a software which communicates directly with the heterogeneous networks and consists of three layers. The dedicated Interface, the lowest layer, directly receives all the incoming data from the devices, regardless of communication protocols, hardware or network topology. Each technology needs a specific software Interface, which interprets environmental data (e.g. Temperature, Humidity, Power Consumption, etc.) and stores them in an integrated database, which is in the second layer. Since data are stored locally, the database makes the whole infrastructure flexible and reliable with respect to backbone network failures. Finally, the SEEMPubS Web Services layer interfaces the different technologies to other components of the infrastructure, easing remote management and control, and enabling the interoperability between heterogeneous devices. From this layer, trough the Event Manager, real-time data collected by sensors are sent to other applications, such as the *Measurements Database*, which collects data coming from the district's devices.

In particular, we developed proxies for IEEE 802.15.4, ZigBee and EnOcean protocols, which are wireless technologies. Moreover, about wired technologies, it was developed a specific proxy to allow the interoperability with the OPC Unified Architecture[3], which incorporates all the features provided by different standards, such as SCADA or BACnet.

3.2   Abstracting Underlying Data Sources

Different databases store district data. Unfortunately, the integration to a unique database is not feasible, because of heterogeneity (different formats) and conflicting values (the same key can be used to identify different objects in different databases). Furthermore, the update of such database would be laborious.

In our distributed infrastructure, each database is accompanied with an interface (Database-proxy), which provides data retrieval from the database publishing a Web Service. Simultaneously, a master node of the infrastructure stores the relationships between the available proxies into an ontology. In this way, the user queries a single entry point (the master node) to receive proxies URIs. Afterwards, s/he receives the Web Service URIs of the proxies and the relationships between them. Finally, s/he retrieves the data using the proxies' Web Services and is able to integrate them.

---

[3] https://www.opcfoundation.org/UA/.

3.3   Information Modeling and Data Export

To export the models behind the Database-proxies in the DIMCloud, it was necessary to use Autodesk Revit and ESRI ArcGIS 10. The Level of Development and the Level of Detail were carefully chosen before the modeling step, referring to the American Institute of Architects (A.I.A.)[4]. In Revit we developed the model of the building with *Local Masses*. Afterwards, we enriched the BIM model with semantic information. The building and the context models were oriented and located appropriately. In addition, more informations could be inserted using *Shared parameters*. Working on ArcGIS, we defined the geographic coordinates' system and we made shapefiles (.shp) of buildings and of addresses. Shapefiles are used to store non-topological geometries and attribute informations [1], such as construction typology or data, and were developed to describe the GIS model.

   Parametric models need an export/import process, to share data between different applications. Therefore, several formats have to be tested to avoid errors and data losses. For instance, IFC[5] and CityGML[6] are two predominant standard exchange formats in the building industry. We decided to export BIM and GIS models by means of relational databases.

3.4   Exploiting Ontologies to Relate District Entities

When the master node search for the Web Service's URI of data source, it refers to an ontology. The ontology stores a model for the whole district. This model is a tree, in which the root node identifies the district and its global properties (e.g. Web Services for GIS Database-Proxy URI), and defines the relationships between different data sources. In the ontology each node connected to the root node describes a building or an energy distribution network, and it is labeled with a unique id. Each node stores:

- the Web Service's URIs for both BIM or SIM Database-Proxy;
- the ID of the BIM or SIM in the GIS Database-Proxy;
- a dictionary containing, for each sensor, its ID in the measurements' database.

Figure 2 depicts the ontology's schema. From the root node, it is possible to reach every data source in the district. Each found leaf node discloses the necessary references to query the related data sources.

3.5   Use Case: District Data Query

Figure 3 depicts the sequence diagram to retrieve the data related to a district, which can include real-time measurements, BIM and SIM models for N selected buildings and energy distribution networks respectively. The Client, for instance an application for simulation or data visualization, asks the Master (step 1) for

---

[4] http://www.aia.org/groups/aia/documents/pdf/aiab095711.pdf.
[5] http://www.buildingsmart.org/standards/ifc.
[6] http://www.citygml.org.

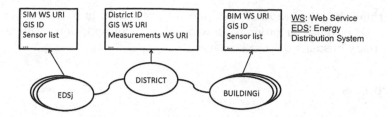

Fig. 2. Ontology schema

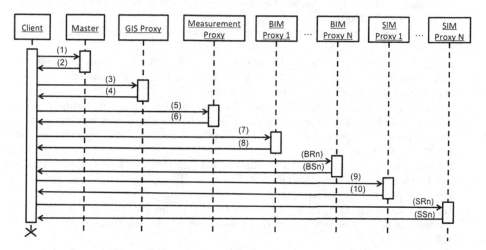

Fig. 3. District data query sequence diagram

data and Web Services URIs (proxies). The Master checks the ontology and returns (2) all the information for the requested GIS, BIM, SIM and their relative measurements. In (3) the Client asks for geographical data for the required BIM and SIM IDs to the GIS proxy, which responds in (4). Afterwards, the Client retrieves measurements data from the Measurements Proxy (5, 6). Finally, in (7) and (8), in (9) and (10) and, generically, in (BRn) and (BSn) and in (SRn) and (SSn), the Client retrieves the data from the N BIM and SIM models invoking the Web Services for the related proxies.

4   Conclusions

The CDIM approach [16] showed that a district-based simulation can be beneficial to optimize energy consumption, with respect to BIM simulations. In our work, we introduced a different model for the district, i.e. DIMCloud, in which each data source is reachable by means of a Web Service proxy. The underlying hardware is available as a service, and the user can query in the same way heterogeneous sources, to monitor real-time energy consumption in the district.

We think that the proposed system can be of crucial importance to manage district energy data, in order to develop energy consumption awareness and sustainability in smart district scenarios.

References

1. Esri shapefile tecnical description. ESRI White paper (1998)
2. Candido, G., Colombo, A.W., Barata, J., Jammes, F.: Service-oriented infrastructure to support the deployment of evolvable production systems. IEEE Trans. Ind. Inf. **7**, 759–767 (2009)
3. Chen, G., Kotz, D.: A survey of context-aware mobile computing research. Technical report TR2000-381, pp. 1–16 (2000)
4. Choi, J.W., Kim, S.A., Lertlakkhanakul, J., Yeom, J.H.: Developing ubiquitous space information model for indoor gis service in ubicomp environment. In: Proceedings of 4th IEEE NCM 2008, pp. 381–388 (2008)
5. de Pina Filho, A.C., Lima, F.R., Dias Calado do Amaral, R.: Computational Tools applied to Urban Engineering, Methods and Techniques in Urban Engineering
6. Del Giudice, M., Osello, A., Patti, E.: Bim and gis for district modeling. In: ECPPM 2014 Conference, Vienna (2014)
7. Eastman, C., Teicholz, P., Sacks, R., Liston, K.: Bim Handbook: A Guide to Building Information Modeling for Owners, Managers, Designers, Engineers, and Contractors. Wiley, New Jersey (2008)
8. Irizarry, J., Karan, E.P., Jalaei, F.: Integrating BIM and GIS to improve the visual monitoring of construction supply chain management. Autom. Constr. **31**, 241–254 (2013)
9. Isikdag, U., Underwood, J., Aouad, G.: An investigation into the applicability of building information models in geospatial environment in support of site selection and fire response management processes. Adv. Eng. Inf. **22**(4), 504–519 (2008)
10. Karnouskos, S.: The cooperative internet of things enabled smart grid. In: Proceedings of the 14th IEEE ISCE, Braunschweig, Germany, June 2010
11. Osello, A.: The Future of Drawing with BIM for Engineers and Architects. Dario Flaccovio Editore, Palermo (2012)
12. Patti, E., Acquaviva, A., Jahn, M., Pramudianto, F., Tomasi, R., Rabourdin, D., Virgone, J., Macii, E.: Event-driven user-centric middleware for energy-efficient buildings and public spaces. IEEE Syst. J. (2014)
13. Patti, E., Acquaviva, A., Macii, E.: Enable sensor networks interoperability in smart public spaces through a service oriented approach. In: Proceedings of 5th IEEE IWASI, pp. 2–7, June 2013
14. Stavropoulos, T.G., Gottis, K., Vrakas, D., Vlahavas, I.: aWESoME: a web service middleware for ambient intelligence. Expert Syst. Appl. **40**(11), 4380–4392 (2013)
15. Tomlinson, R.F.: A geographic information system for regional planning. J. Geogr. (Chigaku Zasshi) **78**(1), 45–48 (1969)
16. Wolisz, H., Böse, L., Harb, H., Streblow, R., Müller, D.: City district information modeling as a foundation for simulation and evaluation of smart city approaches. In: Proceedings of Building Simulation and Optimization Conference. UCL, London (2014)

Model-Driven Development for Internet of Things: Towards Easing the Concerns of Application Developers

Arpan Pal, Arijit Mukherjee$^{(\boxtimes)}$, and Balamuralidhar P.

Innovation Labs, Tata Consultancy Services, Kolkata, Bangalore, India
{arpan.pal,mukherjee.arijit,balamurali.p}@tcs.com

Abstract. Internet-of-Things (IoT) is poised for a disruptive growth in near future with wide and easy deployments of sensor connected to Internet. Horizontal service platforms for IoT are increasingly gaining prominence for quick development and deployment of IoT applications. However, IoT application development needs diverse skill and knowledge from domain, analytics, infrastructure and programming, which is difficult to find in one application developer. In this paper we introduce a Model-driven-development (MDD) framework that tries to address the above issue by separating out the concern of different stakeholders through models and knowledgebases.

Keywords: Iot · MDD · Knowledgebase · Meta model · Service platform

1 Introduction

The Internet of Things (IoT) has already been recognized by researchers and analysts as one of the most disruptive technologies that will transform human lives and have major economic impact. People foresee lot of penetration of IoT technology in large-scale, complex applications such as Smart Cities, Smart Transportation, Smart Manufacturing, Smart Healthcare etc. Given the complexity of the system, there is increasing requirement for IoT development platforms providing different services.

In this paper we present the case for a model-driven framework to develop and deploy IoT applications and services on top of an IoT platform. In Sect. 2, we present the requirements of such a framework and provide a technology gap analysis. In Sect. 3, we present the proposed Model-driven-development (MDD) framework for IoT platforms. Finally we summarize and conclude in Sect. 4.

2 Need for Model-Driven-Development in IoT

IoT applications, traditionally, like all other embedded applications, are built bottom up as per vertical requirements. It starts with sensor integration, moving into sensor data collection using sensor networking, storing the collected data and finally analyzing the stored data to draw actionable insights [1, 2].

However, instead of taking the bottom-up vertical approach for application development, it is beneficial to have a horizontal, platform-driven approach [3].

© Institute for Computer Sciences, Social Informatics and Telecommunications Engineering 2015
R. Giaffreda et al. (Eds.): IoT360 2014, LNICST 150, pp. 339–346, 2015.
DOI: 10.1007/978-3-319-19656-5_46

A model-driven-development (MDD) approach that can abstract out the meta-model of the IoT system and automate much of the application development process allowing the application developer to focus only on domain specific concerns will be of high interest to the industry.

Many of the existing IoT service platforms, support features like user management, resource provisioning, application life cycle management, device management and configuration, connectivity service provisioning and management etc. [3]. Another such platform (TCS Connected Universe Platform - TCUP) [4] tries to address a few of the above concerns by providing an integrated application development platform covering device management, data storage and management, an API based application development framework and a distributed application deployment framework.

However, none of these actually addresses the issues related to ease of application development like code reusability, need for multiple skills in domain, analytics, sensors, programming etc., or visibility of data across application.. These can be addressed through the concept of separation of concerns among different stakeholders – this has been already prevalent in the area of MDD and recently it has been also applied in the context of IoT [5, 6] which provides a framework to specify the requirements at different levels. However, this framework does not address issues like analytics algorithm re-use, distributed execution of analytics, generation of analytics and reasoning workflows, a common ontology and semantics for sensor data etc. needed for a full-fledged MDD.

On MDD systems implementation side, OASIS [12] has brought out a new standard meta model for IT services "The Topology and Orchestration Specification for Cloud Applications" (TOSCA) [13] for improving portability of cloud applications to address the challenges related to heterogeneous application environments. In TOSCA, the structure of a service is defined by the Topology Template, a directed graph, which consists of Node Templates and Relationship Templates. Node Template is an instantiation of Node Type which defines the properties and operations of a component. TOSCA uses plans, a process model defining complex workflows that can be used for the management process of creating, deploying and terminating services. TOSCA specifies an XML based syntax for defining the entities described above. For the plans it relies on existing business process modeling languages such as BPEL [14] and BPMN [15]. Some initial exploration has been reported on using TOSCA as a meta-model for IoT services [11]. From our studies we observe that this approach has a potential for addressing multiple views of the IoT application development and is much suited for offering the services following a Platform-as-a-Service (PaaS) model.

In this paper, we propose an integrated MDD framework as part of an IoT Service Platform.

3   Proposed Model-Driven Framework

A typical IoT platform caters to the needs of four different types of users or stakeholders – Applications Developers, Sensor Providers, End Users and Platform Administrators. Out of these four types of stakeholders, the focus of the proposed MDD framework is the Application Developer and the Sensor Provider. We further sub-divide sensor providers into sensor manufacturers and sensor service providers and application developers into domain experts, application programmers and algorithm experts. In subsequent paragraphs we show how these stakeholders interact with the MDD framework.

3.1   Support Knowledgebase for MDD

Sensor Knowledgebase – The sensor knowledgebase is contributed by multiple stakeholders. The sensor device manufacturer can register the sensor in the system providing information on sensor make/model, features, operating conditions (information that is available in datasheets of sensors) along with details on sensor communication interfaces/protocols, device drivers, sensor data models etc. The sensors are normally instantiated and provisioned in the system by the sensor service provider where they add additional metadata like deployment time/location, user details etc. This knowledge base then can be used by the application developer to query specific sensors via the Sensor Explorer Interface [7].

Analytics Algorithm Knowledgebase – The analytics algorithm knowledgebase is contributed mainly by the algorithm writers and experts. It not only contains the archive of algorithm executables in form of libraries, it also contains metadata about algorithms detailing their application areas, performance parameters, accuracy, CPU complexity, memory load etc. This knowledge base can be used by the application developers to query and look for specific algorithms suitable for their application [8].

Domain-Specific Knowledgebase – Finally the application developers are primarily concerned about solving a specific set of domain problems. They are expected to be having good programming skill but limited domain knowledge, sensor knowledge and algorithm analytics knowledge. The domain-specific knowledgebase that is populated by domain experts intend to bridge this gap by providing knowledge like mapping between physical phenomenon and sensor observation, mapping between sensor application and sensor technology etc.

Infrastructure Knowledgebase – Application developers, after development of applications, need to deploy them – typically part of the applications run on edge or gateway devices collecting sensor data and part of the applications run on the cloud [9, 10]. The infrastructure knowledgebase needs to collect information about the compute/memory/communication capabilities of the available gateway devices, available gateway-to-cloud communication channels, storage capacity of the cloud and detail of available compute hardware in infrastructure of the cloud. All this knowledgebase is typically contributed by the System Administrator.

3.2   Proposed Model Driven Framework

Here we propose a model driven framework for easy development and life-cycle management of IoT applications. The motivation is to use the skills of existing IT workforce to easily understand and develop the IoT applications using an abstract layer hiding the heterogeneity and complexity of underlying diverse technologies.

An IoT application in totality has multiple views and respective design concerns (Fig. 3). Following views can be considered to capture major design dimensions (as illustrated in Fig. 1 with their respective dependencies on knowledgebase):

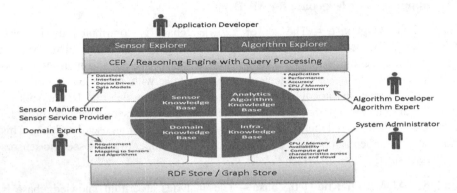

Fig. 1. Support knowledgebase structure for MDD

Information Flow and Evolution – An IoT application can be viewed as a set of data flows from sensor to sinks (actuator, database, reports, visualizer) traversing many computing operations that transforms the data to various information elements. This information flow can be modeled as a directed graph with nodes as computing modules that computes the designated information element. The edges indicate the input/output dependency relation. This also serves as a semantic model for the IoT application. It can also map to domain ontology (Sect. 3.1) through a suitable semantic mapping. Figure 2 depicts the flow graph corresponding to an example vehicle telematics service.

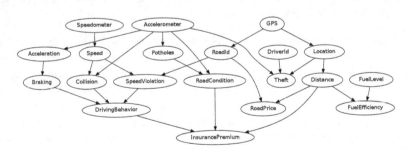

Fig. 2. Information flow graph corresponding to a vehicle telematics application - the raw sensor data is generated at the root nodes (Speedometer, accelerometer, GPS, fuel level)

Each of these nodes requires a specification of the computing model or algorithm to be used for computing the designated information element(s). There could be standard re-usable computing blocks that can be used across applications or there can be application specific algorithms. Some of the computing operations may involve a rule engine or a complex event processing. But in general they are highly domain specific and need to be developed with the help of domain experts. The developer may seek the help of an algorithm explorer tool (introduced in Sect. 3.1) to pick the most suitable algorithm to compute the desired information element and specify it as a node property.

Node Binding to Devices – In a typical IoT application, sensing and computing may span multiple devices/platforms. For example in healthcare application a smartphone may be used to sense the vital parameters and the preprocessing, aggregation and diagnostics may be partitioned across smart phone, and cloud platform. Here we view the partitioning of the computing flow graph into sub-graphs and binding suitable computing devices to execute them. A sub-graph may be assigned to run on a Linux box, or a mobile phone. Further it may use a CEP engine or a JavaME environment to run. Specific device with its detailed specifications can be selected from the Infrastructure Knowledgebase and set the related node property. If it is computing node then the designated algorithm should have compatibility with the device chosen. If it is a sensor node then the selected device should have the required support. The respective knowledgebase (KB) described in Sect. 3.1 will be helpful in ensuring this compatibility.

Communication of Software Modules Within and Across Devices – When the computing operations are modularized, there is need for specifying the communication mechanism between these modules. The connected modules within same computing environment can use standard parameter passing mechanisms, messaging or interprocess communication primitives. Communication across devices will require external interfaces such as USB, Bluetooth, Zigbee, Wi-Fi 2G/3G etc. Further the nature of data exchange may follow models of REST, Pub-Sub, Proxy etc. The edges in the flow graph model can be used to capture the communication interface details. As in the case of device binding, the infrastructure knowledge base will be used to check the compatibility and consistency.

Security Bindings to Devices, Software and Information – The security schemes for data while communicating, storage and transformation are captured in this view. The specification is applied to a path in the sub graph spanning two end-points. Identity, credentials and security keys are also to be specified.

Deployment and Orchestration – This view captures the information to build the executable software modules, test and deploy them to the target devices. Also the specification of operational behaviors of the entire system that need to orchestrate during the operation is also specified in this view.

We need to have an underlying meta-model to represent all of the above dimensions of an IoT service and a user friendly environment to build and deploy the application from its specifications. Recently there is a development framework proposed in [6, 7] which uses Srijan language specifications as a meta-model. In our opinion they have some shortcomings in representing some of the specific contexts of IoT applications including communications, temporal behavior of the system and business process orchestrations. Probably that language can be extended to support

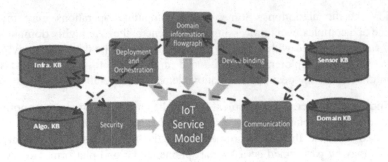

Fig. 3. Different views of an IoT application

these aspects. Here we explore the use of another meta-model specified for cloud applications.

4 Initial Prototype and Experimental Results

We have built an initial prototype which covers some of the aspects mentioned in the paper. The prototype is built and tested on a set of use-cases primarily linked with the healthcare domain. In this section, we explain the principles using one of the use-cases where a mobile phone camera is used as an optical sensor to capture the video of a person's index finger using which the heart-rate is calculated based on the concepts of PPG (photoplethysmogram) [17]. In this method, the video signal from the camera is converted to a PPG signal which is then processed following the steps of a typical signal processing workflow (as shown in Fig. 4).

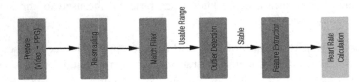

Fig. 4. Workflow showing steps to calculate heart-rate using PPG

To assist the application developer at each stage, several components have been built, although each of these is at a very nascent stage, but are capable of sufficiently underlying the concepts proposed in this paper. As a starting point, an application developer must discover sensors capable of generating a video signal which can be used for PPG. Figure 5 shows a snapshot of the SensorExplorer component (the sensor knowledgebase) which semantically links the sensors and the metadata from which the application developer can discover sensors using temporal/spatial/spatio-temporal queries [18]. We have used standard technologies such as SensorML, RDF to create ontologies for all involved entities such as sensors, algorithms etc. These graph based models enable the development of a visual programming interface where the developer can assemble a flow graph using nodes and relations from a library. With suitable pre-built command they can test and validate the compiled application and deploy over a real infrastructure. The open source tool "Node_RED" [16] is an example of such visual tool for workflow development which we plan to use in our implementation.

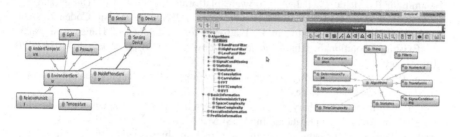

Fig. 5. Semantic linking of sensors and algorithms

Once a sensor and the corresponding data stream is discovered, the application developer creates the signal processing workflow by selecting different algorithms for each workflow step. At this stage, another component, namely the Algopedia (the algorithm knowledgebase), which is an annotated repository of algorithms (shown in Fig. 5), assists the developer to select the algorithms based on the data type, sensor type, and other algorithmic requirements which are available as metadata in the algorithm ontology. The workflow created at this step is then tested and deployed using information from the infrastructure knowledgebase and it has been found that the results are comparable to the output of similar workflows created after numerous experiments and considerable development effort by developers who are experienced in the domain. The sensor and algorithm knowledgebase semantically link information of sensors used to capture information in the healthcare domain and algorithms used to process the signals from such sensors. As of now, the domain knowledgebase is rudimentary in nature, but we plan to build it using information retrieved from several sources available over the Web.

5   Conclusion

In this paper we have introduced a MDD based framework for application development for IoT platforms. The concept of MDD specific to IoT is a recent one. Our proposed framework tries to separate and abstract out concerns of different stakeholders in IoT application development through use of models and knowledgebase, thereby improving the ease of application development. In this paper we present the concept and possible approaches to implement it. As future work, we intend to develop specific applications using the proposed framework and measure the ease of application development experienced by the developer community.

References

1. Gubbi, J., Buyya, R., Marusic, S., Palaniswami, M.: Internet of Things (IoT): a vision, architectural elements, and future directions. Elsevier J. Future Gener. Comput. Syst. **29**, 1645–1660 (2013)
2. Balamurali, P., Misra, P., Pal, A.: Software platforms for Internet of Things and M2M. J. Indian Inst. Sci. Multi. Rev. J. **93**(3), 1–12 (2013). ISSN: 0970-4140 Coden-JIISAD
3. Köhler, M., Wörner, D., Wortmann, F.: Platforms for the Internet of Things – An Analysis of Existing Solutions. http://cocoa.ethz.ch/downloads/2014/02/1682_20140212%20-%20Bocse.pdf
4. Misra, P., et al.: A computing platform for development and deployment of sensor data based applications and services. Patent No. WO2013072925 A2
5. Patel, P., Morin, B., Chaudhary, S.: A model-driven development framework for developing sense-compute-control applications. In: MoSEMInA 2014, 31 May 2014
6. Patel, P., Pathak, A., Cassou, D., Issarny, V.: Enabling high-level application development in the Internet of Things. In: Zuniga, M., Dini, G. (eds.) S-Cube. LNICST, vol. 122, pp. 111–126. Springer, Heidelberg (2013)
7. Dasgupta, R.; Dey, S.; A comprehensive sensor taxonomy and semantic knowledge representation: energy meter use case. In: 7th International Conference on Sensing Technology (2013)
8. Maiti, S., et al.: Repository and Recommendation System for Computer Implemented Functions. Indian Patent Application No: 918/MUM/2014
9. Bonomi, F., Milito, R., Zhu, J., Addepalli, S.: Fog computing and its role in the Internet of Things. In: Proceedings of the First Edition of the MCC Workshop on Mobile Cloud Computing, MCC 2012, New York, NY, USA, pp. 13–16. ACM (2012)
10. Mukherjee, A., Paul, H.S., Dey, S., Banerjee, A.: Angels for distributed analytics in IoT. In: 2014 IEEE World Forum on Internet of Things (WF-IoT), pp. 565–570. IEEE (2014)
11. Li, F., Vögler, M., Claeßens, M., Dustdar, S.: Towards automated IoT application deployment by a cloud-based approach. In: IEEE 6th International Conference on Service-Oriented Computing and Applications (SOCA) (2013)
12. Organization for the Advancement of Structured Information Standards (OASIS) https://www.oasis-open.org/
13. Topology and Orchestration Specification for Cloud Applications, V1.0. November 2013. OASIS. http://docs.oasis-open.org/tosca/TOSCA/v1.0/os/TOSCA-v1.0-os.html
14. Business Process Execution Language (BPEL). https://www.oasis-open.org/committees/wsbpel
15. Business Process Model and Notation (BPMN). http://www.bpmn.org/
16. Node-Red, A visual tool for wiring the Internet of Things. http://nodered.org/
17. Pal, A., Sinha, A., Choudhury, A.D., Chattopadhyay, T., Viswanathan, A.: A robust heart-rate detection using smartphone video. In: 3rd ACM MobiHoc Workshop on Pervasive Wireless Healthcare (2013)
18. Dasgupta, R., Dey, S.: A comprehensive sensor taxonomy and semantic knowledge representation: energy meter usecase. In: 7th International Conference on Sensing Technology (ICST), pp 791–799 (2013)

Domain Specific Modeling (DSM) as a Service for the Internet of Things and Services

Amir H. Moin[✉]

fortiss, An-Institut Technische Universität München, Munich, Germany
moin@fortiss.org

Abstract. In this paper, we propose a novel approach for developing Sense-Compute-Control (SCC) applications for the Internet of Things and Services (IoTS) following the Model-Driven Software Engineering (MDSE) methodology. We review the recent approaches to MDSE and argue that Domain Specific Modeling (DSM) suites our needs very well. However, in line with the recent trends in cloud computing and the emergence of the IoTS, we believe that both DSM creation tools and DSM solutions that are created via those tools should also be provided to their respective users in a service-oriented fashion through the cloud in the IoTS. In this work, we concentrate on the latter, i.e., DSM solutions that are created via a DSM creation tool. We argue that it makes sense for the owners of a DSM solution in a domain to provide their DSM solution as a service, following the well known Software as a Service (SaaS) model, to the interested customers through the IoTS. Our proposed approach concentrates on such a DSM solution for developing SCC applications in the IoTS. However, the idea could be applied to DSM solutions in other domains as well.

Keywords: internet of things and services · model-driven software engineering · domain specific modeling · development as a service · cloud computing

1 Introduction

Similar to the rapid spread of the Internet among human users in the 1990s, the Internet Protocol (IP) is currently rapidly spreading into new domains, where constrained embedded devices such as sensors and actuators also play an important role. This expanded version of the Internet is referred to as the Internet of Things (IoT) [1]. On the other hand, the convergence between Web 2.0 and Service Oriented Architecture (SOA), has led to the creation of a global SOA on top of the World Wide Web (WWW), known as the Internet of Services (IoS) [2]. The combination of the IoT and the IoS is referred to as the Internet of Things and Services (IoTS). This emerging vision together with Cyber Physical Systems (CPS), in which the physical world merges with the virtual world of cyberspace [3], are believed to have sufficient power to trigger the next (i.e., fourth) industrial revolution [4].

© Institute for Computer Sciences, Social Informatics and Telecommunications Engineering 2015
R. Giaffreda et al. (Eds.): IoT360 2014, Part I, LNICST 150, pp. 347–354, 2015.
DOI: 10.1007/978-3-319-19656-5_47

However, with this great power often comes an enormous degree of complexity as well as an extremely high cost of design, development, test, deployment and maintenance for software systems too. One of the main reasons is the multi-disciplinary nature of the field of the IoTS. A number of major challenges in this field are scalability, heterogeneity of things and services, variety of protocols, communication among stakeholders and fast pace of technological advances.

In particular, here we are interested in Sense-Compute-Control (SCC) applications [5], a typical group of applications in the IoTS. A SCC application senses the environment (e.g., temperature, humidity, light, UV radiation, etc.) through sensors, performs some computation (often decentralized, i.e., distributed) and finally prompts to take one or more actions through actuators (very often sort of control) in the environment. There exist two main differences between these applications in the IoTS and the similar ones in the field of Wireless Sensor and Actuator Networks (WSAN), a predecessor of the field of the IoTS. First, the scale of the network is quite different. While WSANs typically have several hundreds or thousands of nodes, SCC applications in the IoTS may have several millions or billions of nodes. Second, the majority of nodes in a WSAN are more or less similar to each other. However, here in the IoTS we have a wide spectrum of heterogeneous devices, ranging from tiny sensor motes with critical computational, memory and energy consumption constraints to highly capable servers for cloud computing. Heterogeneity is a property inherited from another predecessor field, known as Pervasive (Ubiquitous) computing [6].

A recent trend in software engineering for dealing with complexity through raising the level of abstraction is Model-Driven Software Engineering (MDSE). In this paper, we advocate Domain Specific Modeling (DSM), a state-of-the-art approach to the MDSE methodology, for addressing the above mentioned challenges. DSM not only provides a very high level of abstraction by letting domain experts model the design specifications in their own technical jargon (i.e., the domain vocabulary), but also lets complete code generation in a fully automated manner.

The paper makes three main contributions:

1. It reviews the three mainstream recent approaches to the MDSE methodology.
2. It proposes MDSE in general, and DSM in particular, for addressing the above mentioned challenges and increasing the development productivity in the domain of SCC applications in the IoTS.
3. In line with the recent trends in cloud computing, i.e., Software as a Service (SaaS), Platform as a Service (PaaS), Infrastructure as a Service (IaaS), data model as a service, etc., and with the emergence of the Internet of Things and Services (IoTS), also Sensor/Actuator as a Service, Integrated Development Environments (IDEs) as well as integrated Model-Driven Software Engineering (MDSE) tools have also got the opportunity to expose themselves to users in a service-oriented fashion through the cloud, called Development as a Service (DaaS), IDE as a Service or Modeling tool as a Service. We propose DSM solution as a Service.

The rest of this paper is structured as follows: Section 2 reviews the three major recent approaches to the Model-Driven Software Engineering (MDSE) methodology. In Sect. 3, we propose our novel approach for addressing the above mentioned challenges. This is followed by a brief literature review in Sect. 4. Finally, we conclude and mention our future work in Sect. 5.

2 Model-Driven Software Engineering (MDSE)

In fact, the idea of applying models with different levels of abstraction in order to develop software according to the design intent rather than the underlying computing environment [7], a field that used to be better known as model-based software engineering (or model-based development), has a long tradition in software engineering [8], which dates back to over five decades ago. Computer-Aided Software Engineering (CASE) tools of the 1980s and the 1990s are the famous examples of such efforts. However, although those tools were attractive and interesting at their time, in practice, they did not really affect the software industry too much. One major reason was that they mapped poorly to the underlying platforms. Moreover, they were not scalable enough to support large projects [7]. Also, their modeling language as well as code generators were all hard-coded (fixed) by tool vendors. Thus, the user of those tools had no control on the modeling language nor on the generators in order to adapt them to his or her needs and evolving requirements. Unfortunately, this is true for many existing CASE tools in the present time too.

In this section, we briefly review the three major recent approaches to the MDSE methodology.

2.1 Model-Driven Architecture (MDA)

In 2001, the Object Management Group (OMG) adopted a standard architectural framework for MDSE known as Model-Driven Architecture (MDA) [9], which was a key step towards standardization and dissemination of MDSE. MDA defines three default levels of abstraction on a system in order to address Separation of Concerns (SoC) among the stakeholders. Firstly, a Computation Independent Model (CIM) defines the business logic independent of any kind of computational details and system implementation concerns. Secondly, a Platform Independent Model (PIM) is created based on the CIM. The model transformation from CIM to PIM is often done manually or in a semi-automated manner by information technology and computer science experts. A PIM defines a set of parts and services of the system independently of any specific technology and platform. Finally, a Platform Specific Model (PSM) defines the concrete implementation of the system on a specific platform and is generated from a PIM by means of model-to-model transformations in an automated manner. Later, a number of (model-to-model and) model-to-text transformations generate the implementation including the source code out of the PSM for that specific platform. The generated implementation is usually not complete and still needs some manual development.

MDA uses Meta-Object Facility (MOF) for its metamodeling architecture. The modeling languages that are used on the PIM and PSM levels are either UML (or UML profiles) or other MOF- or EMOF-based Domain Specific Modeling Languages (DSMLs).

Although the separation of concerns through different levels of abstraction for models in MDA is very interesting, in practice since iterative model refinements are typical and model transformations are very often not bidirectional, i.e., one cannot automatically go up in the modeling layers, e.g., from PSM to PIM, due to modifications in models on the PSM level, we will easily end up in inconsistencies in the models and serious maintenance problems in the long term. Moreover, another drawback of the MDA approach is that the generated code is often not complete and still needs manual development in order to become the final usable product.

2.2 Model-Driven Software Development (MDSD)

Model-Driven Software Development (MDSD) [10] prevents the crucial maintenance problem that we mentioned for MDA by avoiding iterative model refinements. In other words, no round-trip engineering is performed. A model in MDSD should have all required platform-specific details (for one or more platforms), so that it could be directly transformed to the source code through model-to-code transformations. Moreover, any modifications to the system should be done on the model level.

The main concentration of a model in MDSD is on the architecture of the software. However, the business logic is implemented manually in handwritten code rather than being generated out of the model. Following this approach could lead to about 60 % to 80 % of automatically generated code [11]. Furthermore, the source code of the final product in the MDSD approach consists of three main parts [11]:

1. *Generic code:* This part of the source code is specific to each platform. The idea is to generate this part automatically for each platform.
2. *Schematic code:* This part of the source code is generated out of the platform-independent architecture model of an application through model-to-text transformations. Depending on the target platform, the model is transformed differently.
3. *Individual code:* This part is specific to each application and contains its business logic. This part should be written by developers manually.

Similar to the MDA approach, the MDSD approach could not lead to 100 % code generation either. Therefore, one needs to keep the generated code separated from the handwritten code.

2.3 Domain Specific Modeling (DSM)

About five decades ago, software development was mainly shifted from the Assembly language to high-level third-generation programming languages (3GLs) like BASIC. This shift led to about 450 % of productivity leap on average. However, the migration from BASIC to Java has only caused an improvement of about 20 % in the development productivity on average. This is due to the fact that almost all the third-generation programming languages such as BASIC, FORTRAN, PASCAL, C, C++, Java, etc. are more or less on the same level of abstraction. Furthermore, although models are abstract representations that should hide complexity and one expects modeling languages to provide a higher level of abstraction than programming languages, however, in practice, general-purpose modeling languages such as the Unified Modeling Language (UML) often have a one-to-one correspondence between modeling elements and code elements. Therefore, they cannot hide the complexity so much. In fact, with both programming languages and general-purpose modeling languages, developers must first try to solve the problem in the problem domain using the domain's terminology, then they should map the domain concepts to development concepts, i.e., to source code elements in case of programming languages and to modeling elements in case of general-purpose modeling languages without any tool support [12].

In contrast, Domain Specific Modeling (DSM) is based upon two pillars: domain specificity and automation. The first one means DSM lets one specify the solution in a language that directly uses concepts and rules from a specific problem domain rather than the programming concepts and rules (i.e., concepts and rules of the solution domain). Thus, it tremendously increases the productivity. According to many industrial reports, employing DSM solutions in various domains has led to an average productivity leap of between 3 to 10 times (i.e., 300 % to 1000 %) comparing the general-purpose modeling and manual programming approaches. The second one means complete and automated generation of the final product, including the source code in a programming language, out of models without any need for further development and manual modifications. This is somehow analogous to the role that compilers play for 3GLs. Unlike domain specificity, which is also the case in some other MDSE approaches (e.g., in some MDA- and MDSD-based approaches which use DSMLs instead of general-purpose modeling languages such as UML), automation is an essential property of DSM that distinguishes it from other MDSE approaches [12].

3   DSM as a Service

Recall from the mentioned major challenges for developing SCC applications for the IoTS in Sect. 1 (i.e., scalability, heterogeneity of things and services, variety of protocols, communication among stakeholders and fast pace of technological advances), we believe that DSM is the best choice to address those challenges. Firstly, due to providing full automation and complete code generation (not only source code, but even other artifacts such as documentation, build scripts, configuration files, etc.), it helps a lot in dealing with the scalability challenges. Secondly, different code generators (i.e., model-to-text transformations) can generate the implementation and APIs for different heterogeneous hardware and software platforms as well as various communication protocols out of the same model. The code generators are developed once, but work for as many times as one needs to generate the implementation out of a model. Furthermore, since the modeling languages use the terms, concepts and rules of the problem domain instead of software development (i.e., the solution domain's) terms, concepts and rules, the communication among stakeholders will be definitely much easier, comparing using general purpose modeling or programming languages. Last but not least, to cope with the fast pace of technological advances, one needs to maintain the code generators over time to adapt the old ones or create new ones that can generate the implementation for new platforms, protocols, etc. As mentioned, DSM creation tools give full control to their users over their modeling languages and code generators in order to adapt them to their evolving needs. This latter feature is also a property of MDA and MDSD.

Complete and automated code generation is possible in DSM mainly because of two reasons. First, because DSM is specific to a very narrow problem domain. For instance, the automotive domain is too broad as a domain in DSM, whereas the infotainment system of a particular car manufacturer could be a proper candidate to be a domain in DSM. Second, because unlike in the CASE tools of the 1980 s and the 1990s (and many other existing ones in the present time), meta-modeling tools (e.g., the free open source Eclipse Modeling Framework (EMF)) which are used to create DSM solutions let their users have full control over their modeling languages as well as code generators, whereas in CASE tools both were hardcoded (i.e., fixed) by the tool vendors in advance. Hence, in DSM's view, there is no one-size-fits-all solution. Instead, every organization should come up with its own solution either by developing it from scratch or by tailoring an existing one (if it is publicly available) to its needs. Moreover, as time goes on, due to changes in the requirements, business logic, technologies, etc. one needs to maintain and adapt the DSM solution [12].

However, not all organizations can afford the cost of building their own DSM solution from scratch. One option would be to reuse a free open source one, if there is any in the exact particular narrow target domain, and tailor it to one's needs. But, this is not really a realistic option, since those companies who own a good DSM solution consider it as their key asset. Therefore, they often do not disclose it. In this paper, we propose a novel idea to address this issue. We argue that it actually makes sense for the owners of a DSM solution in a domain to provide their DSM solution as a service, following the well known Software as a Service (SaaS) model (more specifically Development as a Service, IDE as a Service and Modeling tool as a Service), to the interested customers through the IoTS. This will not only help the customer of the DSM solution save costs, but will also let the DSM solution owner make money out of it. Moreover, comparing traditional DSM solutions (i.e., non-SaaS), this will be much easier to use (no need for installation, configuration, etc.) and also more friendly to collaboration via model repositories, since everything is basically stored on the cloud.

However, the key point here is that if the provided DSM solution service does not allow its users to access the modeling languages or change the code generators in order to adapt them to their needs, then we are, unfortunately, back to the traditional CASE tools, where the modeling languages and code generators were hardcoded (i.e., fixed) by tool vendors. It is clear that such a tool can support complete and fully automated code generation only in very rare cases, where the narrow application domains have 100 % overlap with each other. Therefore, in order to make the service more valuable and useful to a broader range of audience, the service must at least allow the users to write new code generators of their own on demand. Of course, this requires having (read) access to the metamodel of the modeling language.

This way, users may either use the DSM solution, as it is, as a service, or they could write their own code generators and may still use some of the provided ones as services. Moreover, one could compose these services from different DSM solution service providers. In any case, the service provider does not have to disclose the source code of the code generators.

4   Related Work

The general concept of providing software that is used for creating other software as a service on the cloud already exists in a number of web-based tools ranging from web-based IDEs such as the Cloud9 IDE[1], Arvue[2], etc. to various web-based tools for creating composite SOA applications, web-based mashup development tools, etc. Similarly, the idea is recently also proposed for Model-Driven Engineering (MDE) tools, e.g., (data) Model as a Service (MaaS)[3] or (software) modeling as a service (a.k.a. MDE in the cloud)[4]. Most recently, the idea is also applied to DSM creation tools [13]. The essential difference of this contribution with our proposed approach is that our work is about the DSM solutions that have been created via a DSM creation tool for particular narrow domains, e.g., SCC applications in the IoTS. However, their work is about providing the DSM creation tool itself as a service for creating DSM solutions.

5   Conclusion and Future Work

In this paper, we proposed a novel approach for developing Sense-Compute-Control (SCC) applications for the Internet of Things and Services (IoTS) based on the Model-Driven Software Engineering (MDSE) methodology, a paradigm in software engineering for dealing with complexity. First, we briefly reviewed the three main recent approaches to MDSE. Second, according to the challenges and requirements for developing SCC applications for the IoTS, we advocated Domain Specific Modeling (DSM) among the MDSE approaches. Finally, we proposed the idea of providing the DSM solutions as services through the IoTS. Implementation and validation of the proposed ideas remained as future work.

---

[1] https://c9.io/.

[2] http://www.cloudsw.org/under-review/31a7a63b-856a-488f-9ce1-1ed5e6cfe63e/ designing-ide-as-a-service/at_download/file.

[3] http://cloudbestpractices.wordpress.com/2012/10/21/maas/.

[4] http://modeling-languages.com/maas-modeling-service-or-mde-cloud/.

References

1. Ishaq, I., Carels, D., Teklemariam, G.K., Hoebeke, J., Van den Abeele, F., Poorter, E.D., Moerman, I., Demeester, P.: IETF standardization in the field of the internet of things (IoT): a survey. J. Sens. Actuator Netw. **2**(2), 235–287 (2013)
2. Cardoso, J., Voigt, K., Winkler, M.: Service engineering for the internet of services. In: Filipe, J., Cordeiro, J. (eds.) ICEIS 2008. LNBIP, vol. 19, pp. 15–27. Springer, Heidelberg (2009)
3. Broy, M.: Cyber Physical Systems (Part 1). it-Information Technology **54**(6), 255–256 (2012)
4. Zukunftsprojekt Industrie 4.0: Website of the German Federal Ministry of Education and Research - Bundesministerium für Bildung und Forschung (BMBF). http://www.bmbf.de/de/19955.php
5. Patel, P., Morin, B., Chaudhary, S.: A Model-driven development framework for developing sense-compute-control applications. In: MoSEMInA 2014 Proceedings of the 1st International Workshop on Modern Software Engineering Methods for Industrial Automation, pp. 52–61. ACM, New York, NY, USA (2014)
6. Patel, P., Pathak, A., Teixeira, T., Issarny, V.: Towards application development for the internet of things. In: MDS 2011 Proceedings of the 8th Middleware Doctoral Symposium, pp. 5:1–5:6. ACM, New York, NY, USA (2011)
7. Schmidt, D.C.: Guest editor's introduction: model-driven engineering. IEEE Comput. **39**(2), 25–31 (2006)
8. Schaetz, B.: 10 years model-driven - what did we achieve? In: IEEE Eastern European Conference on the Engineering of Computer Based Systems. p. 1 (2011)
9. Miller, J., Mukerji, J.: MDA Guide Version 1.0.1. Technical report, object management group (OMG) (2003)
10. Völter, M., Stahl, T., Bettin, J., Haase, A., Helsen, S., Czarnecki, K., von Stockfleth, B.: Model-Driven Software Development: Technology, Engineering, Management. Wiley Software Patterns Series, Wiley, Chichester (2013). http://books.google.de/books?id=9ww_D9fAKncC
11. Küster, J.: The model-driven software engineering (MDSE) lecture slides, IBM research Zurich. http://researcher.watson.ibm.com/researcher/files/zurich-jku/mdse-01.pdf
12. Kelly, S., Tolvanen, J.: Domain-Specific Modeling: Enabling Full Code Generation. Wiley, Chichester (2008)
13. Hiya, S., Hisazumi, K., Fukuda, A., Nakanishi, T.: clooca: web based tool for domain specific modeling. In: Demos/Posters/StudentResearch@MoDELS, pp. 31–35 (2013)

QoS Optimization for Cloud Service Composition Based on Economic Model

Hisham A. Kholidy[1,5], Hala Hassan[2(✉)], Amany M. Sarhan[3],
Abdelkarim Erradi[1], and Sherif Abdelwahed[4]

[1] Department of Computer Science and Engineering, College of Engineering,
Qatar University, Doha, Qatar
{hkholidy, erradi}@qu.edu.qa
[2] Department of Computer Engineering and Systems, Faculty of Engineering,
Mansoura University, Mansoura, Egypt
Hala_h62@yahoo.com
[3] Faculty of Engineering, University of Tanta, Tanta, Egypt
amany_m_sarhan@tanta.edu.eg
[4] Electrical and Computer Engineering,
Mississippi State University, Starkville, MS, USA
sherif@ece.msstate.edu
[5] Faculty of Computers and Information, Fayoum University, Fayoum, Egypt

Abstract. Cloud service composition is usually long term based and economically driven. Services in cloud computing can be categorized into two groups: Application services and Computing Services. Compositions in the application level are similar to the Web service compositions in Service-Oriented Computing. Compositions in the computing level are similar to the task matching and scheduling in grid computing. We consider cloud service composition from end users perspective. We propose Genetic Algorithm-based approach to model the cloud service composition problem. A comparison is given between the proposed composition approach and other existing algorithms such as Integer Linear Programming. The experiment results proved the efficiency of the proposed approach.

Keywords: Cloud service composition · Cloud computing · Genetic algorithm · Quality of service

1 Introduction

Cloud computing is emerging as the new paradigm for the next-generation distributed computing. Big companies such as Amazon, Microsoft, Google and IBM are already offering cloud computing solutions in the market. A fast increasing number of organizations are already outsourcing their business tasks to the cloud, instead of deploying their own local infrastructures [1]. A significant advantage of cloud computing is its economic benefits for end users and service providers.

Services in cloud computing can be categorized into application services and computing services [2]. Almost all the software/applications that are available through the Internet are application services, e.g., flight booking services. Computing services

R. Giaffreda et al. (Eds.): IoT360 2014, Part I, LNICST 150, pp. 355–366, 2015.
DOI: 10.1007/978-3-319-19656-5_48

are software or virtualized hardware that supports application services, e.g., virtual machines, CPU services and storage services. Service compositions in cloud computing include compositions of application services and computing services. Compositions in the application level are similar to the Web service compositions in SOC. Compositions in the computing level are similar to the task matching and scheduling in grid computing. Cloud service composition is usually long-term based and economically driven. Traditional QoS (Quality of Service)-based composition techniques usually consider the qualities at the time of the composition [3]. This is fundamentally different in cloud environments where the cloud service composition should last for a long period.

In this paper, a genetic-algorithm-based cloud service composition approach is proposed. We focus on the selection of composition plans based solely on non-functional or QoS attributes. The comparisons between the proposed approach and other existing ones show the effectiveness and efficiency of the proposed approach. The rest of the paper is structured as follows: Sect. 2 illustrates the preliminaries of service composition in cloud computing. Section 3 provides an overview of cloud service composition problem. Section 4 highlights the related work of the cloud service composition models. Section 5 describes in details the proposed composition approach. Section 6 tests and evaluates the proposed approach and presents the experiment results. Section 7 draws a conclusion and highlights the future work.

2 Preliminaries

In this section we present basic knowledge about cloud computing, service compositions in cloud computing and QoS model.

2.1 Cloud Computing System

Cloud computing provides two types of services, application and computing services. Application services are the most visible services to the end users (i.e. Google Apps), Cloud systems provide these services to the end users through the software providers in SaaS (Software as a Service) layer. Computing services are the hardware and system software in the datacenters that provide those services [2] see Fig. 1.

Some vendors use terms such as PaaS (Platforms a Service) or IaaS (Infrastructure as a Service) to describe their products. In this paper, PaaS and IaaS are considered together as Computing Services. PaaS are platforms that are used to develop, test, deploy and monitor application services. For example, Google has Google App Engine that works as the platform to develop, deploy and maintain Google Apps. IaaS services provide fundamental computing resources, which can be used to construct new platform services or application services. Computing Services include computation services, i.e., Virtual Machines (VMs); storage services, i.e., Databases; and network services. Computing Services Vendors are these companies or organizations that make their computing resources available to the public such as Amazon EC2.

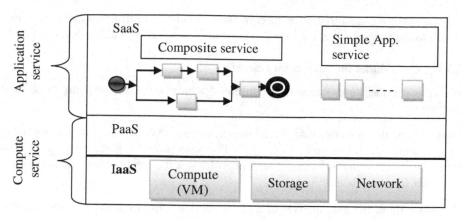

Fig. 1. Cloud system

2.2 Service Composition in Cloud Computing

A composite service is specified as a collection of abstract application services according to a combination of control-flow and data-flow. Similar to traditional service composition, cloud service composition is conducted in two steps. First, a composition schema is constructed for a composition request. Second, the optimal composition plan is selected. Control-flow graphs are represented using UML activity diagrams. Each node in the graph is an abstract application service. There are four control-flow patterns for defining a composite cloud service (composition schema), such as sequential, parallel, conditional and iterative (loop) patterns [8] (Fig. 2). Directed acyclic graphs (DAGs) are used to represent composition schema.

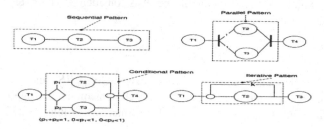

Fig. 2. Basic composition patterns

Any solution to a composition problem in cloud computing includes: (1) Map the abstract application services to concrete application services and corresponding compute service (VM, database and network services). (2) Schedule the execution order of the application services. In this research we introduce only the selection of the composition plan (abstract application services) based solely on user's QoS attributes.

2.3 QoS Model

QoS-based cloud service selection is a critical process that directly determines the QoS values of the composite cloud service. The ultimate goal of the selection process is to find the best composition plan for the composite cloud service that provides the optimal choice to the end user. We use a QoS model that is applicable to all the SaaS and IaaS.

2.3.1   QoS Model for Elementary Services

We consider the three major QoS attributes which are: cost, response time, and throughput.

Cost: the amount of money that the end user has to pay to the service provider for using a cloud service S, it is denoted as $Q_{cost}(S)$. For SaaS provider, it is the execution cost for using a single request SaaS, for IaaS provider it is the computation cost for using a unit IaaS for one second.

Response time: the time interval of a cloud service S from request to response, it is denoted as $Q_{resp}(S)$. For SaaS provider SP, response time is the expected delay in seconds between the moment when a request is sent and the moment when the results are received. For IaaS provider IP, the response time is the number of CPU (network, storage) units used for processing a computation (data transfer, storage) request.

Throughput: the rate at which a cloud service S can process requests, it is denoted as $Q_{th}(S)$. For SaaS provider SP, the throughput is the number of requests the SaaS provider is able to process per second. For IaaS provider IP, the service rate is the number of CPU (network, storage) requests IaaS provider is able to process per sec.

2.3.2   QoS Model for Composite Services

In addition to the QoS attributes of each individual service, the composition pattern and corresponding aggregate functions should be also considered. The overall QoS can be defined as shown in Eq. 1.

$$QoS_{total}(S) = \left[Q_{cost}(S), \ Q_{resp}(S), \ Q_{th}(S) \right] \tag{1}$$

where S is a single path composite cloud service; $QoS_{total}(S)$ indicates the overall quality of a composed cloud service S. Each dimension is the aggregation of all services which is calculated by the aggregation functions (Table 1) [18].

Table 1. Aggregation functions

	Sequential	Parallel	Conditional	Loop
Cost	$\sum\limits_{i=1}^{n} Q_{cost}(i)$	$\sum\limits_{i=1}^{n} Q_{cost}(i)$	$\sum\limits_{i=1}^{n} (P(i) * Q_{cost}(i))$	$K * Q_{cost}(i)$
Response Time	$\sum\limits_{i=1}^{n} Q_{resp}(i)$	$\max\limits_{i=1...n} (Q_{resp}(i))$	$\sum\limits_{i=1}^{n} (P(i) * Q_{resp}(i))$	$K * Q_{resp}(i)$
Throughput	$\min\limits_{i=1...n} (Q_{th}(i))$	$\min\limits_{i=1...n} (Q_{th}(i))$	$\sum\limits_{i=1}^{n} (P(i) * Q_{th}(i))$	$Q_{th}(i)$

3 System Model

In this section, we highlight the service composition model, the problem formulation, and the cloud service composition problem.

3.1 Cloud Service Composition Model

The service composition model introduced in this paper is similar to the one given in [6]. In this model we identify four components: IaaS (Infrastructure as a Service) Providers, SaaS (Software as a Service) Providers, Composer and End users, see Fig. 3. Platform as a Service (PaaS) layer is omitted because we assume that this layer is included in the IaaS layer. The IaaS Providers supply IaaS, i.e., CPU services, storage services, and network services, to SaaS providers and end users. The SaaS providers supply SaaS to end users. The end users are usually large companies and organizations, e.g., universities, governments. The Composer is the proposed composition model that acts on behaves of the end users to form composite services that contain services from multiple SaaS providers and IaaS providers. The main functions of composer are: (1) construct composition schema. (2) Select optimal composition plan. Since the main concern in this research is the selection of optimal composition plan based solely on user's preferences (QoS attributes). We assume that existing composition techniques such as the one introduced in [7] to generate composition schema.

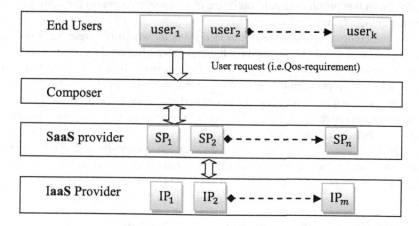

Fig. 3. The proposed composition model

3.2 Problem Formulation

This section introduces the cloud service composition problem as follow:
  Given

1. A set of abstract cloud services (or tasks) T involved in a cloud service composition, where $T = \{T_1, T_2, \ldots, T_n\}$ and n is the total number of abstract cloud services in the composition.

2. For task T_i, a set of K_i candidate SaaS providers can be used to implement the task, $SP_i = \{ SP_i(1), SP_i(2), \ldots, SP_i(K_i) \}$. A set of P_p candidate IaaS providers supply IaaS to composite services: $SP_0 = \{ SP_0(1), SP_0(2), \ldots, SP_0(P_p) \}$

3. A candidate composition plan (denoted as Plan $[\{SP_0(K_0), SP_1(K_1), SP_2(K_2) \ldots SP_0(K_0)\}]$ is formed by selecting certain SaaS providers and IaaS providers for the end user.

4. In the composition plan, the composite service is supported by the IaaS provider $SP_0(K_0)$. Task T_i is implemented by SaaS provider $SP_i(K_i)$.

5. We assume sequential composition pattern is used for composition and user's QoS attributes are numbered from 1 to 3, with 1 = cost, 2 = response time and 3 = throughput. The QoS values for a composition plan using the aggregation functions stated above is denoted as: $QoS_{total}(plan) = [Q(1), Q(2), Q(3)]$

6. Since Service composition in cloud is long-term based economically driven user's QoS requirement, The end users would have different QoS requirements (cost, response time, throughput) on the composite service during long period, i.e., the end user may prefer composite service that has less cost, while in another period the end user may find that the cost is less important than decreasing the response time as much as possible.

The Composite Cloud Service (CCS) is the problem whose goal is to choose one or more composition plan (execution plan) that have a good performance on most of the QoS factors and meet user requirements. [19] The CCS problem based on multiple QoS criteria is a combinational optimization problem that is known to be an NP-Hard [12]. The solution to this problem should optimize (minimize/ maximize) the components of the vector $QoS_{total}(plan)$.

When the composition system makes decisions on which concrete SaaS providers and IaaS providers should be selected for the end user, it has no idea about how will the ultimate composite service behave during a long period. To enable long-term cloud service composition, economic models are needed to predict the long-term preferences of the end users. An economic model is defined as "a theoretical construct that represents economic processes by a set of variables and a set of logical and quantitative relationships between them". [9].

The final objective is to find a fully cloud service composition that minimizes the cost and time, and improves the throughput. We model the cloud service composition problem as a multi-objective optimization problem (MOP).

3.3 Cloud Service Composition Optimization Problem

In this problem, we consider the three user objectives, the lowest cost, the shortest response time, and the highest throughput. This makes it infeasible to find an optimal composition as these objectives can conflict with each other. One way to address this problem is to convert the composition problem to a single-objective problem by asking users to give weights to each objective. The end user presents these preferences through a Score Function [3]. We denote the QoS requirements of the end user as: $W_a(t) = [w1(t), w2(t), w3(t)]$, where $W_a(t)$ denotes the weight of QoS attribute (a) for the composite service at period t. Each composition plan is associated with a score from the end user's perspective. A commonly used score function is the weighted sum of QoS values of the composite service. The main objective is to find an optimal composition plan S *(plan)* that provides the maximum score value.

$$S \text{ (plan)} = W_1(t) * + W_2(t) * Q_2(t) + W_3(t) * Q_3(t) \tag{2}$$

4 Related Works

Service composition problem can be categorized into two groups. One group focuses on the functional composition among component services. The other group aims to make optimal decisions to select the best Component services based on non-functional properties (QoS).

Functional-driven service composition approaches typically adopt semantic descriptions of services. Examples of automatic approaches include Policy-based approach proposed by [14]. Other functional-driven composition approaches use AI planning methods. Most of them [15] assume that each service is an action which alters the state of the world as a result of its execution. The inputs and outputs parameters of a service act as preconditions and effects in the planning context. Users only need to specify the inputs and the outputs of the desired composite service, a plan (or a composite service) would automatically generated by the AI planners. Different users may have different requirements and preferences regarding QoS. Therefore, QoS-aware composition approaches are needed. QoS-aware service composition problem is usually modeled as a Multiple Criteria Decision Making [3] problem. The most popular approaches include integer linear programming and genetic algorithms. An Integer Linear Program (ILP) consists of a set of variables, a set of linear constraints and a linear objective function. After having translated the composition problem into this formalism, Specific solver software such as LPSolve [13] can be used. References [16, 17] use Genetic Algorithms (GA) for service composition.

Most of the existing composition approaches are not well suited for cloud environment [17]. They usually consider the qualities at the time of the composition [4]. The proposed composition approach considers the problem from a long-term perspective.

5 Genetic Algorithm – Based Approach

Genetic Algorithms (GAs) [12] are heuristic approaches that iteratively find the nearest optimal solution in large search solutions. Any possible solution to the optimization problem is encoded as a Chromosome (genome). A set of chromosomes is referred to as a Population. The first step of a GA is to derive an initial population. A random set of chromosomes is often used as the initial population. This initial population is the first generation from which the evolution starts. The second step is the selection process, each chromosome is eliminated or duplicated (one or more times) based on its relative quality. The population size is typically kept constant. The next step is the Crossover process. Some pairs of chromosomes are selected from the current population and some of their corresponding components are exchanged to form two valid chromosome. After crossover, each chromosome in the population may be mutated with some probability. The mutation process transforms a chromosome into another valid one. The new population is then evaluated and each chromosome is associated with a fitness value, which is a value obtained from the objective function. The objective of the evaluation is to find a chromosome that has the optimal fitness value. If the stopping criterion is not met, the new population goes through another cycle (iteration) of selection, crossover, mutation, and evaluation. These cycles continue until the stopping criterion is met [4].

5.1 Algorithm Implementation

The Proposed Approach Consists of the Following Process:

1. **Define Chromosome:** For genetic algorithms, one of the key issues is to encode a solution of the -problem into a chromosome (individual). In our model, the chromosome is encoded by an integer array with a number of items equals to the number of distinct abstract services that compose our service. Each item, in turn, contains an index to the array of the concrete services matching that abstract service.
2. **Generate Initial Population:** a predefined number of chromosomes are generated to form the initial generation. The chromosome in a generation is first ordered by their fitness values from the best to worst.
3. **Apply Genetic Operator:** To apply this process we define the operator of each step as following:

   - **Selection Operator:** We use the binary tournament selection as the selection operator. The binary tournament selection runs a tournament between two individuals and selects the winner. In this way, the individuals that formed the next generation are determined. The population size of each generation is always P.
   - **Crossover Operator:** We use the single-point crossover as the crossover operator. The crossover point is a random value from 1 to N_t (the number of genes in one chromosome).
   - **Mutation Operator:** We randomly select an abstract service and randomly replace the corresponding concrete service with another one among those available. Clearly, we select the abstract service for which only one concrete service is available.

4. **Evaluate the Chromosomes Using Fitness Function:** The fitness function should maximize some QoS attributes (i.e. throughput), minimize some other attributes (i.e. cost and response time). In addition, the fitness function must penalize solutions that do not meet the QoS constraints and drive the evolution towards constraints satisfaction. Let us suppose that the composite service has a set of constraints defined as QC [10]. we define $D(c)$, the distance from the constraint satisfaction of a chromosome (solution) *c,* as following :

$$D(c) = \sum_{i=1}^{l} QC^i(c) * e_i * weight^i, e_i = \left\{ \begin{array}{l} 0 \, QC^i(c) \leq 0 \\ 1 \, QC^i(c) > 0 \end{array} \right\} \tag{3}$$

where,

- $weight^i$ indicates the weight of the QoS constraint.
- l is number of constraints that composite service has for a specific chromosome (solution) c.

The fitness function for a chromosome c is then defined as:

$$F(c) = \sum_{i=1}^{a} w^i * Q^i(c) + weight_p * D(c) \tag{4}$$

where,

- w^i is the weight corresponding to each QoS attribute i.
- $weight_p$ is the penalty factor.
- A is number of Qos attributes which is 3 in our case.

The stop criterions of the proposed approach are:

(1) Iterate until the constraints are met (i.e. $D(c) = 0$).
(2) If this does not happen within a defined maximum number of generation, 'MAXGEN', then iterate until the best fitness value remains unchanged for a given number 'MAXGEN' of generations.
(3) If neither (1) nor (2) happened within 'MAXGEN' generations, then no solution will be returned.

6 Experiments and Evaluation

We run our experiments on a Dell laptop with 2.3 GHz Intel Core i7 processor and 6G Ram under Windows 7 operating system. We have used Jmetal [11] which is Java framework for implementing multi-objective and single-objective algorithms. We implement the Genetic Algorithm-based approach in this framework that allows us to define each problem by defining each chromosome (variable) to point to a cloud service candidate. After that, we define the fitness functions for all defined objectives and choose the algorithm that solves the problem. We first conduct one experiment to show the effect of changing available concrete services for each abstract service on the execution time, Fig. 4 shows that the execution time increases quickly at the beginning of the experiment, but it keeps nearly constant when the number of concrete services for each abstract service becomes larger than 200. We conduct the experiment that shows the effect of selection operator on reaching to the optimal fitness value. Figure 5 shows the comparison between the tournament selection operator used in the proposed approach and the random selection operator. As shown in Fig. 5, the proposed approach will always reach an optimized fitness value while random selection seldom

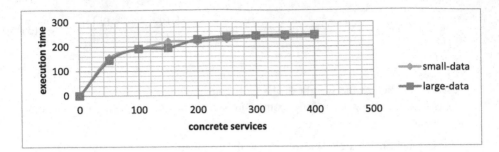

Fig. 4. Concrete services against execution time

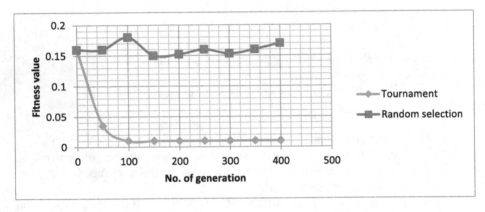

Fig. 5. Tournament selection against random selection

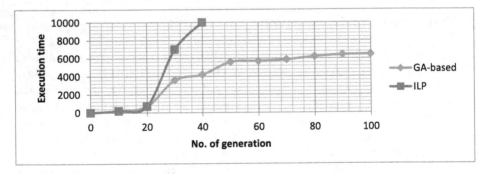

Fig. 6. GA-based against ILP

converges. The proposed GA based approach will always reach an optimal fitness value and the converged point becomes very close to the actual optimal point. We conduct a comparison experiment with another approach such Integer Programming. The Integer Programming (IP) approaches have been proposed to solve QoS-aware service composition. The IP approaches implemented using LPSolve [13], which is an open source integer programming system. Figure 6 shows that the IP approach performs as good as the GA based approach at the beginning. Notice that, when the number of abstract services becomes more than 40, the execution time cost of the IP approaches will increase exponentially to solve composition problems.

7 Conclusions and Future Work

This paper discusses the cloud service composition problem as multi-objective optimization to satisfy the requirements of user's QoS requirements and presents an approach to solve the multi-objective problem by converting it to a single objective problem. We have proposed an approach that uses the Genetic Algorithm to solve this problem. The experiment results proved the efficiency of the proposed approach.

For the future work, we intend to solve the multi-objective composition problem using multi-objective algorithms such NSGA II (Non-dominated Sorting Genetic Algorithm), SPEA-II (Strength Pareto Evolution Algorithm) [20] and other meta-heuristics algorithm which is based on swarm intelligence such as Particle Swarm Optimization (OMOPSO) [21] and compare the efficiency of these algorithms.

Acknowledgments. This work was made possible by NPRP grant # 7 - 481-1 - 088 from the Qatar National Research Fund (a member of Qatar Foundation). The statements made herein are solely the responsibility of the authors.

References

1. Youseff, L., Butrico, M., Da Silva, D.: Toward a unified ontology of cloud computing. In: Grid Computing Environments Workshop (2009)
2. Armbrust, M., Fox, A., Griffith, R., Joseph, A.D., Katz, R., Konwinski, A., Lee, G., Patterson, D., Rabkin, A., Stoica, I., Zaharia, M.: Above the clouds: a Berkeley view of cloud computing. Technical report, February 2009
3. Zeng, L., Benatallah, B., Ngu, A., Dumas, M., Kalagnanam, J., Chang, H.: QoS-aware middleware for web services composition. IEEE Trans. Softw. Eng. **30**(5), 311–327 (2004)
4. Srinivas, M., Patnaik, L.: Genetic algorithms: a survey. Comput. **27**(6), 17–26 (1994)
5. Canfora, G., Di Penta, M., Esposito, R., Villani, M.: An approach for QoS-aware service composition based on genetic algorithms. In: Proceedings of the 2005 Conference on Genetic and Evolutionary Computation, pp. 1069–1075. ACM, New York (2005)
6. Ye, Z., Bouguettaya, A., Zhou, X.: QoS-aware cloud service composition based on economic models. In: Liu, C., Ludwig, H., Toumani, F., Yu, Q. (eds.) Service Oriented Computing. LNCS, vol. 7636, pp. 111–126. Springer, Heidelberg (2012)
7. Medjahed, B., Bouguettaya, A., Elmagarmid, A.: Composing web services on the semantic web. VLDB J. **12**(4), 333–351 (2003)
8. Wu, B., Chi, C., Chen, Z., Gu, M., Sun, J.: Workflow-based resource allocation to optimize overall performance of composite services. Future Gener. Comput. Syst. **25**(3), 199–212 (2009)
9. Baumol, W., Blinder, A.: Economics: Principles and Policy. South-Western Pub, Mason (2011)

10. Canfora, G., Di Penta, M., Esposito, R., Villani, M.: An approach for QoS-aware service composition based on genetic algorithms. In: Proceedings of the 2005 Conference on Genetic and Evolutionary Computation, pp. 1069–1075 (2005)

11. Durillo, J., Nebro, A.: jMetal: a java framework for multi- objective optimization. Adv. Eng. Softw. **42**(10), 760–771 (2011)

12. De Jong, K., Spears, W.M.: Using genetic algorithms to solve NP complete problems. In: Proceedings of the Third International Conference on Genetic Algorithm, pp. 124–132. Morgan Kaufman, Los Altos, CA (1989)

13. Berkelaar, M., Eikland, K., Notebaert, P., et al.: lpsolve: Open source (mixedinteger) linear programming system. Eindhoven U. of Technology

14. Chun, S.A., Atluri, V., Adam, N.R.: Using semantics for policy-based web service composition. Distrib. Parallel Databases **18**(1), 37–64 (2005)

15. Wu, D., Parsia, B., Sirin, E., Hendler, J., Nau, D.S.: Automating DAML-S web services composition using SHOP2. In: Fensel, D., Sycara, K., Mylopoulos, J. (eds.) ISWC 2003. LNCS, vol. 2870, pp. 195–210. Springer, Heidelberg (2003)

16. Canfora, G., Di Penta, M., Esposito, R., Villani, M.: An approach for QoS-aware service composition based on genetic algorithms. In: Proceedings of the 2005 Conference on Genetic and Evolutionary Computation, pp. 1069–1075 (2005)

17. Ye, Z., Zhou, X., Bouguettaya, A.: Genetic algorithm based QoS-aware service compositions in cloud computing. In: Yu, J.X., Kim, M.H., Unland, R. (eds.) DASFAA 2011, Part II. LNCS, vol. 6588, pp. 321–334. Springer, Heidelberg (2011)

18. Lie Q., Yan, W., Orgun, M. A.: Cloud service selection based on the aggregation of user feedback and quantitative performance assessment. In: Services Computing (SCC). IEEE (2013)

19. Jula, A., Sundararajan, E., Othman, Z.: Cloud computing service composition: a systematic literature review. Expert Syst. Appl. J. **41**, 3809–3824 (2014). Elsevier

20. Zitzler, E., Thiele, L.: Multiobjective evolutionary algorithms: a comparative case study and the strength pareto approach. IEEE Trans. Evol. Comput. **3**(4), 257–271 (1999)

21. Sierra, M.R., Coello, C.A.: Improving PSO-based multi-objective optimization using crowding, mutation and ε-dominance. In: Coello Coello, C.A., Hernández Aguirre, A., Zitzler, E. (eds.) EMO 2005. LNCS, vol. 3410, pp. 505–519. Springer, Heidelberg (2005)

To Run or Not to Run: Predicting Resource Usage Pattern in a Smartphone

Arijit Mukherjee[1][✉], Anupam Basu[2], Swarnava Dey[1], Pubali Datta[1],
and Himadri Sekhar Paul[1]

[1] Innovation Labs, Tata Consultancy Services, Kolkata, India
mukherjee.arijit@tcs.com
[2] Department of Computer Science and Engineering, IIT Kharagpur,
Kharagpur, India

Abstract. Smart mobile phones are vital to the Mobile Cloud Computing (MCC) paradigm where compute jobs can be offloaded to the devices from the Cloud and vice-versa, or the devices can act as peers to collaboratively perform a task. Recent research in IoT context also points to the use of smartphones as sensor gateways highlighting the importance of data processing at the network edge. In either case, when a smart phone is used as a compute resource or a sensor gateway, the corresponding tasks must be executed in addition to the user's normal activities on the device without affecting the user experience. In this paper, we propose a framework that can act as an enabler of such features by classifying the availability of system resources like CPU, memory, network usage based on applications running on an Android phone. We show that, such app-based classifications are user-specific and app usage varies with different handsets, leading to different classifications. We further show that irrespective of such variation in classification, distinct patterns exist for all users with available opportunity to schedule external tasks, without affecting user experience. Based on the next to-be-used applications, we output a predicted set of system resources. The resource levels along with handset architecture may be used to estimate worst case execution time for external jobs.

Keywords: Smart phone · Usage prediction · Resource utilisation · Machine learning · Mobile cloud computing · IoT · Sensor data

1 Introduction

With the advancement of technology more people are using high end mobile phones with increased hardware capabilities. Though such phones are being used for functionalities more than just communication, they remain idle for majority of the time. One of the focus areas of Mobile Cloud Computing (MCC) is to explore possibilities of utilizing mobile phones as compute resources to augment the Cloud infrastructure. In [1], jobs are executed on mobile phones using a map-reduce framework. Authors in [2,3] propose offloading jobs between mobiles where the phones act as compute peers. More recently, in the context of Internet of Things (IoT), the idea of edge devices being used to precess data at

© Institute for Computer Sciences, Social Informatics and Telecommunications Engineering 2015
R. Giaffreda et al. (Eds.): IoT360 2014, Part I, LNICST 150, pp. 367–375, 2015.
DOI: 10.1007/978-3-319-19656-5_49

the network edge was introduced in Fog Computing [4] and the present authors
have implemented a preliminary prototype which is outlined in [5]. The authors
believe that in a *smart city* scenario, with numerous sensors and edge devices
emitting highly fluctuating volume of data, an MCC framework augmenting the
cloud may indeed be useful. Recent works by McCann *et al.* have also pointed
towards the use of personal devices as sensor gateways and data-forwarding
entities [6,7]. We are of the belief that during such phases, the devices may
also be utilised for small amounts of computation in order to reduce the cost
incurred in pushing the data to the cloud and in turn save energy (as apart from
incurring a communication cost, any network transfer is energy intense). However, to effectively schedule jobs on available phones and other edge devices, the
cloud servers would require an estimation of available cpu, memory and other
parameters for those devices as the execution time of an externally assigned computation will vary depending on the foreground(user) and background activities
running on the phone. The same is true if the devices are used as sensor gateways. This implies that the user experience must not get affected while executing
the assigned job or transfering sensor data to the cloud. In other words, it can
be said that the user experience is not affected if such tasks are scheduled at
the right time, when the device is relatively idle. Figure 1 explains the context
described herein.

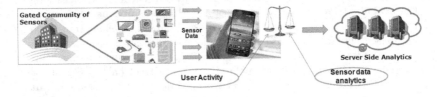

Fig. 1. Using mobile phones in an IoT context

A number of studies have attempted to classify android applications based
on android package details, power consumption and static code analysis. Commercial and free benchmark tools have also been used to measure relative performance of a handset and profile apps. The diversity of smartphone app usage
behavior among users was highlighted in [8,9]. These approaches showed that
unique usage patterns exist, albeit on a per user basis. With this idea of *user
specific patterns*, we propose to predict system resources influencing the performance of an android mobile, based on the currently running android apps,
per user.

Our work focuses on analyzing the CPU, memory etc. resource usage, when
apps are running on the devices to detect phases when the system resources are
relatively free for external job execution. We classify CPU and RAM based on
android apps used on a handset by the user of the handset by analysing the log
containing running apps snapshots, overall idle CPU time, available memory etc.
using machine learning techniques and decide whether *to run* or *not to run* any

externally assigned task. We also show the variation of the classification results with user and handset and present the result of our field-study showing the correlation of our prediction with benchmark scores from a well known benchmark tool, AndEbench [10].

The rest of the paper is organized as follows. We analyze the previous work done in android app classification and android benchmarking in Sect. 2. In Sect. 3, we describe our approach regarding data collection, preprocessing, feature selection classifier selection and field study. We present the results in Sect. 4 and conclude with a summary of the contributions and some pointers for future work.

2   Related Work

Not many systems exist for classifying smart-phone system resources based on app usage. A number of research works have focused on classifying android apps based on android package details, power consumption and static code analysis. The main focus of such analysis is to segregate apps from malwares. Several commercial tools benchmark system resources at both app and handset levels.

Zefferer *et al.* [11] presented a scheme of malware detection by classifying android apps based on power consumption. They found that the power-consumption signature for a given application or phone state could not be determined uniquely and the signature for the same app was analogous to wide pitch and frequency variance of the different speech records from the same person. Sanz *et al.* [12] developed a new app classification scheme using extracted features from said app and the Android Market. They worked with a large set of 820 apps categorizing them into seven categories by using classification techniques and providing a comparative evaluation using the Area Under ROC Curve (AUC). Shabtai *et al.* [13] focussed on app classification using framework methods and classes used by the app, user interface widgets etc. and identified the optimum combination for feature selection method, top features selected and the classifier.

Several commercial tools are available for benchmarking. Notable among these is the Trepn Profiler [14] from Qualcomm which provides system or app specific cpu profiling. AndEBench is another tool that we used extensively in this work and it shows a native and java score for each phone. However, none of the benchmark tools however categorize apps based on the system resource usage or provide a relative scoring for each app. Our work aims to classify system resources based on android apps per user per phone, leveraging the unique usage pattern.

3   Approach

A logging application for android devices was deployed on the mobile phones of several users which was used to gather data over a period of two weeks for each user. This application gathers last app, last service component, data transfer and memory available using android APIs. For system CPU usage and process details, the system parses the `top` command output which outputs processes like `system_server`, `uevent` and several other system activities that are not available using android APIs. As the logger logs data in a very precise form, with only the required values for our analysis, the log file size (at most 2MB in two weeks) is never a concern for the volunteers.

To determine the cpu availability, we used the jiffy values from android `top` output and calculated the percentage of time the cpu was idle. For the two class classification (in this case, *high* and *low*), we applied *k-means clustering technique* [15] on the idle cpu percentage values. For multiprocessor systems, `top` provides a measure of summation over (number of cores x percentage utilized in each core). We scaled the overall value for all cores by dividing it by the number of cores for that phone System On Chip (SoC). We collected available memory information using the `getMemoryInfo` API of android *ActivityManager* and the system memory information from `/proc/meminfo`. An equally weighted average of the two values was used to express the memory free percentage. Similar to the cpu values, k-means clustering was applied on the free memory percentage values, to create two clusters *high* and *low*.

One pertinent note at this point may be that - out of a myriad of available android applications (as per [16] the latest number is 1175286) we are classifying on the basis of only a small subset. To justify our approach, it may be said that as we apply our system on a per user basis, the applications usually running on the phone of the user determines the classification of system resources. The analysis using Principal Component Analysis (PCA) and the ranker algorithm also proves that only a subset of all the apps installed in a phone have any visible effect on the resources as is shown in Table 1, which lists the top-6 ranked features for two different users using two different handsets.

Table 1. Table of top ranked features in phones A110q and Xperia L

A110 top features	Xperia L top features
surfaceflinger	surfaceflinger
mediaserver	system_server
mediatek.bluetooth	mediaserver
android.chrome	king.candycrushsaga
android.systemui	textinput.uxp
android.youtube	android.systemui

We used *machine learning* concepts to depict the dependency between application running in a phone and the level of the available system resources. However, we haven't yet implemented a full-fledged online app prediction system and rather have taken cues from [17] to create a Naïve Bayes classification of offline data from the mobile phones on which we evaluated the current system. We built a prediction model using the WEKA [18] tool and evaluated using test data for top four apps being used in the system, during a 5 second interval. To evaluate our system on real mobile phones we used the *Weka-for-Android* [19] implementation for the Naïve bayes classifier along with the offline model created for that phone using desktop WEKA. With the next four running app prediction at hand along with all other features required for system resource classification, we used a modification of the *LibSVM-androjni* [20] project to run our Logistic Regression classifier. We chose the Logistic Regression classifier for the field study as an android port was easily available and it performed reasonably well, as detailed in the Sect. 4. We mapped the output of the classifier (system resource level high or low) to our final decision - *to run* or *not to run* the external task.

As the MCC frameworks ANGELS [5] is still under development, we decided to use a different innovative measure to evaluate the output. We designed a set of experiments (a snapshot of which is given in Fig. 2a) to obtain a correlation between the AndEBench score and the underlying activities. In each experiment,

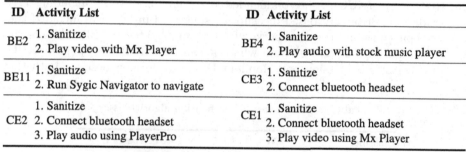

ID	Activity List	ID	Activity List
BE2	1. Sanitize 2. Play video with Mx Player	BE4	1. Sanitize 2. Play audio with stock music player
BE11	1. Sanitize 2. Run Sygic Navigator to navigate	CE3	1. Sanitize 2. Connect bluetooth headset
CE2	1. Sanitize 2. Connect bluetooth headset 3. Play audio using PlayerPro	CE1	1. Sanitize 2. Connect bluetooth headset 3. Play video using Mx Player

(a) Test Scenarios

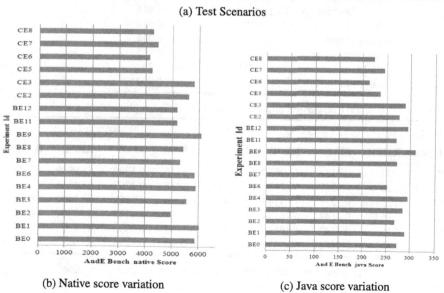

(b) Native score variation   (c) Java score variation

Fig. 2. Experimental scenario and AndEBench scores for native & Java on A110q

the *sanitize* step kills user processes, cleans the cache from task manager, starts AndEBench, performs test scenarios and finally records the scores. We observed this and triggered a run of AndEBench, based on recommendation output from the system resource classifier. As a single AndEBench run takes around one minute, we kept the prediction cycles separated by five minutes for evaluation. Our aim was to correlate the prediction of system resource level for the next cycle to the score from AndEBench in the next cycle. For a *high* level for system resource prediction, if the score of AndEBench is also high, we considered the prediction to be accurate. The apparent correlation between the benchmark score and underlying activities for a snapshot of the experiments is shown in Fig. 2b and c.

4   Results

We used two sets of comparisons to differentiate the classifiers the area under the ROC curve (AUC), as recommended in several literatures including [21] and traditional error rate based measure as suggested in [22]. We included the latter keeping in mind the drawbacks of AUC, highlighted in [23]. The results are shown in Tables 2a and b[1] from where it can be seen that as per the AUC measure Logistic Regression and Random Forest performed best for both the

Table 2. Result from classification algorithms

Classifier	AUC A110	AUC Xperia L
Bayesian networks (K2)	0.921	0.948
J48	0.869	0.944
Naïve Bayes	0.911	0.944
Random Forest	0.937	0.955
SVM	0.838	0.79
Logistic	0.937	0.957

(a) Comparison of AUC measures on different phone data

Error	A110Q				Xperia L			
Measure	RMSE	MAE	RRSE	RAE	RMSE	MAE	RRSE	RAE
BN	0.2825	0.1262	71.9829	40.6613	0.3316	0.1394	85.9909	46.8816
J48	0.2639	0.1359	67.2456	44.1284	0.2485	0.1207	64.4535	40.5967
NB	0.2981	0.1279	75.9787	41.5427	0.4303	0.3209	86.1084	64.2394
RF	0.2526	0.1147	63.8559	37.2491	0.2467	0.1147	63.9711	38.5694
SVM	0.2506	0.1147	63.855	37.2491	0.3155	0.0995	81.825	33.4757
L	0.2534	0.1252	63.9517	64.5846	0.2466	0.1195	63.951	40.1906

(b) Comparison of error rates of different classifiers on A110Q and Xperia L

---

[1] RMSE: Root mean-squared error, MAE: Mean absolute error, RRSE: Root relative squared error, RAE: Relative absolute error.

phones. On the other hand, based on the error rate measure Random Forest and SVM gave better results than all other classifiers for A110q phone. For the Xperia L phone Random Forest, SVM and Logistic Regression performed well. During the classification effort, we also observed from the training data that the system resource availability level is *high* 81 % of time in the A110q phone and 82 % of the time in Xperia L phone. Thus we are able to observe distinct patterns (from classification accuracy) for both the users with available opportunity to schedule external jobs, without affecting user experience.

As stated before in Sect. 3, we triggered a run of AndEBench after a 5 min interval based on the recommendation from our system resource prediction system. The actual run happens only when the system resources are classified as high. We present a snapshot run in Fig. 3a to depict the correctness of recommendations. We also profiled our own app using the Trepn profiler [14] and the result is given in Fig. 3b which shows a fairly good performance measure, although we will consider the optimization of this prediction app as a future work.

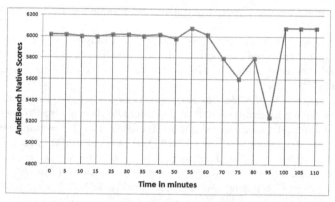

(a) A sample run of the AndEBench tool for our evaluation scheme

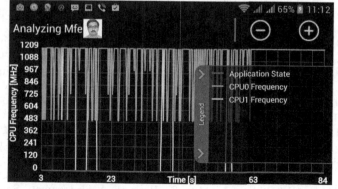

(b) An execution profile of our system using Trepn profiler

Fig. 3. Results of the prediction system

5   Conclusion

In this work we have addressed the issue of predicting the available system resources in the face of a set of apps to be executed. We have applied Logistic regression to classify the availability of resources. We have further showed that the resultant classification correlates with the scores from a well known benchmark tool. The major contribution of the work is the demonstration of the efficacy of the classification approach to predict the resource availability. This can be fruitfully employed while selecting mobile phones where MCC based jobs can be executed in a *smart city* context. As a sidebar of this research we have also found that android system and background tasks are particularly useful in predicting the resource availability and those can be predicted using data from android phones and past execution history of such tasks.

References

1. Marinelli, E.E.: Hyrax: Cloud Computing on Mobile Devices using MapReduce (2009)
2. Shi, C., Ammar, M.H. Zegura, E.W., Naik, M.: Computing in cirrus clouds: the challenge of intermittent connectivity. In: Proceedings of the First Edition of the MCC Workshop on Mobile Cloud Computing, MCC 2012, New York, NY, USA, pp. 23–28. ACM (2012)
3. Shi, C., Lakafosis, V., Ammar, M.H., Zegura, E.W.: Serendipity: enabling remote computing among intermittently connected mobile devices. In: Proceedings of the 13th ACM International Symposium on Mobile Ad Hoc Networking and Computing, MobiHoc 2012, New York, NY, USA, pp. 145–154. ACM (2012)
4. Bonomi, F., Milito, R., Zhu, J., Addepalli, S:. Fog computing and its role in the internet of things. In: Proceedings of the First Edition of the MCC Workshop on Mobile Cloud Computing, MCC 2012, New York, NY, USA, pp. 13–16. ACM (2012)
5. Mukherjee, A., Paul, H.S., Dey, S., Banerjee, A.: Angels for distributed analytics in IoT. In: 2014 IEEE World Forum on Internet of Things (WF-IoT), pp. 565–570. IEEE (2014)
6. Adeel, U., Yang, S., McCann, J.A.: Self-optimizing citizen-centric mobile urban sensing systems. In: 11th International Conference on Autonomic Computing (ICAC 2014), Philadelphia, PA, pp. 16–1167. USENIX Association, June 2014
7. Yang, S., Adeel, U., McCann, J.: Selfish mules: social profit maximization in sparse sensornets using rationally-selfish human relays. IEEE J. Sele. Areas Commun. **31**, 1124–1134 (2013)
8. Falaki, H., Mahajan, R., Kandula, S., Lymberopoulos, D., Govindan, R., Estrin, D.: Diversity in smartphone usage. In: Proceedings of the 8th International Conference on Mobile Systems, Applications, and Services, MobiSys 2010, New York, NY, USA, pp. 179–194. ACM (2010)
9. Xu, Q., Erman, J., Gerber, A., Mao, Z., Pang, J., Venkataraman, S.: Identifying diverse usage behaviors of smartphone apps. In: Proceedings of the 2011 ACM SIGCOMM Conference on Internet Measurement Conference, IMC 2011, New York, NY, USA, pp. 329–344. ACM (2011)
10. An EEMBC Benchmark for Android Devices. http://www.eembc.org/andebench/

11. Zefferer, T., Teufl, P., Derler, D., Potzmader, K., Oprisnik, A., Gasparitz, H., Hoeller, A.: Power Consumption-based Application Classification and Malware Detection on Android Using Machine-Learning Techniques (2009)
12. Sanz, B., Santos, I., Laorden, C., Ugarte-Pedrero, X., Bringas, P.G.: On the automatic categorisation of android applications. In: CCNC, pp. 149–153. IEEE (2012)
13. Shabtai, A., Fledel, Y., Elovici, Y.: Automated static code analysis for classifying android applications using machine learning. In: 2010 International Conference on Computational Intelligence and Security (CIS), pp. 329–333, December 2010
14. Trepn Profiler. https://developer.qualcomm.com/mobile-development/increase-app-performance/trepn-profiler
15. MacQueen, J.: Some methods for classification and analysis of multivariate observations (1967)
16. Number of Android applications. http://www.appbrain.com/stats/number-of-android-apps
17. Shin, C., Hong, J.-H., Dey, A.K.: Understanding and prediction of mobile application usage for smart phones. In: Proceedings of the 2012 ACM Conference on Ubiquitous Computing, UbiComp 2012, New York, NY, USA, pp. 173–182. ACM (2012)
18. Garner, S.R.: Weka: The waikato environment for knowledge analysis. In: Proceedings of the New Zealand Computer Science Research Students Conference, pp. 57–64 (1995)
19. Weka-for-Android. https://github.com/rjmarsan/Weka-for-Android
20. Libsvm-androidjni. https://github.com/cnbuff410/Libsvm-androidjni
21. Ling, C.X., Huang, J., Zhang, H.: AUC: a better measure than accuracy in comparing learning algorithms. In: Xiang, Y., Chaib-draa, B. (eds.) Canadian AI 2003. LNCS (LNAI), vol. 2671, pp. 329–341. Springer, Heidelberg (2003)
22. Witten, I.H., Frank, E.: Data Mining: Practical Machine Learning Tools and Techniques. Morgan Kaufmann Series in Data Management Systems, 2nd edn. Morgan Kaufmann Publishers Inc., San Francisco (2005)
23. Hand, D.J.: Measuring classifier performance: A coherent alternative to the area under the roc curve. Mach. Learn. **77**, 103–123 (2009)

Human-Computer Interface Based on IoT Embedded Systems for Users with Disabilities

Davide Mulfari$^{(\boxtimes)}$, Antonio Celesti, Maria Fazio, and Massimo Villari

DICIEAMA, University of Messina, Messina, Italy
{dmulfari,acelesti,mfazio,mvillari}@unime.it

Abstract. This paper investigates how low-cost embedded systems can be tailored to support the interaction between users with disabilities and computers. The main idea is to implement several software solutions for assistive technology to deploy on the user embedded device. When such a device is connected to a whichever computing system (e.g. through an USB connection), it acts as HID (Human Interface Device) peripheral (e.g., mouse and keyboard), so that the user can work on the computer without any previous configuration setup to adapt the behavior of the computing system to the user disability. The proposed solution exploits Cloud-based services to adapt the device firmware to the user's needs and preferences. To test the whole system, we discuss the design of an alternative input device based on MEMS accelerometers and the Atmega32u4 microcontroller and it is currently intended for individuals with motor disabilities.

Keywords: Human-computer interface · Users with disabilities · IoT devices · Programmable embedded systems

1 Introduction

The Internet of Things (IoT) aims to interconnect everything into the Internet, from daily life devices to more complex networked systems exploiting global network infrastructures, linking physical and virtual objects, using Cloud computing resources, processing sensor data, and adopting advances communication technologies [2]. Here we consider IoT equipments based on programmable low-cost embedded systems and microcontroller boards which are currently available on the market. Some of these devices (e.g., the Raspberry Pi) come with a tailored Linux operating system able to execute pieces of software implemented in a high-level programming language (such as Python or Java). Generally, they also have an integrated network connection to access the Internet and exchange data with external smart objects. A classic deployment of these embedded devices implies that they manage heterogeneous wireless sensor networks and process data over the Cloud. Multiple application scenarios can be imagined for this approach [3,9]. This paper discusses a different approach to exploit Cloud computing for IoT purposes. It focuses the attention on how such IoT devices are able

© Institute for Computer Sciences, Social Informatics and Telecommunications Engineering 2015
R. Giaffreda et al. (Eds.): IoT360 2014, Part I, LNICST 150, pp. 376–383, 2015.
DOI: 10.1007/978-3-319-19656-5_50

to interface a generic computer and to act as alternative input devices. Specifically, we discuss how a microcontroller board can support external sensors and peripherals in order to work as Human Computer Interface (HCI).

Typically, disable users interacts with a computing environment by means of personalized Assistive Technology (AT) hardware and software solutions. For example, users with motor disabilities cannot use standard keyboards or mouses and rely on alternative input devices (e.g., joysticks, switches, special keyboards, voice recognition systems) and mouse emulation software. Similarly, people with low vision work using screen reader programs to manage a Personal Computer (PC), or executing screen magnification pieces of software in order to better navigate a visual interface. Regardless the type of used AT equipment, such an equipment requires a specific configuration process in order to accomplish the end user's needs. This task has to be performed by an AT expert, who works close to the person with the disability in order to properly adapt the computing environment to its user. The configuration task has to be carried out on any user PC, and it can become an hard task on specific system, such as in an Internet point or in a laboratory, where the user cannot install tailored pieces of software or drivers. In general, a very difficult situation occurs every time an user has to work on a computing environment that does not support his/her personal assistive solutions.

To address the aforementioned issues, we suggest to provide the end user with a smart AT hardware device, that is an IoT embedded system able to interface the user with any computer without any installation of drivers or specific applications. To this aim, the device includes a specific firmware to interface sensors and other AT standard devices (e.g., reduced keyboard or special mouse), converting the produced input data into native input command for a computer. Therefore, if the disable user is usual to work with specific AT tools (e.g., voice recognition application, webcam-based eye tracker), our solution allows him to use the same AT equipment to interact with different computing devices, such as PCs or smartphones. Such embedded system has a built-in wireless network interface and its functionalities can be customized using a Cloud-based service. This is an important feature, since a remote AT expert may support a user by updating the firmware on the embedded HCI platform he/she is going to use to access a computer.

The aforementioned setup process needs to be performed only once and it will make accessible any computer able to interact with the HCI system. To show a concrete adoption of an HCI, in the next sections we discuss the development of a prototype, based on a tri-axial accelerometer, working as mouse emulator for computer users with motor disabilities. The device has an Atmega32u4 microntroller with an USB device connection, while we use a different processor to run our software controller on a Linux embedded operating system.

The rest of the paper is structured as follows. Section 2 presents the architecture of the proposed HCI prototype and describes the configuration process based on Cloud services. Related works in the field of AT are presented in Sect. 3. Finally, conclusion and future works are summarized in Sect. 4.

2   HCI System Description

The proposed human computer interface consists of two key components. First, an Atmega32u4 microcontroller is required to appear as a native mouse (or keyboard) when the device is attached to a generic computer with an USB host port. More specifically, the same microcontroller executes a custom version of the Arduino bootloader that supports the Mouse/Keyboard libraries. Another main hardware component of our HCI system is a second processor allowing to boot a Linux embedded operating system equipped with a Python runtime. Therefore we use a standard Python high - level programming language to acquire and to process data from external devices and sensors. Additionally, our embedded system needs to manage a network connection to access the Internet and an USB host port able to interface external peripherals.

To fulfill these conditions, currently our prototype is based on an Arduino Yun board, a microcontroller board based on the Atmega32u4 and the Atheros AR9331 procesor which supports a Linux distribution based on OpenWrt named Linino. The board has built-in Ethernet and WiFi support, a USB host port, micro-SD card slot, 20 digital input/output pins and a micro USB connection for connecting a computer. Moreover, the YUN itself from other Arduino boards in that it can communicate with the Linux distribution onboard, offering a powerful networked computer with the ease of Arduino. In addition to Linux commands like cURL, the Atheros processor is able to execute shell and Python scripts for robust interactions.

From a technical point of view, we have interfaced the Yun board with several kinds of sensor node, available on the market. Each sensor node consists of an accelerometer, a dedicated microcontroller, and an interface which enables the communication with a computing device, like an embedded system. This interface can be a wireless (bluetooth or zigbee) or wired. Sensor nodes can be powered by using a coin cell battery or a rechargeable battery. So, these devices are very small and non invasive; for example, they can easily be attached on the head. Furthermore, this hardware solution does not impair the natural movement of the body: examples of possible placements of the sensor nodes are given in Figs. 1 and 2.

Here we focus on head movements, since the head is the highest body segment and in consequence, the last affected in spinal cord injury patients. Additionally, many people are unable to use a standard computer mouse because of disabilities affecting their hands or arms. Head controls offer one alternative by allowing people to use head movements to control the computer cursor. Human head-movements can be characterized in movements for any other two dimensional device. By using an accelerometer attached on the head, we are able to detect four kinds of movements, as described in the Fig. 3.

2.1   The Mouse Emulator

According to the proposed mouse emulator, the movements made with the hand to move the mouse pointer are substituted by head movements. Specifically, up

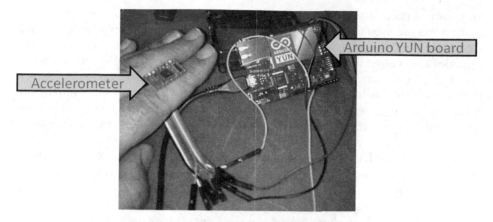

Fig. 1. Arduino Yun and an accelerometer-based sensor node placed on a finger.

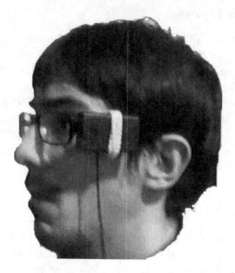

Fig. 2. A wireless accelerometer-based sensor node attached on the head. In this case, it is connected to the Arduino Yun wirelessly.

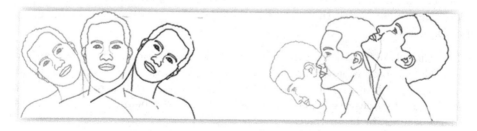

Fig. 3. On the left, there is a roll head movement. On the right, there is a pitch head movement.

and down vertical movement (pitch) is used for up down displacement while roll movements are used for left right displacement. So the end user can fully control a computer: for example, he/she can use an on-screen keyboard. Such a solution provides also a novel interaction method for controlling a computing environment through very intuitive body movements given that a sensor node can detect measurement of inclination changes less than 1.0 °. This is a very important feature which can be a key element for independence and autonomy of people with disabilities: in these cases, enabling alternative and simple interaction with a standard personal computer becomes critical for these kinds of users.

Moreover, our HCI system is based on signal processing algorithms which enable to classify gestures: for these purpose we have marked two kinds of movements: fast and slow. A slow gesture features low acceleration values and it can be used for typical mouse pointer movement; a fast gesture features high acceleration values, so these signal peaks can perform click or double click events.

2.2   Configuration Process

Considering the Arduino YUN environment, all the algorithms for interacting with external sensors or devices have been implemented in Python. This also allows us to create a system service to synchronize all the applications and their options with a Cloud-based service. By using a simple web application running on each Arduino boards, it is possible to configure all the parameters of AT tools running on the board.These data are stored into a user profile available on a remote server. Such feature may allow a remote AT expert to support a user with a disability by adjusting the firmware running on the embedded system used by the person to access to a computer.

3   Related Works

AT can be viewed as technology used by individuals with disabilities in order to perform functions that might otherwise be difficult or impossible. AT can include mobility devices such as walkers and wheelchairs, as well as hardware, software, and peripherals that assist people with disabilities in accessing computers or other information technologies [5].

In this field, alternative input devices allow end users to control their computers through means other than a standard keyboard or pointing device. Examples include [1]:

- Alternative keyboards featuring larger- or smaller-than-standard keys or keyboards, alternative key configurations, and keyboards for use with one hand.
- Electronic pointing devicesused to control the cursor on the screen without use of hands. Devices used include ultrasound, infrared beams, eye movements, nerve signals, or brain waves.
- Sip-and-puff systemsactivated by inhaling or exhaling.
- Wands and sticksworn on the head, held in the mouth or strapped to the chin and used to press keys on the keyboard.

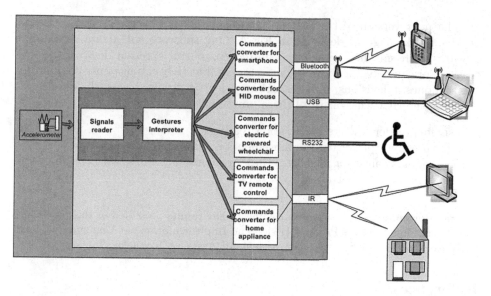

Fig. 4. Block diagram of an universal HCI system based on accelerometers.

- Joysticks manipulated by hand, feet, chin, etc. and used to control the cursor on screen.
- Trackballs movable balls on top of a base that can be used to move the cursor on screen.
- Touch screens allow direct selection or activation of the computer by touching the screen, making it easier to select an option directly rather than through a mouse movement or keyboard. Touch screens are either built into the computer monitor or can be added onto a computer monitor.

Several novel method for supporting the interaction between users with disabilities and computers are available in literature [7]. In [4], the authors describe a prototype based on RGB-D sensors able to support a multimodal human computer interaction and to replace some existing AT solutions. A particular table-top keyboard is discussed in [6], it is mainly designed for stroke patients. EMG sensors can be used to design new types of HCI systems, as discussed in [10]. Also, interesting studies about BCI (brain computer interface) are available in [8].

4   Conclusion

This paper dealt with the usage on embedded systems and IoT devices in order to achieve alternative human-computer interfaces for users with disabilities. The proposed solution exploits Cloud-based services to adjust its functions according users' needs and preferences. To demonstrate a possible usage of the HCI system, a mouse emulator has been developed using an Arduino YUN with a MEMS accelerometer sensor.

The next version of the HCI system discussed in this paper will be based on the block diagram depicted in Fig. 4. Our software will relate recognized gestures with specific commands required to control external devices; the low cost sensor can detect a few of the movements, but they can fit to use computers, smartphones, televisions, cameras, robots, electric powered wheelchairs etc.

Also, the HCI will consist of three functional blocks:

- a signals reader collects acceleration readings;
- a gestures interpreter detects movements on the base of sensor values;
- a commands converter associates these recognized gestures with specific commands needed to control many devices.

Acknowledgments. The research leading to the results presented in this paper has received funding from the Project "Design and Implementation of a Community Cloud Platform aimed at SaaS services for on-demand Assistive Technology".

References

1. Types of Assistive Techonology Products. http://www.microsoft.com/enable/at/types.aspx. Accessed June 2014
2. Benazzouz, Y., Munilla, C., Gunalp, O., Gallissot, M., Gurgen, L.: Sharing user IoT devices in the cloud. In: 2014 IEEE World Forum on Internet of Things (WF-IoT), pp. 373–374, March 2014
3. Fazio, M., Celesti, A., Puliafito, A., Villari, M.: An integrated system for advanced multi-risk management based on cloud for IoT. In: Gaglio, S., Re, G.L. (eds.) Advances onto the Internet of Things. AISC, vol. 260, pp. 253–269. Springer International Publishing, Heidelberg (2014). http://dx.doi.org/10.1007/978-3-319-03992-318
4. Fuentes, J.A., Oliver, M., Fernández-Caballero, A.: Towards a unified interface in the field of assistive technologies. In: Proceedings of the 13th International Conference on Interaccion Persona-Ordenador, INTERACCION 2012, pp. 33:1–33:2. ACM, New York (2012). http://doi.acm.org/10.1145/2379636.2379668
5. ISO: 9999–2007: Assistive Products for Persons with Disability - Classification and Terminology (2007)
6. Khademi, M., Mousavi Hondori, H., Dodakian, L., Lopes, C.V., Cramer, S.C.: An assistive tabletop keyboard for stroke rehabilitation. In: Proceedings of the 2013 ACM International Conference on Interactive Tabletops and Surfaces, ITS 2013, pp. 337–340. ACM, New York(2013). http://doi.acm.org/10.1145/2512349.2512394
7. Mulfari, D., Celesti, A., Puliafito, A., Villari, M.: How cloud computing can support on-demand assistive services. In: Proceedings of the 10th International Cross-Disciplinary Conference on Web Accessibility, W4A 2013, pp. 27:1–27:4. ACM, New York (2013). http://doi.acm.org/dx.doi.org/10.1145/2461121.2461140
8. Poli, R., Cinel, C., Matran-Fernandez, A., Sepulveda, F., Stoica, A.: Towards cooperative brain-computer interfaces for space navigation. In: Proceedings of the 2013 International Conference on Intelligent User Interfaces, IUI 2013, pp. 149–160. ACM, New York (2013). http://doi.acm.org/10.1145/2449396.2449417

9. Tei, K., Gurgen, L.: Clout : Cloud of things for empowering the citizen clout in smart cities. In: 2014 IEEE World Forum on Internet of Things (WF-IoT), pp. 369–370, March 2014
10. Zhang, D., Wang, Y., Chen, X., Xu, F.: EMG classification for application in hierarchical FES system for lower limb movement control. In: Jeschke, S., Liu, H., Schilberg, D. (eds.) ICIRA 2011, Part I. LNCS, vol. 7101, pp. 162–171. Springer, Heidelberg (2011)

Author Index

Printed in the United States
By Bookmasters